Interventional Pericardiology

Bernhard Maisch · Arsen D. Ristić · Petar M. Seferović ·
Teresa S. M. Tsang

Interventional Pericardiology

Pericardiocentesis, Pericardioscopy,
Pericardial Biopsy, Balloon Pericardiotomy
and Intrapericardial Therapy

With contributions of

Sabine Pankuweit
Ružica Maksimović
Heinz Rupp
Jae K. Oh
James B. Seward
A. Jamil Tajik

With 85 Figures

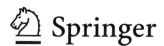 Springer

Reviewers:
Ralph Shabetai, San Diego, CA, USA
David H. Spodick, Worcester, MA, USA

ISBN 978-3-642-11334-5 Springer Medizin Verlag Heidelberg

Bibliografische Information der Deutschen Bibliothek
The Deutsche Bibliothek lists this publication in Deutsche Nationalbibliographie;
detailed bibliographic data is available in the internet at http://dnb.ddb.de.

Springer Medizin Verlag
springer.com
© Springer Medizin Verlag Heidelberg 2011

Planning: Renate Scheddin, Heidelberg
Projectmanagement: Ulrike Dächert, Heidelberg
Copy-Editing and typesetting: Hilger VerlagsService, Heidelberg
Cover design: deblik Berlin
Printer: Stürtz GmbH, Würzburg

SPIN: 11012160

Printed on acid free paper   18/5135/UD – 5 4 3 2 1 0

Foreword

This is the first book dedicated to pericardial interventional procedures joining a long-term clinical and research experience of the leading experts in the field from both sides of the Atlantic. It comes a decade after the book "Pericardiology: Contemporary answers to continuing challenges" edited by Seferovic, Spodick, and Maisch, and many important publications on pericardial disease, function and pathophysiology, as well as several excellent international conferences on myocardial and pericardial disease, and the first international guidelines on pericardial diseases, authored by the same group.

Professors Maisch, Seferović, and Ristić have built over the years a fruitful cooperation and a strong, comprehensive program for the study of myocardial and pericardial diseases. Several new interventional techniques have been developed or improved, above all the use of a flexible pericardioscopy through which "targeted biopsies" of the pericardium and epicardium are obtained. Thus, the random nature of endomyocardial biopsy and its comparative irrelevance to pericardial pathology are largely eliminated. Evaluation of biopsy specimens including PCR, immunological staining and analysis by other molecular techniques is an essential part of this program, and in this respect, PD Dr. Pankuweit, Marburg, is an important co-author of this book. Recognizing the landmark contributions in the field of pericardial diseases made by physicians at the Mayo clinic, Professors Tsang, Oh, Seward, and Tajik were invited to give the "American view" on the development and application of echo-guided pericardiocentesis.

Anybody with a major interest in pericardial disease, or should I say pericardiology, will benefit from this book which will also be an aid to electro-physiologists, investigators working to improve myocardial perfusion by non-surgical means, and directors of cardiac catheterization laboratories. For those interested in the history of pericardiology, there is a good chapter on the history of pericardial interventions.

With this book, the authors introduce us to a new specialty in cardiology, interventional pericardiology, including standard and alternative techniques for pericardial access as well as the pericardioscopy, epicardial and pericardial biopsy, intrapericardial therapy, and percutaneous balloon pericardiotomy, paving the way for future investigation and treatment. These techniques are described along with their applications and are detailed in several of the chapters. The book is accompanied by internet links to nine group of videos demonstrating epicardial halo phenomenon, pericardiocentesis guided by fluoroscopy, pericardioscopy, pericardial, and epicardial biopsy, pericardiocentesis guided by echocardiography, pericardiocentesis with the PerDUCER device, percutaneous balloon pericardiotomy, rescue pericardiocentesis in cardiac tamponade due to a complication of percuteneous coronary intervention, drainage of a large pericardial cyst, and the new interventional procedure, intrapericardial thrombolysis for a large, postoperative intrapericardial hematoma. This comprehensive video collection would be precious for all colleagues interested to learn the techniques or expand their knowledge on interventional procedures in pericardial diseases.

Ralph Shabetai, M.D.
La Jolla, CA, USA

August 2010

Foreword

For decades pericardial basic and clinical research, publication and scientific meetings were mainly centered in the United States (Fowler; Shabetai; Spodick). Pericardiology is now centered in Europe (Maisch; Seferovic; Ristic; Imazio; Soler-Soler) with outstanding results, including many diagnostic and therapeutic innovations presented in Interventional Pericardiology. Here, Maisch, Ristic, and Seferovic have co-opted selected colleagues from theMayo Clinic as contributors to produce an exceptional volume that combines the pericardium's medical history, its anatomy (including superb imaging) and its macrophysiology – notably of tamponade – in magnificent support of the book's main thrust: pericardial intervention to make diagnoses and directly treat pericardial conditions, as well as cardiac disorders like arrhythmias and coronary lesions. Thus, the pericardium is increasingly a transit route for scopes and electronics and a depot for pharmaceuticals. Epicardial mapping and ablation are already well established. Safe intrapericardial delivery of high concentrations of antiarrhythmic and coronary dilating drugs are under further development as are intrapericardial gene therapy, applications of growth factors and stem cells, and even intrapericardial robotics.

In achieving this remarkable text and reference book, the distinguished authors describe every possible method of safely entering the pericardium nonsurgically, from familiar anterior needle drainage to even transbronchial pericardiocentesis (for strictly posterior effusions) and pericardioscopy via the effusive and noneffusive pericardium for inspection, biopsy, drainage, and direct treatment of the pericardial contents; indeed, three of the principal authors: Maisch, Seferovic, and Ristic are masters of this technique. An outstanding example is Maisch's breakthrough to successfully manage the most daunting and stubborn of all pericardial problems: recurrent, presumably autoimmune (autoreactive), pericarditis via a scope-delivered, poorly absorbed corticosteroid. Practical instructions accompany all techniques making this both a learned textbook and a how-to-do-it manual.

Anyone dealing with pericardial problems will welcome this magnificent work enthusiastically. Indeed, its current and potential applications in diseases of the heart itself will interest any cardiologist. Accordingly, Interventional Pericardiology belongs in every medical library. It would make a superb gift for favorite colleagues and trainees.

David Spodick, M.D.
Worcester, MA, USA

Preface

For many years the diagnosis of pericardial disease has been primarily made non-invasively. Our understanding was based on pathophysiology and the impairment of function. The assessment of the etiology was, when at all, left to the pathologist at the time of necropsy. Invasive and interventional procedures were questioned and neglected and therefore not available in the majority of the institutions.

Due to the development of new technologies to access the pericardium and obtain samples of effusion or tissue, refined diagnostic procedures could be applied including molecular and immunological methods. They have opened a new window to the heart and to the pericardium. To open this window for clinical cardiologists is one of the major aims of this book, the first one entirely focused on interventional procedures related to diagnosis and management of pericardial diseases, accompanied by a collection of educational video recordings.

In this pioneering intention, the book is following the path of the recently published guidelines of the European Society of Cardiology, the first official international document on pericardial diseases, also mainly written by the lead authors of this book. It is a result of a long-term co-operation and common efforts of two European centers with extensive clinical experience and profound research interest in the area of pericardial diseases, the Departments of Cardiology of Marburg and of Belgrade University Medical Centers. The input by the authors from the Mayo Clinic provides a broader view and adds an American perspective to the European perception of this frequently forgotten, but yet important topic in interventional cardiology.

Although the book is dedicated to interventions, we are well aware that the indications for an interventional procedure should be carefully balanced and based on the risk/benefit ratio for each procedure and each individual patient. In cases in which a safe and efficient non-invasive alternative is available, non-invasive procedures should be taken first. Nevertheless, there is a substantial subset of patients in whom the pericardial diseases are either acutely (as cardiac tamponade or purulent infection) or chronically life threatening (e.g. neoplastic or constrictive pericarditis) and prompt intervention and etiological diagnosis are essential and determine prognosis and outcome. These patients unquestionably benefit from the invasive and interventional procedures. It is the aim of this book is to provide comprehensive and detailed information for the physicians and researchers interested to extend their knowledge and skill in this challenging area of cardiology.

Bernhard Maisch   Marburg, Germany
Arsen D. Ristić   Belgrade, Serbia
Petar M. Seferović Belgrade, Serbia
Teresa S.M. Tsang Vancouver, Canada

January 2011

Acknowledgment

Much of our current knowledge on pericardial disease is based on the landmark contributions made by two outstanding scientists: Professor David Spodick (Worcester, Massachusetts) and Professor Ralph Shabetai (San Diego, California). We had the privilege of learning from their brilliant publications and lectures, and we are continuously inspired by their work. We are especially grateful to Professor Shabetai and to Professor Spodick for they review and kind foreword of this book.

Our friend Prof. Ralph Shabetai has died at the end of last year after an academic life with many precious contributions dedicated to Pericardiology in the past decades. We will keep him a very special memory.

The authors also appreciate the support of the Working group on Myocardial and Pericardial Diseases of the European Society of Cardiology and the former Council of Cardiomyopathies of the World Heart Federation. We would also like to acknowledge the support from the Tempus project JEP 19046 and should like to thank all sponsors of the book. We are particularly grateful to Prof. Dr. Dr. h.c. mult. Reinfried Pohl and the cardiac promotions society Marburg for their continuous support of our academic work in the field of pericardial disease.

Acknowledgment

Authors

Bernhard Maisch, MD, FESC, FACC
Professor of Internal Medicine – Cardiology,
Director, Department of Internal Medicine – Cardiology
Philipps University Marburg, Germany

Arsen D. Ristić, MD, PhD, FESC
Associate Professor of Internal Medicine – Cardiology,
Belgrade University School of Medicine,
Department of Cardiology, Institute of Cardiovascular Diseases,
Clinical Center of Serbia, Belgrade, Serbia

Petar M. Seferović, MD, PhD, FESC, FACC
Professor of Internal Medicine – Cardiology,
Belgrade University School of Medicine
Deputy Director for Education, Clinical Center of Serbia
Head, Cardiology 2, Department of Cardiology
Clinical Center of Serbia, Belgrade, Serbia

Teresa S. M. Tsang, MD, FACC
Professor of Medicine, University of British Columbia
Diamond Health Care Centre, 2775 Laurel Street
Vancouver, BC V5Z 1M9, Canada

Co-Authors

Sabine Pankuweit, PhD
Priv.-Doz., Laboratory of Cardioimmunology,
Department of Internal Medicine – Cardiology,
Philipps University Marburg, Germany

Ružica Maksimović, MD, PhD
Associate Professor of Radiology,
Belgrade University School of Medicine
MRI Center, Clinical Center of Serbia, Belgrade, Serbia

Heinz Rupp, PhD
Professor of Medical Physiology
Laboratory for Experimental Cardiology,
Department of Internal Medicine – Cardiology,
Philipps University Marburg, Germany

Jae K. Oh, MD, FACC
Professor of Medicine, Mayo Clinic College of Medicine
Co-Director, Echocardiography Laboratory,
Consultant, Division of Cardiovascular Diseases and Internal Medicine,
Mayo Clinic, Rochester, MN, USA

James B. Seward, MD, FACC
Division of Cardiovascular Diseases and Internal Medicine,
Mayo Clinic, Rochester, MN, USA

John M. Nasseff, Sr.
Professor of Cardiology in Honor of Dr. Burton Onofrio,
Professor of Medicine and of Pediatrics, Mayo Clinic College of Medicine,
Consultant, Division of Cardiovascular Diseases,
Internal Medicine, and Pediatric Cardiology, Mayo Clinic, Rochester, MN, USA

A. Jamil Tajik, MD, FACC
Division of Cardiovascular Diseases and Internal Medicine,
Mayo Clinic, Rochester, MN, USA

Thomas J. Watson, Jr.
Professor in Honor of Dr. Robert L. Frye,
Professor of Medicine and of Pediatrics, Mayo Clinic College of Medicine;
Chairman (Emeritus) Zayed Cardiovascular Center,
Mayo Clinic, Rochester, MN;
Consultant, Division of Cardiovascular Diseases,
Internal Medicine, and Pediatric Cardiology,
Mayo Clinic, Scottsdale, AZ, USA

Content

Accompanying DVD

Video 1: Epicardial halo phenomenon
        1a – grade 0.5/AP view
        1b – grade 0.5/lateral view
        1c – grade 1/AP view
        1d – grade 1/lateral view
        1e – grade 2/AP view
        1f – grade 2/lateral view

Video 2: Pericardiocentesis guided by fluoroscopy, pericardioscopy, pericardial, and epicardial biopsy (Marburg experience)

Video 3: Pericardiocentesis guided by echocardiography

Video 4: Pericardiocentesis guided by fluoroscopy, pericardioscopy, pericardial, and epicardial biopsy (Belgrade experience)

Video 5: Pericardiocentesis with PerDUCER device

Video 6: Percutaneous balloon pericardiotomy

Video 7: Rescue pericardiocentesis in cardiac tamponade due to a complication of percutaneous coronary intervention

Video 8: Drainage of a large pericardial cyst

Video 9: Intrapericardial thrombolysis for a large, postoperative intrapericardial hematoma

A Historical Perspective

Introduction

… then my lord Gawan dismounted. There lay a man pierced through, with his blood rushing inward. He asked the hero's lady whether the knight was still alive … "You would soon see and hear him in health, he is not mortally wounded, the blood is only pressing on his heart." He grasped a branch of the linden tree, slipped the bark off like a tube … and inserted it into the body through the wound. Then he bade the woman suck on it until the blood flowed toward her. The hero's strength revived so that he could speak and talk again.

Parzival's Pericardial Puncture
Wolfram von Eschenbach, 1200 A.D. [1]

Pericardium was first described by Hippocrates (460–370 B.C.) but its diseases remained neglected in the history of medicine for many centuries. Galen (131–201 AD) was the first to discover the pericardial effusion in a monkey and made probably the first pericardial resection in a man with anterior mediastinitis [2–4]. In injured gladiators dying from pericardial infections he noted similarities with heart failure, but has also recognized that if the pericardium is inflamed, the disease does not inevitably affects the myocardium. More than 900 years later, Avenzoar, a famous physician from Eshbeelia (now Seville, Andalusia, Spain), known in the Arabic world under the name of Ibn Zuhr, described in his book "Al Taisir", "water, which is collected in the pocket of the heart or pericardial sac" [5]. His classification of pericardial diseases into serous, fibrinous, and purulent forms is kept until the present time. In the middle ages, pericardial diseases have attracted attention of many prominent physicians. Richard Lower in his "Tractatus de corde" (1669) and Jean Baptiste Senac in his "Traité de la Structure du Coeur" (1774) dedicated extensive chapters to pericardial diseases. Recognizing the complexity of the problem Laënnec was writing in 1819 that "there are few diseases attended by more variable symptoms and more difficult diagnosis than this". Although changes in precordial dullness on percussion were noted by Auenbrugger in 1761, the pericardial rubs were described much later by Collins in 1824. Distinctive features of rheumatic and tuberculous pericarditis were first described by Jean Cruveilhier (1828) and Jean-Baptiste Bouillaud (1835) in their anatomic textbooks (Fig. 1.1). Norman Chevers was the first physician striking the importance of diastole in diagnosis of constrictive pericardial diseases (1842). Richard Bright from the Guy's Hospital in London described pericardial effusion in renal failure [6]. A German surgeon, Edmund Rose, introduced the term "cardiac tamponade" in 1884 after the analysis

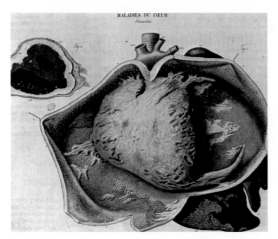

□ **Fig. 1.1.** "Hydropericarditis". Illustration by Jean Cruveilhier, Anatomie pathologique du corps humain, Paris (1828). Reproduced with permission from Villey et al. (1978) [14]

of the series of cases of fatal heart wounds in which the patients have died due to the compression by a relatively small intrapericardial hemorrhage [7]. One of the famous victims of traumatic cardiac tamponade was Empress Sissi of Austria who died due to the small stab wound in the left ventricle after an attack in Geneva, Switzerland [8].

William Osler wrote a statement in 1892 stressing that the pericardial diseases are insufficiently acknowledged "Probably no serious disease is so frequently overlooked by the practitioners. The experience based on post-mortem examinations show how often pericarditis remains unrecognized or goes on to resolution and adhesion without attracting notice" [9].

Diagnostic and Therapeutic Pericardial Interventions

Pericardiocentesis and Pericardial Drainage

Although Galen described first drainage of purulent pericardial effusion and an improvised pericardial drainage was also described in the above quoted lyrical text from 1200, the first pericardial puncture was proposed in the scientific literature by Jean Riolan, professor of surgery from Paris [10, 11]. In his treatise *Encheiridion anatomicum et pathologicum*

(1653) he suggested trepaning of the sternum as an approach to drain the pericardial effusion. However, it is not know if he actually ever performed this procedure.

Giovanni Battista Morgagni in the text "De Sedibus" (1756) has observed that the outcome of soldiers with heart wounds depended on the rate of pericardial filling. However, he feared the injury of coronary arteries and did not attempt to perform drainage of the pericardial effusion in his patients. Jean Baptiste de Sénac, the personal physician to the Louis XVth, described clinical findings in pericarditis in detail in his "Traité de la coeur et les maladies" and associated it with mediastinitis, pneumonia, and pleurisy. He recognized pain and pericardial distress as symptoms of a "hydrops pericardii" and advocated parasternal drainage.

Corvisart, one of the most prominent physicians of the Napoleon's time, distinguished various forms of „dry" pericarditis and was able to differentiate them from pericardial effusion by means of percussion. Despite this achievement, the French school in the XIXth century was still reluctant to take the risk of performing pericardial punctures. Percussion of the thorax revealing dullness beyond the cardiac apex was assumed as diagnostic for large pericardial effusions (Ewart's sign or Bamberger-Pins-Ewart's sign, 1896)[12]. However, he considered the probability of an accurate diagnosis too uncertain to permit incision or blind puncture of the pericardium and drained pericardial effusions by surgical pericardiotomy [13].

For the same reason, Laënnec rejected pericardiocentesis despite his extensive correlation of auscultatory and necropsy findings. On the contrary he was advising the use of blistering agents on the precordium under the hypothesis, that they would draw pericardial fluid through the chest wall into the blister. The preferred agent was cantharides – „the Spanish fly" [4]. Similar unsuccessful attempts have been made with the ventusa technique, a form of acupressure that uses heated glasses with the idea to remove the effusion through the chest wall. Even in the XXI century in the middle of Europe, the authors of this book had the opportunity to see skin injuries from ventusa glasses made by an "alternative medicine practitioner" in a disastrous attempt to remove the pericardial effusion.

Direct, Surgical Approach to Pericardial Drainage

Francisco Romero performed the first successful drainage of pericardial effusion in three patients in Barcelona most probably in 1801 or 1803. His approach involved an incision into the chest wall and into the pericardium itself under direct vision [10]. Two patients completely recovered from their pericardial effusion. The cases were reported to the faculty of the Paris Medical School in a paper "Sur l'hydropéricarde" in 1814, but the original report was unfortunately lost later on [10, 12].

Another early record of pericardial incision for relief of effusion and cardiac tamponade was made by the chief surgeon of Napoleon's Grande Armée, Dominique-Jean Larrey. He reported a case of a pericardial section in 1829. His patient had stabbed himself in the left side of the chest and wounded both pericardium and the lung. The knife, having passed through the fifth costal cartilage, was still in the wound when the man was brought to the hospital in Paris. Prompt local care was followed by slowly progressive dyspnea and pain. Forty-five days after injury, an incision was made into the pericardium and a liter of fluid was removed. Marked relief of symptoms resulted for several days, but a post-operative infection caused the patient's death 23 days after the operation. The autopsy revealed suppurative mediastino-pericarditis. Larrey conducted further experiments on the cadaver to determine the best surgical approach to the heart.

Ludwig Rehn was the first surgeon who successfully performed suture of the wound on the heart and saved from cardiac tamponade a 22-year-old gardener stabbed in the fourth left intercostal space. Although there was no external bleeding after the injury, two days later his condition deteriorated and the area of cardiac dullness increased. Rehn explored the wound through the fourth intercostal space, evacuated a large clot from the pericardium and sutured the 1.5-cm wound in the right ventricle [15].

Indirect, Blind Pericardiocentesis

The first successful technique for the evacuation of pericardial effusion, without making incisions at the chest wall, was introduced by Franz Schuh (1840) in Vienna. He effectively performed a blind tap, similar to the pericardiocentesis procedure as we know today, with a trocar (third intercostal space, at the left sternal margin, without previous incision) in a 24-years-old woman with dyspnea and tachycardia, who suffered from a mediastinal tumor. Drainage of large amounts of blood-stained fluid through the fourth left intercostal space resulted in a complete relief. The patient survived 5 months after the procedure and autopsy confirmed mediastinal neoplasm [13, 16, 17]. Schuh's trocar and cannula were initially designed, with help from Josef Skoda, for thoracentesis rather than for pericardiocentesis [16], but with minor modifications could have been used for both.

Indirect, blind pericardiocentesis, using Schuh's trocar and cannula became slowly a generally accepted technique, due to the lower incidence of infection in comparison to the open, surgical procedures. Later, Dieulafoy established aspiration as preferable to pericardial incision in his "Pneumatic aspiration of morbid fluids. The same practice was successfully carried out by Karawajew [18] in Russia in a patient with scorbutic hemopericardium (outbreak of Scurvy during the Crimean War, Sevastopol, 1847). A few accidents were reported, including the Callender's case (death during blind pericardiocentesis due to the rupture of the right ventricle in 1874 at Guy's Hospital in London) but the procedure was generally regarded as safe for the standards of the time [10]. Some authors have mentioned the danger of puncturing the dilated heart instead of distended pericardium with a large effusion. The procedure therefore had some strong and well-respected opponents, led by Theodore Billroth, who wrote in 1875 that pericardial paracentesis was "a prostitution of surgical skill" or "madness" and that "any surgeon who would attempt to suture a wound of the heart is not worthy of the serious consideration of his colleagues" [19]. French military surgeons Delorme and Mignon [20] put forth some serious objections and reviewed the technique for pericardiocentesis providing a list of their own severe complications including lesion and contamination of the pleura, damaging the lung, and wounding of the heart itself. Out of 82 cases of blind pericardiocentesis that they collected in 1896, lethal outcome of the procedure occurred in 54 patients (65.9%). Then again, among

18 cases in which an open pericardial incision was done "only" 7 died (38.9%). Accepting the fact that the comparison was inconclusive they developed their own, semi-direct approach.

A different approach to the pericardial interventions was made by Ludolf Brauer from the Philipps-University of Marburg. He advocated resections of contiguous ribs and costal cartilages in cases of mediastino-pericarditis in which adhesions extended to the thoracic wall. Improvement after surgery in two patients, performed by Petersen and Simon in Heidelberg were reported by Brauer in the Münchener Medizinische Wochenschrift in 1902 [11].

Roberts, Hindenlang, and West were the first to practice pericardiocentesis in the United States and analyzed the reports on 41 cases published in the literature of that time (1876) [21, 22]. However, the procedure was regarded as successful in only one third of the cases.

Despite frequently observed complications, by 1915, blind pericardiocentesis was the accepted technique for diagnosing and treating pericardial effusion. The open surgical drainage was reserved for purulent forms. The subxiphoid approach was suggested by Marfan 1911 [23] but five other alternative approaches were also practiced. To demonstrate the safety of the subxiphoid approach, Marfan's associate Blechmann has punctured one patient 17 times [11].

Volkmann applied pericardiocentesis and instillation of air for drainage of purulent pericardial effusions. He was also the first to apply contrast imaging of the pericardium with instillation of air or iodine contrast solution (pericardiography and pneumopericardiography) [24]. He also measured the average distance from the Larrey's spot to the pericardium during pericardiocentesis. The obtained distance in 36 patients was 4–8 cm, with a median value of 5.5 cm.

Advances Through the Development of Technology

With the development of radiology, "bottle-like" and "tent-like" heart, as well as the calcifications of the pericardium were described as radiological signs of pericardial disease (Holmes, 1920–1924). At the same time first surgical pericardiectomies were performed by Rehn in Germany [25] and by Churchill in the United States [26]. Changes in the electrocardiogram typical for acute pericarditis were first published in 1938 by Max Winternitz and Richard Langendorf [27]. After the introduction of heart catheterization, Picquet (1939) first measured the increase of venous pressure, and Bloomfield and Cournand underlined the importance of the "dip and plateau phenomenon" in the pressure curves of the right ventricle and jugular vein [10].

Later on, major contributions to the area were made by Ralph Shabetai regarding the physiology of the pericardium, pericardial effusion, and cardiac tamponade [28–31] and by David Spodick through the codification of ECG stages in acute pericarditis, characteristics of pericardial rubs, and numerous other important issues [32–35]. Both Shabetai and Spodick authored or co-authored several major textbooks on pericardial diseases and provided precious scientific support for other centers and younger authors during their initial steps in "pericardiology" [12, 36–40].

Since the introduction of echocardiography, this noninvasive technique has become the method of choice in the diagnosis of pericardial effusion and constriction as well as for the guidance of pericardiocentesis. Edler published the first investigation on application of echocardiography in detection of pericardial effusion in 1955 [41]. Feigenbaum [42], Horowitz [43], D'Cruz [44], Popp [45], and Teichholz [46] have made important contributions. Hatle et al. [47] superbly described impeded flow in late diastole in pericardial effusion and constriction. Several milestone contributions on constrictive pericarditis [48–50] and echocardiography-guided pericardiocentesis [51–53] were made by the authors from the Mayo clinic.

Important studies on acute pericarditis, tuberculous pericarditis, large pericardial effusion, and effusive-constrictive pericarditis were published by authors from Barcelona under the leadership of Jordi Soler-Soler that remained for decades one of the most prestigious world centers for pericardial diseases [54–63].

Maisch and coworkers in Marburg were the first to implement pericardiocentesis guided by the epicardial halo phenomenon in fluoroscopy [64, 65] and to perform the endoscopically guided pericardiocentesis

◻ Table 1.1. Various techniques for pericardiocentesis: modifications of the approach, guidance or puncturing devices

Pericardiocentesis		Technique
Guidance	State of the art	▬ Echocardiography [51–53] ▬ Fluoroscopy [67]
	Emerging/ alternative	▬ Halo phenomenon guidance [65] ▬ Tuohy needle approach to normal pericardium [68, 69] ▬ Simultaneous RV/puncturing needle contrast injection [67] ▬ Pacing capture [70] ▬ CT-guided pericardiocentesis [71] ▬ CT-fluoroscopy [72] ▬ Computer-assisted pericardiocentesis [73, 74]
	Obsolete	▬ No guidance – 4% mortality [75] ▬ ECG (ST elevation) [70]
Approach	Standard	▬ Subxiphoid [76, 77] ▬ Intercostal (apical) [51–53]
	Emerging/ alternative	▬ Paracardial [76] ▬ Transatrial [78, 79] ▬ Transright ventricular [80] ▬ Transbronchial [81] ▬ Transcardiac [82, 83]
Devices	Standard	▬ 16- or 18-gauge (5.1 to 8.3-cm) polytef-sheathed venous "intracath" needles (Deseret Medical – Nogales, AZ, USA) ▬ 17-gauge Tuohy needle ▬ Thin-walled 18-gauge needle
	Emerging/ alternative	▬ PerDUCER® device [66, 84–88] ▬ Peri-Attacher® (see Chapter 5) ▬ FLEXview® system (Boston Sci., St. Clara, CA) [89]

with the PerDUCER device in patients with myopericarditis [66]. State of the art approaches, alternative and emerging techniques for pericardiocentesis are listed in the Table 1.1.

After 200 years of clinical practice in modern medicine, pericardiocentesis remains an important procedure in diagnosis and treatment of pericardial disease. However, it is routinely carried out only in patients with large symptomatic pericardial effusions or cardiac tamponade. When the amount of pericardial effusion is small (no hemodynamic compromise) the diagnostic and therapeutic value of pericardial puncture has to be balanced with the possible procedural risk. Despite notable advances introduced with fluoroscopic and echocardiographic guidance, pericardiocentesis is still associated with the risk of serious complications, higher than during cardiac catheterization and most of the invasive procedures [51–53, 64, 67]. In addition, improvement of pericardial fluid diagnostics and introduction of

flexible pericardioscopy for aimed pericardial and epicardial sampling could change contemporary indications for this procedure. In institutions in which diagnostic procedures additional to pericardiocentesis are available (pericardioscopy, epicardial/pericardial biopsy, molecular biology and immunology techniques for pericardial fluid and biopsy analyses) pericardiocentesis of small pericardial effusions yields valuable diagnostic results, which are relevant for intrapericardial or systemic treatment.

Pericardioscopy

The term pericardioscopy was introduced by a German surgeon Johannes Volkmann in 1957 (Fig. 1.2, left) [24]. He used a rigid and rather short instrument produced by C.G. Heymann in Leipzig and Munich (Germany), previously applied in 1923 for endoscopic investigations of the brain ("Encephaloscopy") and

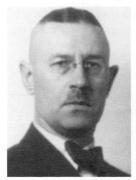
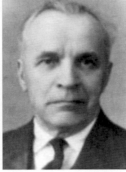

◘ **Fig. 1.2.** Johannes Volkmann (*left*), professor of surgery at the University of Ulm, Germany, was the first to apply rigid endoscopic instruments for pericardiocopy [24]. Nikolai Petrovich Sinitsyn (*right*), professor of pharmacology from Moscow, developed the first transthoracic optical system for the examination of the heart and pericardium [95]

cystoscopy [24]. A simple pocket battery lamp was used as a light source. The device had the working channel for rinsing of the cavities and optics was protected by a cover during the introduction of the endoscope into the pericardium. The procedure was performed in general endotracheal anesthesia after thoracotomy. Instillation of air or 60–100 ml 0.5% procaine solution enabled good endoscopic view. Procaine was applied to prevent arrhythmias during manipulation with the endoscope. Volkmann's pericardioscopy studies were inspired by the experimental work of Russian pharmacologist N.P. Sinitsyn (Fig. 1.2, right) who developed an transthoracic optical system for examination of the heart and pericardium "in

vivo" (Fig. 1.3) [95]. However, the procedure was radical and included resection of the segments of the 6–8th left ribs, removal of the muscles of the chest wall from the spine to the sternum and the extirpation of the middle segment of the left lung.

More recently, the technique was further developed by Kondos in United States [96, 97] and in Europe by Maisch (Marburg) [90–94] (Fig. 1.4), Wurtz, Millaire, Nugue, and Ponte (Lille) [98–102] as well as Seferovic and Ristic (Belgrade) (Fig. 1.5) [103, 104]. Maisch introduced a comprehensive protocol for the etiological diagnosis of pericardial disease comprising aimed, endoscopically guided epicardial and pericardial biopsy, PCR detection of (peri)cardiotropic viruses and bacteria, and immunological analyses to establish autoreactive pericarditis and implement intrapericardial treatment with cisplatin in neoplastic pericardial effusions and with triamcinolone in autoreactive ones [93, 94].

Pericardial Biopsy

Janovsky and coworkers [105] in 1952 as well as Williams and Soutter [106] in 1954 were the first to perform surgical pericardial biopsy. Blind-needle biopsy was first reported by Sanghvi and Samuel [107] in 1958 and by Bawa and co-workers in Lancet in 1959 [108].

Pericardial biopsy has opened a new perspective for establishing the etiology of pericardial diseases. However, its diagnostic value has been initially re-

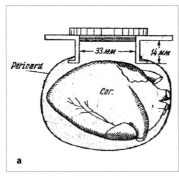
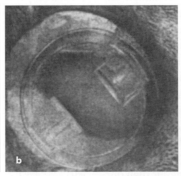
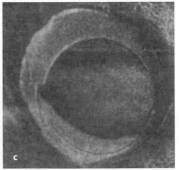

◘ **Fig. 1.3.** Transthoracic optical system for examination of the heart and pericardium "in vivo" introduced by N.P. Sinitsyn in the 1950s [95]. The drawing (**a**) demonstrates the position of the optical system on the thoracic wall in the cross-section. **b** Implanted device with covers closing the optical system, **c** the device without covers enabling visualization of the heart and the pericardium. Reproduced with permission from Sinitsyn et al. (1978) [95]

reported clinically relevant results using flexible percutaneous pericardioscopy to guide epicardial biopsies [91–94] and emphasized its diagnostic superiority in comparison with parietal pericardial biopsy. The endoscopic guidance was also shown to enable a safe approach for taking a very large number of samples (up to 20) reducing the sampling error inherent to all biopsy procedures [104].

The introduction of new techniques in investigating pericardial diseases, including pericardial biopsy and tissue analyses, has opened a whole new perspective in understanding the pathophysiology of the disease and making specific diagnoses.

However, apart from pericardiocentesis, other interventional procedures such as pericardioscopy, pericardial/epicardial biopsy, and percutaneous balloon pericardiotomy have not yet been accepted in many major medical centers. It is the intention of this book is to provide additional instructions and to review our experience that may warrant the adoption of the procedure by tertiary cardiology institutions willing to develop the required facilities and staff, and where large numbers of patients with pericardial disease are evaluated and treated.

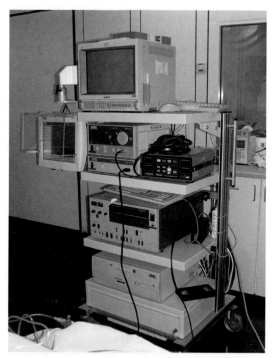

◘ **Fig. 1.4.** Contemporary system for video-pericardioscopy currently applied at the Department of Internal Medicine-Cardiology of the Philipps-University Marburg including 16F flexible endoscope AF1101B1 and AIDA video archiving system (both by Karl Storz, Tuttlingen, Germany)

ported as unsatisfactory [90, 91, 109]. Advances in instrumentation [110] and introduction of targeted sampling under visual control during pericardioscopy [91–94, 98–104] have improved the diagnostic yield.

Several studies have confirmed the diagnostic value of targeted pericardial biopsy guided by surgical pericardioscopy [98-103]. Other investigators have

Percutaneous Balloon Pericardiotomy

Percutaneous balloon pericardiotomy was introduced by Palacios et al. in 1991 for the prevention of recurrences of neoplastic pericardial effusions [111]. In the further application, the procedure was also safely performed in recurrent non-malignant, non-infectious large pericardial effusions/cardiac tamponade [112] and also in children [113]. The final report of the US percutaneous balloon peri-

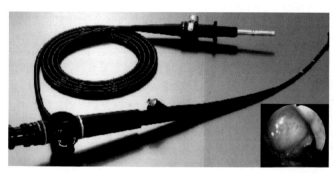

◘ **Fig. 1.5.** Flexible hysterosalpingoscope HYF-1T (Olympus, Japan) used for pericardioscopy and targeted pericardial biopsy at the Department of Cardiology, Institute for Cardiovascular Diseases of the Clinical Center of Serbia, Belgrade [100, 101]. Reproduced with permission from the Olympus Medical Systems Corp., Tokyo, Japan

cardiotomy Registry [114] included 130 patients (110 with neoplastic pericardial effusion) studied in eight centers. The procedure was successful in 91% of patients, with no recurrent effusion during the mean follow-up of 4.2 months.

Iaffaldano et al. [115] were the first to apply double balloon pericardiotomy in patients with significant pericardial stiffness, and Hsu et al. [116] implemented the double-balloon technique with one longer and one shorter balloon. Trefoil (triple) balloon catheter was also successfully applied for prevention of recurrences in patients with neoplastic pericardial effusion [117]. This concept was further developed by Sochman et al. [118] who used a cutting pericardiotome to achieve a pericardiopleural shunt in patients with recurrent pericardial effusion.

Intrapericardial Treatment of Pericardial Disease

Johannes Volkmann was the first investigator who announced in 1957 the potential application of intrapericardial therapy in patients undergoing pericardiocentesis [24]. The application of intrapericardial steroids was for the first time proposed by Spodick in 1964 [119] for the prevention of constriction after tuberculous pericarditis and later on by Zeman and Scovern [120] in 1977 for the treatment of rheumatoid pericardial tamponade.

Further intrapericardial application of crystalloid steroids was, however, mostly dedicated to uremic and dialysis-associated pericardial effusion [121, 122] until the study of Maisch et al. [93] showed high efficacy and safety of intrapericardial treatment of patients with autoreactive pericardial effusion.

For intrapericardial treatment of neoplastic pericardial effusion, instillation of cisplatin was highly efficient in patients with secondary neoplastic pericarditis due to lung cancer [94, 123]. Thiotepa was successful in intrapericardial treatment of metastatic breast cancers [124-126]. Furthermore, favorable results were reported after the intrapericardial application of radioactive chromium phosphate [127]. The application of tetracycline is efficient and inexpensive, but requires multiple instillations and is painful in up to 70% of patients [64]. Other agents such as mitomycin C, bleomycin, mitoxantrone,

vinblastine, interferon-α, -β, and interleukin-2 were also sporadically used for intrapericardial treatment (see Chapter 10).

Intrapericardial Treatment of Non-Pericardial Disease

The development of novel techniques for percutaneous access to the pericardial space (see Table 1.1) is changing our view on its potential usefulness for treatment of cardiovascular disease. However, the idea of non-surgically entering the normal pericardial sac for diagnostic or therapeutic purposes was unrealistic until recently and is still far from the wide clinical application. In addition to the potentials of intrapericardial treatment for pericardial disease, several investigations have indicated the therapeutic potential of intrapericardial therapy for coronary artery disease, heart muscle disease, and arrhythmias (see Chapter 12). The instillation of an agent in the pericardial space to be slowly taken up by the myocardium causes less systemic effects than injecting it into the coronary or general circulation, and enables achievement of high local concentrations. Importantly, the intrapericardial application of various therapeutic agents so far has resulted in no demonstrable toxicity both in experimental and clinical setting.

Another important area for intrapericardial therapy of non-pericardial diseases is electrophysiology and radiofrequent ablation. Epicardial mapping and ablative therapy have been successfully performed with advantages in comparison to endocardial ablation for epicardial arrhythmogenic zones in a subset of patients with epicardial arrhythmogenic foci (see Chapter 12).

For the research of pericardial physiology and pathophysiology, the ability to develop a bank of pericardial fluid from different disease states may provide an as yet unexplored resource for investigation of the fluid content and range of normal values, as well as the changes in various cardiac diseases.

An additional potential application is the stimulation of the pericardium to produce greater quantities of substances that it naturally releases into the normal pericardial fluid in relatively small amounts [128]. A promising possibility is receptor-specific therapy, targeting both the coronary vessels and the pericardial mesothelium with an antibody carrier for the anti-arrhythmic agent. Successful angiogenesis has been accomplished via basic fibroblast growth factor (FGF), which targets the coronary vessels increasing myocardial vascularity in chronic ischemia and acute myocardial infarction. Infarct-avid agents have successfully decreased excessive intracellular calcium accumulation. Hypothermia-inducing agents delivered intrapericardially reduced epicardial temperature and with it the degrees of ischemia and ischemic myocardial damage. Nitric oxide donors and L-arginine (a nitric oxide precursor), delivered in concentrations that could be toxic systemically, have successfully reduced or prevented not only acute and chronic ischemia but also the development of atherosclerotic lesions in the porcine overstretch model of experimental atherosclerosis [128]. Initial results of investigation of intrapericardial therapy in non-pericardial diseases had stimulated new series of studies, attempting to provide the most efficient technique for pericardial access in the presence of moderate or small pericardial effusion or even in the absence of effusion. Several new procedures and different technical modifications of pericardiocentesis are reviewed in this book (see Table 1.1). Further experimental and clinical trials should clarify their feasibility, safety, and clinical value.

Future Perspectives and Recommendations

For many years, investigations of the etiology of pericardial disease were primarily non-invasive and often "per exclusionem" or post-mortem. Invasive procedures were questioned as insufficiently informative and risky and interventional procedures were not available. With the development of new technology, refined diagnostic approaches became possible. They synthesize the achievements of modern imaging with molecular biology and immunology techniques. Comprehensive implementation of new techniques of pericardiocentesis, pericardial fluid analysis, pericardioscopy, epicardial and pericardial biopsy have opened new windows to the pericardial diseases, permitting early specific diagnosis and creating foundations for etiology-based treatment in previously unresolved cases. However, the entire field is still investigational and there is a lot of research, especially randomized studies, which need to be done in order to obtain final confirmation of the diagnostic and therapeutic value of various procedures and therapeutic approaches. Recommendations for the routine clinical practice were recently summarized in the European Society of Cardiology guidelines on diagnosis and management of pericardial diseases [129]. These guidelines are the first official international document on pericardial diseases and the authors of this book were the leading authors of the guidelines as well.

Although the book is dedicated to interventions, we are very well aware that the indications for the interventional procedures should be strict and carefully balanced based on the risk/benefit ratio for each procedure in each individual patient. In cases in which a safe and efficient non-invasive alternative is available, it would certainly have the advantage over the invasive procedures. A good example is the treatment of recurrent pericarditis with colchicine. Guindo et al. [130] and Adler et al. [131] were the first to document the efficacy of colchicine in the treatment of recurrent pericarditis. This concept was only recently finally proven both for acute and recurrent forms in two elegant randomized trials (COPE – COlchicine for acute PEricarditis) [132] and CORE (COlchicine for REcurrent pericarditis) by Imazio and coworkers [133]. Nevertheless, we would like to stress that there is a subset of patients in whom the pericardial effusion is life threatening and prompt etiological diagnosis is essential and strongly determines the selection of treatment and final prognosis. These patients unquestionably benefit from the invasive and interventional procedures and the aim of this book is to provide comprehensive and detailed information for the physicians and researchers interested to extend their knowledge and skill in this challenging area of cardiology.

References

1. Farrar WE Jr. Parzival's pericardial puncture. Ann Intern Med 1980; 92(5): 640
2. Maisch B. Pericardial diseases, with a focus on etiology, pathogenesis, pathophysiology, new diagnostic imaging methods, and treatment. Curr Opin Cardiol 1994; 9(3): 379–388

3. Spodick DH. Historical cornerstones in pericardial disease. In: Seferović PM, Spodick DH, Maisch B, Maksimović R, Ristić AD (eds) Pericardiology: contemporary answers to continuing challenges. Belgrade: Science, 2000, pp 1–8

4. Spodick DH. The hairy hearts of hoary heroes and other tales. Medical history of the pericardium from antiquity through the twentieth century. In: Fowler NO (ed) The pericardium in health and disease. Futura Publishing Company, Mount Kisco, NY, 1985, pp 1–17

5. Abdel-Halim RE, Elfaqih SR. Pericardial pathology 900 years ago. A study and translations from an Arabic medical textbook. Saudi Med J 2007; 28(3): 323–325

6. Bright R. Tabular view of the morbid appearances in 100 cases connected with albuminous urine: with observations. Guys Hosp Rep 1836; 1: 380–400

7. Rose E. Herztamponade. Dtsch Z Chir 1884; 13: 329–410.

8. Meyer P, Keller P-F, Spodick DH. Empress Sissi and cardiac tamponade: an historical perspective. Am J Cardiol 2008; 102(9): 1278–1280

9. Osler W. The principles and practice of medicine. New York: Appleton Co., 1892, 1079

10. Kilpatrick ZM, Chapman CB. On pericardiocentesis. Am J Cardiol 1965; 16: 722–728

11. Rogers FB. Historical review of pericardial diseases. In: Reddy PS, Leon DF, Shaver JA (eds) Pericardial disease. New York: Raven Press, 1982, pp 3–21

12. Shabetai R. The pericardium. Boston (MA): Kluwer Academic Publishers, 2003

13. Dumreicher J. Zur Erinnerung an Prof. Franz Schuh. Wien Med Wochenschr 1866: 16: 409

14. Villey R, Brunet F, Valette G, et al. Histoire de la Médicine, de la Pharmacie, de l'Art Vétéinaire. Société française d'éditions professinnelles, médicales et scientifiques. Albin Mitchel-Laffont-Tchou, Paris, 1978

15. Hurt R. The history of cardiothoracic surgery from early times. New York, New York: Parthenon, 1996, pp 399–423

16. Schuh F. Erfahrungen über die Paracentese der Brust und des Herzbeutels. Medzinisches Jahrbuch Kaiserlichen Königlichen Staates Wien 1841; 33: 388

17. Schuh F. Erfarungen über die Paracentese der Brust und des Herzbeutels. Schmidt´s Jahrsb 1842: 33: 329

18. Karawajew WK Paracentese des Brustkastens und des Pericardiums. Med Zeitung Berlin 1840; 9: 251

19. Dupre M, O'Leary JP. The first successful closure of a laceration of the pericardium. Am Surg 1997; 63(4): 372–374

20. Delorme E, Mignon A. Sur la ponction et l´incision du péricarde. Rev Chir 1895; 16: 56

21. Roberts JB. Paracentesis of the pericardium with an analysis o forty-one cases. New York Med J 1876; 24: 585

22. Hindenlang C. Ein Fall von Paracentesis pericardii. Deutch Arch Klin Med 1879; 24: 452

23. Marfan AB. Ponction du péricarde par l'epigastre. Ann de Méd et Chir Inf 1911; 15: 529

24. Volkmann J. Perikardioskopie und Kontrastdarstellung des Herzbeutels mit anatomischen Grundlagen. Z Aerztliche Fortb 1957; 24: 1105–1108

25. Rehn L. Zur experimentellen Pathologie des Herzbeutels. Verhandl Deutch Gesellsch Chir 1913; 42: 339–352

26. Churchill ED. Decortication of the heart (Delorme) for adhesive pericarditis. Arch Surg 1929; 19: 1457–1465

27. Winternitz M, Langendorf R. Das Elektrokardiogramm der Perikarditis. Acta Med Scand 1938; 94: 141–188

28. Shabetai R, Fowler NO, Fenton JC. Restrictive cardiac disease, pericarditis and the myocardiopathies. Am Heart J 1965; 69: 271–280

29. Shabetai R, Fowler NO, Guntheroth WG. The hemodynamics of cardiac tamponade and constrictive pericarditis. Am J Cardiol 1970; 26(5): 480–489

30. Shabetai R. Measuring pericardial constraint. J Am Coll Cardiol 1986; 7(2): 315–316.

31. Shabetai R. Effect of pericardiocentesis on ventricular function and volume in pericardial effusion. Am J Cardiol 1984; 53(9): 1412

32. Spodick DH. Pericardial friction. Characteristics of pericardial rubs in fifty consecu-tive, prospectively studied patients. N Engl J Med 1968; 278(22): 1204–1207

33. Spodick DH. Differential characteristics of the electrocardiogram in early repolarization and acute pericarditis. N Engl J Med 1976; 295(10): 523–526

34. Spodick DH. Arrhythmias during acute pericarditis. A prospective study of 100 consecutive cases. JAMA 1976; 235(1): 39–41

35. Spodick DH. Diagnostic electrocardiographic sequences in acute pericarditis. Significance of PR segment and PR vector changes. Circulation 1973; 48(3): 575–580

36. Fowler NO, ed. The Pericardium in Health and Disease. Mount Kisco, NY: Futura Publishing Company, 1985

37. Spodick DH. Acute pericarditis. New York, Grune & Stratton, 1959

38. Spodick DH (ed) Pericardial Diseases. Philadelphia, FA Davis, 1976, pp 219–235

39. Shabetai R. The Pericardium. New York, Grune & Stratton, 1981

40. Spodick DH. The Pericardium: A Comprehensive Textbook. New York: Marcel Dekker, 1997

41. Edler I, Lindström K. The history of echocardiography. Ultrasound Med Biol 2004; 30(12): 1565–1644

42. Feigenbaum H. Echocardiographic diagnosis of pericardial effusion. Am J Cardiol 1970; 26: 475–479

43. Horowitz MS, Sehultz CS, Stinson EB, Harrison DC, Popp RL. Sensitivity and speci-ficity of echocardiographic diagnosis of pericardial effusion. Circulation 1974; 50: 239–246

44. D'Cruz IA, Cohen HC, Prabhu R, Glick G. Diagnosis of cardiac tamponade by echocardiography: changes in mitral valve motion and ventricular dimensions, with special reference to paradoxical pulse. Circulation 1975; 52(3): 460–465

45. Popp RL. Echocardiographic assessment of cardiac disease. Circulation 1976; 54(4): 538–552

46. Teichholz LE. Echocardiographic evaluation of pericardial diseases. Prog Cardiovasc Dis 1978; 21(2): 133–140

47. Hatle LK, Appleton CP, Popp RL. Differentiation of constrictive pericarditis and restrictive cardiomyopathy by Doppler echocardiography. Circulation 1989; 79: 357–370

48. Oh JK, Hatle LK, Seward JB, et al. Diagnostic role of Doppler echocardiography in constrictive pericarditis. J Am Coll Cardiol 1994; 23(1): 154–162

49. Oh JK, Tajik AJ, Appleton CP, Hatle LK, Nishimura RA, Seward JB. Preload reduction to unmask the characteristic Doppler features of constrictive pericarditis. A new observation. Circulation 1997; 95(4): 796–799

50. Ha JW, Oh JK, Ling LH, Nishimura RA, Seward JB, Tajik AJ. Annulus paradoxus: transmitral flow velocity to mitral annular velocity ratio is inversely proportional to pulmonary capillary wedge pressure in patients with constrictive pericarditis. Circulation 2001; 104(9): 976–978

51. Tsang TS, Freeman WK, Barnes ME, Reeder GS, Packer DL, Seward JB. Rescue echocardiographically guided pericardiocentesis for cardiac perforation complicating catheter-based procedures. The Mayo Clinic experience. J Am Coll Cardiol 1998; 32(5): 1345–1350

52. Tsang TS, Barnes ME, Hayes SN, et al. Clinical and echocardiographic characteristics of significant pericardial effusions following cardiothoracic surgery and outcomes of echo-guided pericardiocentesis for management: Mayo Clinic experience, 1979–1998. Chest 1999; 116(2): 322–331

53. Tsang TS, Enriquez-Sarano M, Freeman WK, et al. Consecutive 1127 therapeutic echocardiographically guided pericardiocenteses: clinical profile, practice patterns, and outcomes spanning 21 years. Mayo Clin Proc 2002; 77(5): 429–436

54. Soler Soler J, Permanyer G, Sagristà-Sauleda J, Shabetai R. Pericardial disease: new insights and old dilemmas. Dordrecht; Boston: Kluwer Academic Publishers, 1990

55. Sagristà-Sauleda J, Angel J, Sambola A, Alguersuari J, Permanyer-Miralda G, Soler-Soler J. Low-pressure cardiac tamponade: clinical and hemodynamic profile. Circulation 2006; 114(9): 945–952

56. Sagristà-Sauleda J, Angel J, Sánchez A, Permanyer-Miralda G, Soler-Soler J. Effusive-constrictive pericarditis. N Engl J Med 2004; 350(5): 469–475

57. Sagristà-Sauleda J, Angel J, Permanyer-Miralda G, Soler-Soler J. Long-term follow-up of idiopathic chronic pericardial effusion. N Engl J Med 1999; 341(27): 2054–2059

58. Mercé J, Sagristà-Sauleda J, Permanyer-Miralda G, Soler-Soler J. Should pericardial drainage be performed routinely in patients who have a large pericardial effusion without tamponade? Am J Med 1998; 105(2): 106–109

59. Sagristà-Sauleda J, Barrabés JA, Permanyer-Miralda G, Soler-Soler J. Purulent pericarditis: review of a 20-year experience in a general hospital. J Am Coll Cardiol 1993; 22(6): 1661–1665

60. Alió-Bosch J, Candell-Riera J, Monge-Rangel L, Soler-Soler J. Intrapericardial echocardiographic images and cardiac constriction. Am Heart J 1991; 121: 207–208

61. Sagristà-Sauleda J, Permanyer-Miralda G, Soler-Soler J. Tuberculous pericarditis: ten year experience with a prospective protocol for diagnosis and treatment. J Am Coll Cardiol 1988; 11(4): 724–728

62. Galve E, Garcia-Del-Castillo H, Evangelista A, Batlle J, Permanyer-Miralda G, Soler-Soler J. Pericardial effusion in the course of myocardial infarction: incidence, natural history, and clinical relevance. Circulation 1986; 73(2): 294–299

63. Candell-Riera J, García del Castillo H, Permanyer-Miralda G, Soler-Soler J. Echocardiographic features of the interventricular septum in chronic constrictive pericarditis. Circulation 1978; 57(6): 1154–1158

64. Ristić AD. Pericardiocentesis and intrapericardial treatment: Advances of the technique, diagnostic, and therapeutic value. Doctoral Thesis. Faculty of Medicine, Philipps Universtiy Marburg, Germany, 2002

65. Maisch B, Ristić AD. Practical aspects of the management of pericardial disease. Heart 2003; 89: 1096–1103

66. Maisch B, Ristić AD, Rupp H, Spodick DH. Pericardial access using the PerDUCER® and flexible percutaneous pericardioscopy. Am J Cardiol 2001; 88: 1323–1326

67. Seferović PM, Ristić AD, Maksimović R, Mitrović V. Therapeutic pericardiocentesis: Up-to-date review of indications, efficacy, and risks. In: Seferović PM, Spodick DH, Maisch B (eds) Maksimović R, Ristić AD (assoc. eds) Pericardiology: contemporary answers to continuing challenges, Belgrade: Science, 2000, pp 417–426

68. Sosa E, Scanavacca M, d'Avila A. Different ways of approaching the normal pericardial space. Circulation 1999; 100(24): e115–116

69. Brugada J, Berruezo A, Cuesta A, et al. Nonsurgical transthoracic epicardial radiofrequency ablation: an alternative in incessant ventricular tachycardia. J Am Coll Cardiol 2003; 41(11): 2036–2043

70. Tweddell JS, Zimmerman AN, Stone CM, et al. Pericardiocentesis guided by a pulse generator. J Am Coll Cardiol 1989; 14(4): 1074–1083

71. Duvernoy O, Magnusson A. CT-guided pericardiocentesis. Acta Radiol 1996; 37(5): 775–778

72. Bruning R, Muehlstaedt M, Becker C, Knez A, Haberl R, Reiser M. Computed tomography-fluoroscopy guided drainage of pericardial effusions: experience in 11 cases. Invest Radiol 2002; 37(6): 328–332

73. Chavanon O, Carrat L, Pasqualini C, Dubois E, Blin D, Troccaz J. Computer guided pericardiocentesis: experimental results and clinical perspectives. Herz 2000; 25(8): 761–768

74. Marmignon C, Chavanon O, Troccaz J. CASPER, a computer-assisted PERicardial puncture system: first clinical results. Comput Aided Surg 2005; 10(1): 15–21

75. Krikorian JG, Hancock EW. Pericardiocentesis. Am J Med 1978; 65: 808–812

76. Spodick DH. The technique of pericardiocentesis. When to perform it and how to minimize complications. J Crit Illn 1995; 10(11): 807–812

77. Spodick DH. Acute cardiac tamponade. N Engl J Med 2003; 349(7): 684–690

78. Verrier RL, Waxman S, Lovett EG, Moreno R. Transatrial access to the normal pericardial space: a novel approach for diagnostic sampling, pericardiocentesis, and therapeutic interventions. Circulation 1998; 98(21): 2331–2333

79. Waxman S, Pulerwitz TC, Rowe KA, Quist WC, Verrier RL. Preclinical safety testing of percutaneous transatrial access to the normal pericardial space for local cardiac drug delivery and diagnostic sampling. Catheter Cardiovasc Interv 2000; 49(4): 472–477

80. March KL, Woody M, Mehdi K, Zipes DP, Brantly M, Trapnell BC. Efficient in vivo catheter-based pericardial gene transfer mediated by adenoviral vectors. Clin Cardiol 1999; 22 (Suppl 1): I23–29

81. Ceron L, Manzato M, Mazzaro F, Bellavere F. A new diagnostic and therapeutic approach to pericardial effusion: transbronchial needle aspiration. Chest 2003; 123(5): 1753–1758

82. Fisher JD, Kim SG, Ferrick KJ, Gross JN, Goldberger MH, Nanna M. Internal transcardiac pericardiocentesis for acute tamponade. Am J Cardiol 2000; 86(12): 1388–1389

83. Hsu LF, Scavée C, Jaïs P, Hocini M, Haïssaguerre M. Transcardiac pericardiocentesis: an emergency life-saving technique for cardiac tamponade. J Cardiovasc Electrophysiol 2003; 14(9): 1001–1003

84. Macris MP, Igo SR. Minimally invasive access of the normal pericardium: initial clinical experience with a novel device. Clin Cardiol 1999; 22 (Suppl 1): I36–39

85. Seferović PM, Ristić AD, Maksimović R, et al. Initial clinical experience with PerDUCER®: Promising new tool in the diagnosis and treatment of pericardial disease. Clin Cardiol 1999; 22(Suppl 1): I30–35

86. Seferović PM, Ristić AD, Maksimović R, Spodick DH. New Percutaneous Pericardial Access Device: Early Clinical Data. In: Seferović PM, Spodick DH, Maisch B (eds) Maksimović R, Ristić AD (assoc. eds) Pericardiology: Contemporary answers to continuing challenges. Belgrade: Science, 2000, pp 407–416

87. Hou D, March KL. A novel percutaneous technique for accessing the normal pericardium: a single-center successful experience of 53 porcine procedures. J Invasive Cardiol 2003; 15(1): 13–17

88. Tio RA, Grandjean JG, Suurmeijer AJ, van Gilst WH, van Veldhuisen DJ, van Boven AJ. Thoracoscopic monitoring for pericardial application of local drug or gene therapy. Int J Cardiol 2002; 82(2): 117–121

89. Zenati MA, Shalaby A, Eisenman G, Nosbisch J, McGarvey J, Ota T. Epicardial left ventricular mapping using subxiphoid video pericardioscopy. Ann Thorac Surg 2007; 84(6): 2106–2107

90. Maisch B, Drude L. Pericardioscopy-a new diagnostic tool in inflammatory diseases of the pericardium. Eur Heart J 1991; 12 (Suppl D): 2–6

91. Maisch B, Bethge C, Drude L, Hufnagel G, Herzum M, Schönian U. Pericardioscopy and epicardial biopsy – new diagnostic tools in pericardial and perimyocardial disease. Eur Heart J 1994; 15 (Suppl. C): 68–73

92. Maisch B, Pankuweit S, Brilla C, et al. Intrapericardial treatment of inflammatory and neoplastic pericarditis guided by pericardioscopy and epicardial biopsy – results from a pilot study. Clin Cardiol 1999; 22 (Suppl 1): I17–22

93. Maisch B, Ristić AD, Pankuweit S. Intrapericardial treatment of autoreactive pericardial effusion with triamcinolone: the way to avoid side effects of systemic corticosteroid therapy. Eur Heart J 2002; 23: 1503–1508

94. Maisch B, Ristić AD, Pankuweit S, Neubauer A, Moll R. Neoplastic pericardial effusion: efficacy and safety of intrapericardial treatment with cisplatin. Eur Heart J 2002; 23: 1625–1631

95. Sinitsyn NP. Method of implantation of the cannula into the thorax for visual observa-tion of coronary circulation. [Н. П. Синицын. Методика вживления канюли в грудную клетку для визуального наблюдения за коронарным кровообращением][Russian]. Biull Eksp Biol Med 1955; 39(3): 74–76

96. Kondos G, Rich S, Levitsky S. Flexible fiberoptic pericardioscopy for the diagnosis of pericardial disease. J Am Coll Cardiol 1986; 7: 432–434

97. Kondos G, Rich S, Levitsky S. Flexible fiberoptic pericardioscopy. Chest 1986; 90(5): 787–788

98. Millaire A, Wurtz A, Brullard B, et al. Value of pericardioscopy in pericardial effusion. Arch Mal Coeur 1988; 81: 1071–1076

99. Millaire A, Wurtz A, de Groote P, Saudemont A, Chambon A, Ducloux G. Malignant pericardial effusions: usefulness of pericardioscopy. Am Heart J 1992; 124 (4): 1030–1034

100. Wurtz A, Chambon JP, Millaire A, Saudemont A, Ducloux G. Pericardioscopy: techniques, indications and results. Apropos of an experience with 70 cases. Ann Chir 1992; 46(2): 188–193

101. Nugue O, Millaire A, Porte H, et al. Pericardioscopy in the etiologic diagnosis of pericardial effusion in 141 consecutive patients. Circulation 1996; 94(7): 1635–1641

102. Porte HL, Janecki-Delebecq TJ, Finzi L, Metois DG, Millaire A, Wurtz AJ. Pericardoscopy for primary management of pericardial effusion in cancer patients. Eur J Cardiothorac Surg 1999; 16(3): 287–291

103. Seferović PM, Ristić AD, Maksimović R, et al. Flexible percutaneous pericardioscopy: Inherent drawbacks and recent advances. Herz 2000; 25(8): 741–747

104. Seferović PM, Ristić AD, Maksimović R, Tatić V, Ostojić M, Kanjuh V. Diagnostic value of pericardial biopsy: improvement with extensive sampling enabled by pericardioscopy. Circulation 2003; 107: 978–983

105. Janovsky RC, Boettner JF, Van Ordstrand HS, Effler DB. Recurrent tuberculous pericarditis. Ann Intern Med 1952; 37(6): 1268–1274

106. Williams C, Soutter L. Pericardial tamponade; diagnosis and treatment. Arch Intern Med 1954; 94(4): 571–584

107. Sanghvi LM, Samuel KC. Pericardial biopsy with Vim-Silverman needle. Arch Intern Med 1958; 101(6): 1147–1150

108. Bawa YS, Mehta MC, Wahi MC. Pericardial biopsy. Lancet 1959; 2: 1065–1067

109. Fernandes F, Ianni BM, Arteaga E, Benvenutti L, Mady C. Value of pericardial biopsy in the etiologic diagnosis of pericardial diseases. Arq Bras Cardiol 1998; 70(6): 393–395

110. Ziskind AA, Rodriguez S, Lemmon C, Burstein S. Percutaneous pericardial biopsy as an adjunctive technique for the diagnosis of pericardial disease. Am J Cardiol 1994; 74(3): 288–291

111. Palacios IF, Tuzcu EM, Ziskind AA, Younger J, Block PC. Percutaneous balloon pericardial window for patients with malignant pericardial effusion and tamponade. Cathet Cardiovasc Diag 1991; 22: 244–249

112. Ziskind AA, Pearce AC, Lemmon CC, et al. Percutaneous balloon pericardiotomy for the treatment of cardiac tamponade and large pericardial effusions: description of technique and report of the first 50 cases. J Am Coll Cardiol 1993; 21: 1–5

113. Thanopoulos BD, Georgakopoulos D, Tsaousis GS, Triposkiadis F, Paphitis CA. Percutaneous balloon pericardiotomy for the treatment of large, nonmalignant pericardial effusions in children: immediate and medium-term results. Cathet Cardiovasc Diagn 1997; 40: 97–100

114. Ziskind AA, Palacios IF. Percutaneous balloon pericardiotomy for patients with pericardial effusion and tamponade. In: Topol EJ (ed) Textbook of Interventional Cardiology, 5th edn. Philadelphia: W.B. Saunders Company, 2007, pp. 977–985

115. Iaffaldano RA, Jones P, Lewis BE, Eleftheriades EG, Johnson SA, McKiernan TL. Percutaneous balloon pericardiotomy: a double balloon technique. Cathet Cardiovasc Diagn 1995; 36: 79–81

116. Hsu KL, Tsai CH, Chiang FT, et al. Percutaneous balloon pericardiotomy for patients with recurrent pericardial effusion: using a novel double-balloon technique with one long and one short balloon. Am J Cardiol 1997; 80: 1635–1637

117. Ristić AD, Seferović PM, Maksimović R, Ostojić M. Percutaneous balloon pericardiotomy in neoplastic pericardial effusion. In Seferović PM, Spodick DH, Maisch B (eds) Maksimović R, Ristić AD (assoc. eds). Pericardiology: Contemporary answers to continuing challenges. Belgrade: Science, 2000, pp 427–438

118. Sochman J, Peregrin J, Pavcnik D. The cutting pericardiotome: another option for pericardiopleural draining in recurrent pericardial effusion. Initial experience. Int J Cardiol 2001; 77(1): 69–74

119. Spodick DH. Chronic tuberculous and other granulomatous pericarditis. In: Spodick DH (ed) Chronic and constrictive pericarditis. New York: Grune & Stratton, 1964, p 34

120. Zeman RK, Scovern H. Intrapericardial steroids in treatment of rheumatoid pericardial tamponade [letter]. Arthritis Rheum 1977; 20(6): 1289–1290

121. Peraino RA. Pericardial effusion in patients treated with maintenance dialysis. Am J Nephrol 1983; 3(6): 319–322

122. Buselmeier TJ, Davin TD, Simmons RL, Najarian JS, Kjellstrand CM. Treatment of intractable uremic pericardial effusion. Avoidance of pericardiectomy with local steroid instillation. JAMA 1978; 240(13): 1358–1359

123. Tomkowski WZ, Wiśniewska J, Szturmowicz M, et al. Evaluation of intrapericardial cisplatin administration in cases with recurrent malignant pericardial effusion and cardiac tamponade. Support Care Cancer 2004; 12(1): 53–57

124. Bishiniotis TS, Antoniadou S, Katseas G, Mouratidou D, Litos AG, Balamoutsos N. Malignant cardiac tamponade in women with breast cancer treated by pericardiocentesis and intrapericardial administration of triethylenethiophosphoramide (thiotepa). Am J Cardiol 2000; 86(3): 362–364

125. Colleoni M, Martinelli G, Beretta F, et al. Intracavitary chemotherapy with thiotepa in malignant pericardial effusions: an active and well-tolerated regimen. J Clin Oncol 1998; 16: 2371–2376

126. Martinoni A, Cipolla CM, Cardinale D, et al. Long-term results of intrapericardial chemotherapeutic treatment of malignant pericardial effusions with thiotepa.Chest 2004; 126(5): 1412–1416

127. Dempke W, Firusian N. Treatment of malignant pericardial effusion with 32P-colloid. Br J Cancer 1999; 80(12): 1955–1957

128. Spodick DH. Intrapericardial therapeutics and diagnostics. Am J Cardiol 2000; 85: 1012–1014

129. Maisch B, Seferović PM, Ristić AD, et al. Task Force on the Diagnosis and Manage-ment of Pericardial Diseases of the European Society of Cardiology. Guidelines on the diagnosis and management of pericardial diseases. Eur Heart J 2004; 25: 587–610

130. Guindo J, Rodriguez de la Serna A, et al. Recurrent pericarditis. Relief with colchicine. Circulation 1990; 82(4): 1117–1120

131. Adler Y, Finkelstein Y, Guindo J, et al. Colchicine treatment for recurrent pericarditis. A decade of experience. Circulation 1998; 97(21): 2183–2185

132. Imazio M, Bobbio M, Cecchi E, et al. Colchicine in addition to conventional therapy for acute pericarditis: results of the COlchicine for acute PEricarditis (COPE) trial. Circulation 2005; 112(13): 2012–2016

133. Imazio M, Bobbio M, Cecchi E, et al. Colchicine as first-choice therapy for recurrent pericarditis: results of the CORE (COlchicine for REcurrent pericarditis) trial. Arch Intern Med 2005; 165(17): 1987–1991

Anatomy of the Pericardium Relevant for Pericardial Access, Pericardioscopy, and Intrapericardial Interventions

Introduction

Due to the increased interest in the pericardial space for interventional procedures, and intrapericardial therapy the refined knowledge of its precise anatomy becomes more and more important [1–4]. Therefore, the aim of this chapter is to provide all necessary anatomic information for the operators performing pericardioscopy, pericardial/epicardial biopsies or epicardial ablation procedures.

Structures of the Normal Pericardium

The normal pericardium is a double-layered membrane consisting of an outer fibrous cover and an inner serous sac, invaginated by the heart. The serous pericardium has a visceral layer, the epicardium that covers the heart and the great vessels, and a parietal layer lining the inner side of the fibrous pericardium. The epicardium is reflected from the heart onto the parietal pericardium along the great vessels (Fig. 2.1). The thickness of the parietal pericardium varies from 0.8–2.5 mm (up to 3.5 mm on magnetic resonance imaging (MRI) and computed tomography (CT)) [5]. The fibrous pericardium is attached to the diaphragm by loose fibro-alveolar tissue, except for fusion over a small area of the central tendon (phrenicopericardial

ligament or "triangle of safety") [4]. The pericardium is also attached to the posterior surface of the sternum by superior and inferior sterno-pericardial ligaments that securely anchor the fibrous pericardium and maintain the general position of the heart inside the thorax (Table 2.1). The pericardial cavity is a closed virtual space that lies between the two opposite layers of serous pericardium, normally containing 20–50 ml of fluid [13, 14]. In healthy persons, most of the normal fluid is undetectable except in the major sinuses and the atrioventricular (AV) grooves and numerous recesses. In the supine position, this small amount can be detected in the superior and transverse sinus on CT scans.

Pericardial Sinuses and Recesses

Proper catheter manipulation during epicardial electrophysiology studies [3, 15–24] as well as the endoscopic inspection and aimed pericardial or epicardial biopsy [25–28] is not possible without knowing the anatomy of the pericardial recesses, sinuses, and the epicardial fat.

The normal pericardial cavity is a non-uniform, mainly virtual space. Its capacity is limited by the size and extensibility of the pericardial sac and even more by the rate of fluid accumulation over time.

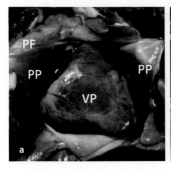 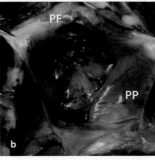

■ **Fig. 2.1a,b.** Opened normal pericardium during autopsy. *VP* visceral serous pericardium (epicardium); *PP* parietal serous pericardium, *PF* parietal fibrous pericardium (outer layer). Images were kindly provided by P. Cocco, MD, and Prof. G. Thiene, MD (Padua)

■ **Table 2.1.** Structures of the normal pericardium [5–12]	

Pericardial layers	▬ Fibrous pericardium
	▬ Serous pericardium
	    ▬ Visceral layer (lining the epicardium)
	    ▬ Parietal layer (lining the fibrous pericardium)

Pericardial sinuses	▬ Superior (SS)
	▬ Transverse (TS)
	    ▬ Anterior vertical,
	    ▬ Middle horizontal, and
	    ▬ Posterior vertical segments
	▬ Oblique (OS)

Pericardial recesses	▬ Superior aortic (SAR)
	    ▬ Anterior portion (aSAR)
	    ▬ Posterior portion (pSAR)
	    ▬ Right lateral portion (rSAR)
	▬ Inferior aortic (IAR)
	▬ Posterior pericardial recess (PPR)
	▬ Postcaval (PCR)
	▬ Left pulmonary (LPR)
	▬ Right pulmonary (RPR)
	▬ Right pulmonary vein (RPVR)
	▬ Left pulmonary vein (LPVR)

Fat tissue	▬ Epicardial fat ▬ Pericardial fat
Nerves	▬ Phrenic nerves ▬ Esophageal plexus (vagal fibers)
Parasympathetic ganglia in fat pads	▬ RA-right superior pulmonary vein (vagal inhibition of the SA node) ▬ VCI-LA fat pad (regulates AV conduction) ▬ VCS-right pulmonary artery fat pad (vagal fibers to both atria and the other fat pads)
Vascularization	▬ Pericardiacophrenic artery ▬ Internal mammary arteries ▬ Small aortic twigs

Lymphatics	▬ Parietal pericardial lymphatics
	    ▬ Drain to anterior and posterior mediastinal nodes
	▬ Visceral pericardial lymphatics
	    ▬ Drain to tracheal and bronchial mediastinal nodes

Ligaments	▬ Phrenicopericardial ligament ▬ Sternopericardial ligament

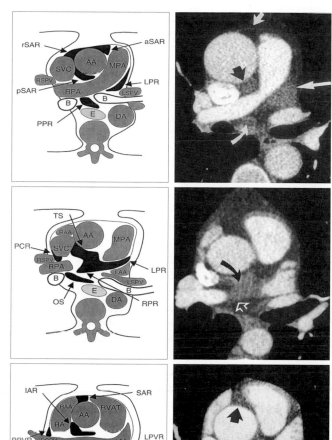

Superior, transverse, and oblique sinus can be recognized (see Table 2.1). CT and MRI disclose numerous smaller recesses not detectable in the open pericardium at surgery or post mortem [12]. The pericardial sinuses and recesses increase its capacity to accommodate fluid (or other contents), thus contributing to the pericardial reserve volume.

At the level of pericardial reflections and at the posterior wall between the great vessels, the pericardial space is divided into several recesses and sinuses. Importantly, all pericardial reflections are located behind the great vessels. Thus, there are no obstacles during intrapericardial catheter manipulation along the anteriorly/apically situated ventricular surface of the heart [3].

Epicardial and Pericardial Fat

Physicians performing invasive epicardial procedures should be aware of the anatomic distribution of fatty tissue located around the heart [3, 29]. Fatty tissue can only be found in two locations:

1. outside the pericardial sac attached to the outer layer of fibrous pericardium (pericardial fat);

2. underneath the visceral layer of the epicardium (epicardial or subepicardial fat).

There is no fatty tissue in the pericardial sac itself. Importantly, epicardial fat may accumulate around the heart and mimic pericardial effusion during CT, MRI, or ultrasonography [30].

The thickness of the epicardial fat is different in the various regions of the heart. The epicardial fat layer on the surface of the right ventricle can be up to 13.6 mm thick (mean 2.19) [31] and frequently increases with age and visceral obesity [32]. The thickness of the epicardial fatty tissue layers and subcutaneous fat correlate well in humans. However, even slim persons can present with a substantial quantity of epicardial fat [32]. The mean thickness of the epicardial fat in front of the middle of the interventricular septum is 0.8 mm but at the base of the heart is 4.12 mm. A thicker fat layer is found along the ventrolateral edge of the right ventricle [31, 33].

However, the amount of subepicardial fat is most remarkable over the anterior wall. In women, the epicardial fat layer in front of the right ventricle is thicker than in men (ratio 1.65:1) [31]. In the area in front of the left ventricle epicardial fat is mostly expressed around and along the epicardial blood vessels. The diaphragmatic wall along the septum is the region where no fat should be observed. Similarly, the area around and between the pulmonary veins is covered by minimal amount of epicardial fat. As described in the further sections, excessive pericardial fat tissue can be a cause for unsuccessful pericardiocentesis with the PerDUCER device [34]. The quantity of epicardial fat has been recently correlated to the likelihood of atherosclerosis and coronary artery disease.

Normal Pericardial Fluid

Normal pericardial fluid is a serous ultrafiltrate of plasma with a lower protein concentration than in plasma but with a relatively high albumin level. However, electrolyte concentrations yield an osmolarity less than plasma [5]. In healthy persons 15–50 ml of this fluid is present in the pericardial space.

Nerves, Arteries, Lymphatics, and Lymph Nodes

The phrenic nerves located over the medial section of the frontal side of the parietal pericardium supply most of the pericardial innervations. It is of great importance to protect phrenic nerves and their nutrient pericardiacophrenic artery during surgery and radiofrequent ablation procedures. The esophageal plexus supplies vagal fibers for the pericardium. Only a small portion of the pericardial surface (approximately one sixth) is directly responsive to the painful stimuli (e.g. in acute pericarditis) and the pain is transmitted via the phrenic nerve to the spinal cord at the C4–C6 segment. The stellate ganglion is also important since its block can stop the pericardial pain [35].

Parietal pericardial lymphatic vessels are drained to the ipsilateral anterior and posterior mediastinal nodes while the superficial plexus of the cardiac lymphatics drains the visceral pericardium to the tracheal and bronchial group of mediastinal nodes. The internal mammary arteries and small aortic twigs contribute the arterial supply [4]. Studies in human cadavers [36], in the macaque monkeys [37], and in the dogs [38] show that the lymphatic drainage of the pericardium is mainly to the anterior mediastinal, tracheobronchial, lateropericardial, and posterior mediastinal (juxta-esophageal) lymph nodes and not into the hilar nodes. This has an important impact on the groups of mediastinal lymph nodes that are enlarged in tuberculous pericarditis. The mediastinal node enlargement does not show up on routine chest radiographs but can be seen only on chest computed tomography or magnetic resonance imaging [39]. In other conditions associated with pericardial effusion and mediastinal lymphadenopathy like lymphomas, malignancy, and sarcoidosis, hilar node involvement is prominent [40].

Pericardial Anomalies

The understanding of normal and abnormal pericardial anatomy, potential anatomical variations and congenital defects is important not only for the proper management of the anomalies but also for utilization of the intrapericardial space for therapeutic purposes. For the physician who is about to perform a pericardial procedure it is essential to know if a patient has a congenital defect or a complete absence of the pericardium [3].

Congenital defects of the pericardium can be detected at 1/10.000 autopsies. Most frequently they comprise partial left (70%), right (17%) or total bilateral (extremely rare) pericardial absence. About 30% of patients have additional congenital abnormalities [41]. Most patients with a total absence of pericardium are asymptomatic. Importantly, homolateral cardiac displacement and augmented heart mobility impose an increased risk for traumatic aortic dissection type A [42]. Partial left side defects can be complicated by cardiac strangulation caused by herniation of the left atrial appendage, atrium or left ventricle through the defect (chest pain, shortness of breath, syncope or sudden death). The chest X-ray is typical but the diagnosis is confirmed by echocardiography, CT, and MRI [43, 44]. Excision of the atrial appendage and surgical pericardioplasty (Dacron, Gore-tex, or bovine pericardium) is indicated for imminent strangulation [45].

Distinction of the Pericardium in Humans and Animals Used for Experimental Studies

In the analysis of feasibility and safety of new techniques or devices used for pericardial access and/or intrapericardial therapy it is essential to keep in mind the important differences between the pericardium in humans and in animals used for experimental studies [4]. The pericardium in dogs is without a venous mesocardium. Their fibrous pericardium is substantially less developed [46]. Moreover, dogs do not have the fibrous triangle of safety and the oblique sinus [4]. The fibrous pericardium is well developed in humans (but also in pigs) and the attachment to the diaphragm is extensive. The horse has a strong attachment to the sternum and in herbivore in general the fibrous layer is thick. The thickness of the pericardium in a horse (calculated on a body surface area) is 15 times higher than in a rabbit, and humans are somewhere in between, with a similar thickness as in swine and cattle [47].

Future Perspectives and Recommendations

Improvement of imaging techniques will in the future certainly contribute to the further advances of our knowledge of pericardial anatomy both in health and disease. Proper interpretation of echocardiography, CT, MRI, and pericardioscopy findings is not possible without a good anatomical orientation. The expanding field of epicardial electrophysiology and ablation might assign even greater importance to the pericardial anatomy in the near future [3].

References

1. Spodick DH. Intrapericardial therapy and diagnosis. Curr Cardiol Rep 2002; 4(1): 22–25
2. Spodick DH. Intrapericardial therapeutics and diagnostics. Am J Cardiol 2000; 85(8): 1012–1014
3. D'Avila A, Scanavacca M, Sosa E, Ruskin JN, Reddy VY. Pericardial anatomy for the interventional electrophysiologist. J Cardiovasc Electrophysiol. 2003; 14(4): 422–430
4. Shabetai R. The pericardium. Kluwer Academic Publishers, Boston (MA), 2003
5. Spodick DH. Pericardial diseases. In: Braunwald E, Zipes D, Libby P (eds) Heart disease: A textbook of cardiovascular medicine. 6th edition. WB Saunders, Philadelphia, 2001, pp 1823–1876
6. Vesely TM, Cahill DR. Cross-sectional anatomy of the pericardial sinuses, recesses and adjacent structures. Surg Radiol Anat 1986; 8: 221–227
7. Choe YH, Im JG, Park JH, Han MC, Kim CW. The anatomy of the pericardial space: A study in cadavers and patients. AJR Am J Roentgenol 1987; 149: 693–697
8. Chaffanjon P, Brichon PY, Faure C, Favre JJ. Pericardial reflection around the venous aspect of the heart. Surg Radiol Anat 1997; 19: 17–21
9. Randall WC, Ardell JL. Selective parasympathectomy of automatic and conductive tissues of the canine heart. Am J Physiol 1985; 248: H61–H68
10. Ardell JL, Randall WC. Selective vagal innervation of sino-atrial and atrioventricular nodes in canine heart. Am J Physiol 1986; 251: H764–H773
11. Chiou CW, Eble JN, Zipes DP. Efferent vagal innervation of the canine atria and sinus and atrioventricular nodes. Circulation 1997; 95: 2573–2584
12. Groell R, Schaffler GJ, Rienmueller R. Pericardial sinuses and recesses: Findings at electrocardiographically triggered electron-beam CT. Radiology 1999; 212: 69–73
13. Spodick DH. The pericardium: A comprehensive textbook. Marcel Dekker, New York, 1997
14. Willians PL, Warmick R (eds) Gray's Anatomy, 36th edn. WB Saunders, Philadelphia, 1980

15. Sosa E, Scanavacca M, d'Avila A, Pilleggi F. A new technique to perform epicardial mapping in the electrophysiology laboratory. J Cardiovasc Electrophysiol 1996; 7: 531–536

16. Sosa E, Scanavacca M, D'Avila A, et al. Endocardial and epicardial ablation guided by nonsurgical transthoracic epicardial mapping to treat recurrent ventricular tachycardia. J Cardiovasc Electrophysiol 1998; 9: 229–239

17. Sosa E, Scanavacca M, d'Avila A, Oliveira F, Ramires JAF. Nonsurgical transthoracic epicardial catheter ablation to treat recurrent ventricular tachycardia occurring late after myocardial infarction. J Am Coll Cardiol 2000; 35: 1442–1449

18. Sosa E, Scanavacca M, D'Avila A, Antonio J, Ramires F. Nonsurgical transthoracic epicardial approach in patients with ventricular tachycardia and previous cardiac surgery. J Interv Card Electrophysiol 2004; 10(3): 281–288

19. Soejima K, Stevenson WG, Sapp JL, Selwyn AP, Couper G, Epstein LM. Endocardial and epicardial radiofrequency ablation of ventricular tachycardia associated with dilated cardiomyopathy: the importance of low-voltage scars. J Am Coll Cardiol 2004; 43(10): 1834–1842

20. d'Avila A, Houghtaling C, Gutierrez P, et al. Catheter ablation of ventricular epicardial tissue: a comparison of standard and cooled-tip radiofrequency energy. Circulation 2004; 109(19): 2363–2369

21. Brugada J, Berruezo A, Cuesta A, et al. Nonsurgical transthoracic epicardial radiofrequency ablation: an alternative in incessant ventricular tachycardia. J Am Coll Cardiol 2003; 41(11): 2036–2043

22. Stevenson WG, Soejima K. Inside or out? Another option for incessant ventricular tachycardia. J Am Coll Cardiol 2003; 41(11): 2044–2045

23. De Ponti R, Tritto M, Marazzi R, Salerno-Uriarte JA. How to approach epicardial ventricular tachycardia: electroanatomical mapping and ablation by transpericardial nonsurgical approach. Europace 2003; 5(1): 55–56

24. Swarup V, Morton JB, Arruda M, Wilber DJ. Ablation of epicardial macroreentrant ventricular tachycardia associated with idiopathic nonischemic dilated cardiomyopathy by a percutaneous transthoracic approach. J Cardiovasc Electrophysiol 2002; 13(11): 1164–1168

25. Seferovic PM, Ristic AD, Maksimovic R, Tatic V, Ostojic M, Kanjuh V. Diagnostic value of pericardial biopsy: improvement with extensive sampling enabled by pericardioscopy. Circulation 2003; 107(7): 978–983

26. Maisch B, Pankuweit S, Brilla C, et al. Intrapericardial treatment of inflammatory and neoplastic pericarditis guided by pericardioscopy and epicardial biopsy – results from a pilot study. Clin Cardiol 22 (1 Suppl 1): I17–22

27. Maisch B, Bethge C, Drude L, Hufnagel G, Herzum M, Schonian U. Pericardioscopy and epicardial biopsy – new diagnostic tools in pericardial and perimyocardial disease. Eur Heart J 1994; 15 (Suppl C): 68–73

28. Maisch B, Drude L. Pericardioscopy – a new diagnostic tool in inflammatory diseases of the pericardium. Eur Heart J 1991; 12 (Suppl D): 2–6

29. d'Avila A, Dias R, Scanavacca M, Sosa E. Epicardial fat tissue does not modify amplitude and duration of the epicardial electrograms and/or ventricular stimulation threshold. (Abstract) Eur J Cardiol 2002; 109

30. Duvernoy O, Larsson SG, Thuren J, Rauschning W. Epicardial fat causing pitfalls in CT and MR imaging of the pericardium. Acta Cardiol 1992; 33: 1–5.

31. Schejbal V. Epicardial fatty tissue of the right ventricle: Morphology, morphometry and functional significance. Pneumologie 1989; 43: 490–499.

32. Nakamura T, Tokunaga K, Shimomura I, et al. Contribution of visceral fat accumulation to the development of coronary artery disease in non-obese men. Atherosclerosis 1994; 107: 239–246.

33. Sons HU, Hoffmann V. Epicardial fat cell size, fat distribution and fat infiltration of the right and left ventricle of the heart. Anat Anz 1986; 161: 355–373

34. Maisch B, Ristic AD, Rupp H, Spodick DH. Pericardial access using the PerDUCER and flexible percutaneous pericardioscopy. Am J Cardiol 2001; 88(11): 1323–1326

35. Weissbein AS, Heller FN. A method of treatment for pericardial pain. Circulation 1961; 24: 607–612

36. Eliskova M, Eliska O, Miller AJ. The lymphatic drainage of the parietal pericardium in man. Lymphology 1995; 28: 208–217

37. Eliskova M, Eliska O, Miller AJ, et al. The efferent cardiac lymphatic pathways in the macaque monkey. Lymphology 1992; 25: 69–74

38. Miller AJ, DeBoer A, Pick R, et al. The lymphatic drainage of the pericardial space in the dog. Lymphology 1988; 21: 227–233

39. Cherian G, Habashy AG, Uthaman B, et al. Detection and follow-up of mediastinal lymph node enlargement in tuberculous effusions using computed tomography. Am J Med 2003; 114: 319–322

40. Pesola G, Teirstein AS, Goldman M. Sarcoidosis presenting with pericardial effusion. Sarcoidosis 1987; 4: 42–44

41. Cottrill CM, Tamaren J, Hall B. Sternal defects associated with congenital pericardial and cardiac defects. Cardiol Young 1998; 8(1): 100–104

42. Meunier JP, Lopez S, Teboul J, Jourdan J. Total pericardial defect: risk factor for traumatic aortic type A dissection. Ann Thorac Surg 2002; 74(1): 266

43. Connolly HM, Click RL, Schattenberg TT, Seward JB, Tajik AJ. Congenital absence of the pericardium: echocardiography as a diagnostic tool. J Am Soc Echocardiogr 1995; 8: 87–92

44. Gassner I, Judmaier W, Fink C, et al. Diagnosis of congenital pericardial defects, including a pathognomic sign for dangerous apical ventricular herniation, on magnetic resonance imaging. Br Heart J 1995; 74: 60–66

45. Loebe M, Alexi-Meskhishvili V, Weng Y, Hausdorf G, Hetzer R. Use of polytetrafluoroetylene surgical membrane as a pericardial substitute in the correction of congenital heart defects. Tex Heart Inst J 1993; 20(3): 213–217

46. Spodick DH. Acute pericarditis. Grune & Stratton, New York, 1959

47. Holt JP. The normal pericardium. Am J Cardiol 1970; 26(5): 455–465

Pericardial Effusion and Cardiac Tamponade

Introduction

Pericardial effusion is defined as the accumulation of fluid in the pericardial space either as transudate (hydropericardium), exudate, pyopericardium or hemopericardium. Large pericardial effusions are most common with neoplastic, tuberculous, cholesterol, uremic pericarditis, myxedema, and parasitoses [1, 2]. Slowly developing pericardial effusions can be asymptomatic even when they are very 1–2 l large, while rapidly accumulating smaller effusions of 150–200 ml can cause fatal tamponade (Fig. 3.1).

Loculated effusions occur after surgery, trauma, radiation and purulent infections. Effusions from a hydropericardium are usually small and occur mainly due to heart failure and fluid retention. Such an effusion produces no significant change in blood pressure or cardiac output and no pulsus paradoxus. Massive chronic pericardial effusions under this condition are rare (2–3.5% of all large effusions) [3].

Patients presenting with a pericardial effusion for the first time should undergo comprehensive evaluation and be followed-up in order to determine the cause of the effusion and to observe for the com-

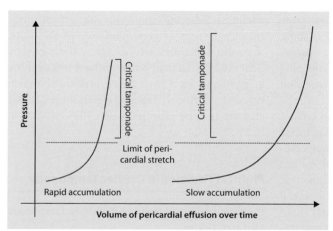

□ **Fig. 3.1.** Pericardial pressure-volume curves in "surgical tamponade" (*left*) – rapidly developing pericardial effusion and "medical tamponade" (right) – slowly accumulating effusion. Adapted with permission from Spodick (2003) [4]

plications such as cardiac tamponade, constriction or complications of the primary disease (e.g. paraneoplastic syndrome). Disease-specific and adjunctive therapy is given to those in whom pericarditis represents one manifestation of a systemic illness. In a recent study Imazio et al. [5] have demonstrated that a significant subset of patients with acute pericarditis can be evaluated and treated as outpatients. Patients without clinical poor prognostic predictors (fever > 38 °C, subacute onset, immunodepression, trauma, oral anticoagulant therapy, myopericarditis, severe pericardial effusion, cardiac tamponade) were considered low-risk cases and assigned to outpatient treatment with high-dose oral aspirin. Patients with poor prognostic predictors or aspirin failure were hospitalized in order to evaluate their potential etiology and apply more intensive treatment. Outpatient treatment was successful in 87% of cases and no serious complications occurred during 38 months of mean follow-up (no cases of cardiac tamponade) [5].

Cardiac tamponade is the hemodynamic consequence of the compression exerted on the outer surface of the heart by accumulating pericardial effusion. Importantly, when cardiac compensatory mechanisms are at the end of its capacities, even a small increase in the volume of effusion or decrease in the systemic pressure (e.g. by i.v. diuretics) can lead to impeded venous return and ventricular diastolic filling raising ventricular diastolic pressure and causing systemic and pulmonary congestion [4, 6, 7]. This decreases the preload, which by itself decreases the cardiac output. If the accumulation of pericardial effusion is progressive and untreated florid tamponade will develop. In "surgical" tamponade (i.e. wounds or iatrogenic perforations causing hemorrhage) intrapericardial pressure is rising rapidly, in the matter of minutes to hours, whereas a low-intensity inflammatory process is developing in days to weeks before critical cardiac compression ("medical" tamponade) (see Fig. 3.1) [4].

Pericardial disease of any etiology can cause a tamponade [6]. "Surgical tamponade," e.g. intrapericardial hemorrhage, can overwhelm compensatory mechanisms in a very short time. With cardiac wounds and intrapericardial rupture of a dissecting aorta as little as 150 ml of blood can be fatal in several minutes. In contrast, in "medical tamponade" fluid exudes not so rapidly and critical cardiac compression may occur at the range from 500–1000 ml or more. The volume of fluid causing tamponade is dependent on pericardial stiffness and thickness. Intense or repeated inflammation causing thickened or scared pericardium can sharply reduce the amount of effusion that can be tolerated before critical cardiac compression occurs. The clinical onset, ranging from subclinical to rapid or sudden, is determined by the balance of exudation rate and pericardial "compliance" permitting compensatory responses to keep effusions tolerable longer than in "surgical tamponade" [4].

Clinical Presentation of Cardiac Tamponade

A careful evaluation of clinical symptoms and signs is essential for the clinicians who should decide which patient with emerging cardiac tamponade is indicated for an emergency procedure and which patients could wait or even be medically treated. Most frequently patients complain about chest discomfort, dyspnea on exertion progressing to orthopnea, occasionally with cough and dysphagia, but also episodes of unconsciousness in the more advanced tamponade. Due to the local compression not only dyspnea, but also dysphagia, hoarseness (recurrent laryngeal nerve), hiccups (phrenic nerve), or nausea (diaphragm) can occur. In the terminal stage of medical tamponade, while reaching the end of their compensation mechanisms, patients complain that they could only sleep in the sitting position or for one or more nights could not sleep at all. Anemia, common in malignancies, exacerbates dyspnea and weakness. Subacute tamponade may initially present with the signs of its complications (renal failure, abdominal plethora, shock liver, and mesenteric ischemia) [8]. In tamponade without two or more inflammatory signs (typical pain, pericardial friction rub, fever, diffuse ST segment elevation) malignant effusion is to be expected with a likelihood ratio of 2.9 [2].

Physical Findings in Cardiac Tamponade

Prominent physical findings in cardiac tamponade are listed below:

1. Tachycardia (> 100 beats/min, but the rate may be lower in hypothyroidism, patients taking beta blockers, and in uremic patients);
2. Pericardial rubs (frequent in uremic acute pericarditis with tamponade);
3. Heart sounds may be distant, owing to insulation by fluid and reduced cardiac function, sometimes with relative accentuation of the pulmonic component of S2.
4. Absolute or relative hypotension. In "surgical tamponade," shock levels are usual; but in early "medical tamponade," systolic blood pressure is commonly greater than 90 mmHg. Occasionally patients with pre-existing hypertension may remain hypertensive [9]. In these patients "normal" blood pressure may be low, too.
5. Fever is related to etiology (subfebrile levels in systemic autoimmune disease, and high fever in acute viral diseases or bacterial infections). Febrile tamponade may be misdiagnosed as septic shock;
6. Jugular venous distension is striking in acute tamponade. However, it may be less prominent in obese and hypovolemic patients or if fluid accumulates slowly. Rapid "surgical tamponade," especially acute hemopericardium after perforations during percutaneous coronary intervention, pacemaker implantation or endomyocardial biopsy, can induce jugular pulsations without distension.

Compression of the base of the lung by large effusions results in a dullness on the precordium and under the left scapula (Bamberger-Pins-Ewart's sign) [1]. An inspiratory increase (or lack of fall) of the pressure in the neck veins (Kussmaul's sign), when verified with tamponade, or more reliable, after pericardial drainage, indicates effusive-constrictive pericarditis [10].

Pulsus Paradoxus

Pulsus paradoxus is a relatively late and therefore very important sign of cardiac tamponade (Fig. 3.2) [11]. It is defined as a decrease in systolic blood pressure greater then 10 mmHg during inspiration. Diastolic blood pressure does not get diminished with

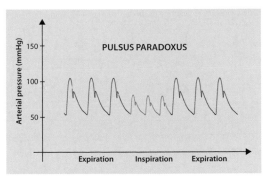

☐ **Fig. 3.2.** Pulsus paradoxus in cardiac tamponade. Note the inspiratory decrease of systolic blood pressure for > 10 mmHg. Adapted with permission from Shabetai (2000) [12]

inspiration and the pulse pressure is getting lower during inspiration in contrast to expiration. Pulsus paradoxus is easily detected by palpation. During inspiration, the pulse may remain palpable, but its volume diminishes significantly. In severe cases, it may disappear altogether. Usually, pulsus paradoxus is detectable at the radial pulse, but before deciding that pulsus paradoxus is absent, the larger arteries such as the brachial or femoral should be checked. Clinically meaningful pulsus paradoxus is apparent when the patient is breathing normally. Caution in interpretation is needed if the sign is present only when the patient breathes very deeply. Pulsus paradoxus is absent in:

1. tamponade complicating a large atrial septal defect [12] (shunt flow is not influenced by respiration); and
2. significant aortic regurgitation (the regurgitant filling is independent of respiration).

Electrocardiogram in Cardiac Tamponade

Electrocardiography may demonstrate diminished QRS and T-wave voltages. Microvoltage is defined as maximum QRS amplitude 0.5 mV in the limb leads and low voltage as the QRS amplitude of 5–10 mm in limb leads. PR-segment depression, ST-T changes, bundle branch block, may also occur. Electrical alternans is especiall important as a late sign of cardiac tamponade indicating the need for the emergency pericardiocentesis in the large majority of patients (Fig. 3.3) [4]. Although low QRS volt-

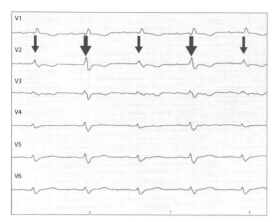

1. Brody's hypothesis – mechanico-electrical alterations of the myocardium (alterations in end-diastolic blood volume will change the magnitude of cardiac electrical potentials recorded at the body surface) [17].
2. Distance of the heart from body surface electrodes.
3. Reduction of cardiac size and volume in large effusions/cardiac tamponade.

However, Bruch et al. [18] have demonstrated that low QRS voltage is characteristic for cardiac tamponade but not for pericardial effusion per se. According to their findings, presence and severity of cardiac tamponade, in addition to inflammatory mechanisms, may contribute to the development of low QRS voltage in patients with large pericardial effusions. In this study, low QRS voltage persisted immediately after successful pericardiocentesis, but QRS amplitude recovered within one week [18]. However, QRS voltage also recovered after successful anti-inflammatory treatment, without pericardiocentesis (Fig. 3.4).

Classic studies on cardiovascular dynamics have shown that the epicardial circumference shortens proportionally less than the endocardial circumference, resulting in different tension distributions [19], with the strong impact of these electrical inhomogeneities on the surface ECG [20]. The rise of intrapericardial and enddiastolic intraventricular pressures during tamponade, leads to compression of the myocardium [21]. As a consequence, the mechanico-electrical

age is indicative of cardiac tamponade, its absence does not rule out the tamponade. Low voltage is most frequent in neoplastic effusions (but also in obese patients). The voltage in ECG generally returns to normal in the time frame from one day to one week after pericardiocentesis. However, in some patients, e.g. 3/25 (12%) in the study of Oliver et al. [13], the voltage remained low after pericardiocentesis.

Different mechanisms have been proposed to explain low QRS voltage associated with pericardial effusion and cardiac tamponade [14–16]:

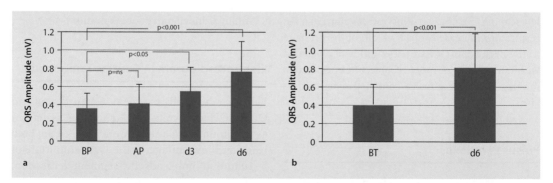

condition of the endocardial and the epicardial myocardium become more alike, offering an explanation for the changes present in the surface ECG [16].

However, Bruch et al. [18] have demonstrated normalization of QRS amplitude six days after initiation of anti-inflammatory treatment, suggesting a potential additional role of inflammation in pathophysiology of electrocardiographic changes in cardiac tamponade.

Chest Radiography

In chest radiography large effusions are depicted as globular cardiomegaly with sharp margins ("water bottle" silhouette, "Bocksbeutel"; Fig. 3.5) [22].

On well-penetrated lateral radiographies, or better on cine films, pericardial fluid is suggested by lucent lines within the cardiopericardial shadow (epicardial halo sign, or various other terms for this phenomenon) [22 31]. Recently, it was suggested that this sign might be useful for fluoroscopic guidance of pericardiocentesis [32] (Video 3.1, 3.2, and 3.3).

Echocardiography

Echocardiography promptly and reliably confirms the presence and hemodynamic impact of pericardial effusion.

The separation of pericardial layers can be detected in echocardiography, when the pericardial fluid exceeds 15–35 ml (Fig. 3.6) [33]. The size of pericardial effusions can be graded as:

1. small (echo-free space in diastole <10 mm),
2. moderate (10–20 mm),
3. large (>20 mm), or
4. very large (>20 mm, often associated with compression of the heart).

In hemodynamically significant effusions and in cardiac tamponade M mode and 2D echocardiography may reveal the diastolic collapse of the anterior right ventricular (RV) free wall (Fig. 3.7), the right atrial (RA) collapse (Fig. 3.8), the left atrial (LA) and rarely the left ventricular (LV) collapse, an increased LV diastolic wall thickness "pseudohypertrophy",

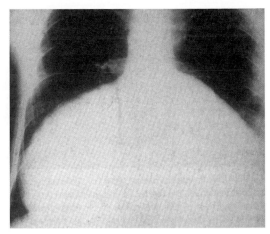

Fig. 3.5. Chest radiography in a patient with a very large pericardial effusion and cardiac tamponade. The cardiac silhouette has a typical "water bottle" ("Bocksbeutel") appearance

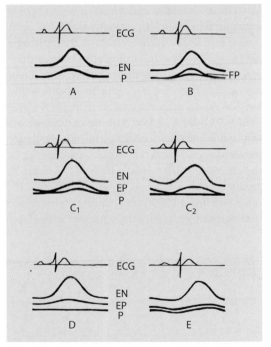

Fig. 3.6. Horowitz classification of pericardial effusions. Type A: No effusion; Type B: Systolic separation of epicardium and pericardium (3–16 ml); Type C1: Systolic and diastolic separation of epicardium and pericardium (small effusion > 16 ml); Type C2: Systolic and diastolic separation of epicardium and pericardium with attenuated pericardial motion; Type D: Pronounced separation of epicardium and pericardium with large echo-free space; Type E: Pericardial thickening (> 4 mm). Modified according to Horowitz et al. (1974) [33]

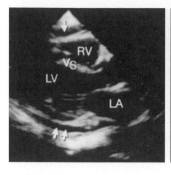 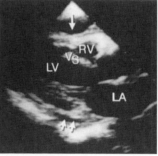

■ **Fig. 3.7.** Two-dimensional echocardiography (parasternal long-axis view) revealing diastolic collapse (*arrow*) of the anterior right ventricular (*RV*) free wall in a patient with a moderately large pericardial effusion. *LV* left ventricle, *LA* left atrium, *VS* interventricular septum. Reproduced with permission from Tsang et al. (2000) [34]

a "swinging heart", and a dilatation with a lack of physiological 50% collapse of the inferior caval vein in inspirium.

M-mode echocardiography detects the right ventricular diastolic collapse more reliably than two-dimensional echocardiography [35]. Compression and inward movements of free walls of right and later of left heart chambers indicate a transient negative transmural pressure (i.e., transiently higher pericardial than intracardiac pressures). These changes can be detected by echocardiography before hemodynamic compromise is clinically detectable. Right cardiac chamber collapse is common in patients with moderate and large pericardial effusion and is correlated weakly with clinical features of tamponade. In a large prospective series in which the reference standard was clinical tamponade, the absence of any chamber collapse had a high (92%) negative predictive value, whereas the positive predictive value was lower (58%) [36]. Cardiac tamponade after surgical procedures may present with atypical features due to adhesions and cardiac disease. Transesophageal echocardiography or CT may be required for the correct diagnosis and selection of treatment [37].

The right ventricular diastolic collapse can be absent in patients with elevated right ventricular pressure and right ventricular hypertrophy, as well as in patients with right ventricular infarction [7]. The mitral diastolic slope also shows a decrease, as well as the separation of mitral leaflets, suggesting decreased mitral valve flow and left ventricular volume. In large pericardial effusions and tamponade the heart may move freely within the pericardial cavity ("swinging heart"; Fig. 3.9). This exaggerated motion of the heart induces "pseudo"-motions like pseudomitral valve prolapse, pseudosystolic anterior motion of the mitral valve, paradoxical motion of the interventricular septum, midsystolic aortic valve closure [38, 39, 40].

Sensitivity and specificity of echocardiographic findings in cardiac tamponade were investigated

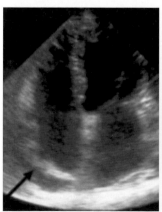 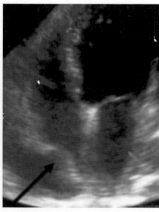

■ **Fig. 3.8.** *Left:* Medium size pericardial effusion without chamber compression. *Black arrow:* no atrial compression with normal atrial expension at this stage. *Right:* Pericardial effusion now with isolated compression of the right atrium (*black arrow*). The effusion has increased and became hemodynamically relevant

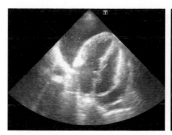 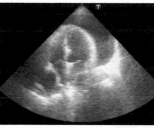

Fig. 3.9. Two-dimensional echocardiography (apical four-chamber view) in a patient with a very large pericardial effusion and pendular, free movements of the heart – "swinging heart". Reproduced with permission from Joffe et al. (1996) [38]

in 50 patients with large pericardial effusions who underwent cardiac catheterization during pericardiocentesis [41]. Diagnosis of cardiac tamponade was established only if both clinical (jugular venous distention, tachycardia, hypotension, pulsus paradoxus) and hemodynamic signs were present (elevation and equilibration of intrapericardial and right atrial (RA) pressures) which was fulfilled in 8/50 patients (16%). The average volume of pericardial effusion evacuated by pericardiocentesis in patients with tamponade was larger but not significantly different in comparison to patients without tamponade (725 ± 344 ml vs. 649 ± 421 ml; $p = 0.317$).

Among the investigated 2D-echocardiographic parameters (Fig. 3.10) RA collapse and sustained inferior vena cava (VCI) congestion had 100% sensitivity, but a low specificity. Right ventricular (RV)

diastolic collapse and "swinging heart" had high sensitivity, but a low specificity. In contrast, left atrial (LA) collapse was highly specific, but had a low sensitivity, with a positive predictive value of 42.9%. Sudden leftward motion of the interventricular septum (IVS) was the only parameter with both high sensitivity and specificity, and a positive predictive value of 80% for the diagnosis of cardiac tamponade.

Doppler echocardiography demonstrates in cardiac tamponade an increase of tricuspid flow and a decrease of mitral flow during inspiration (Fig. 3.11). The reverse process occurs in expiration. Systolic

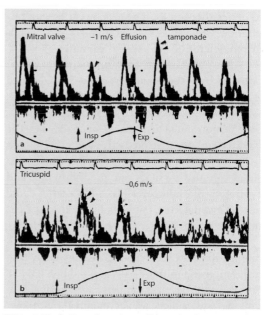

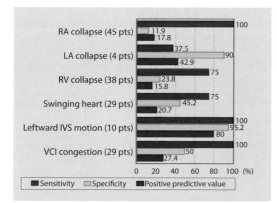

Fig. 3.10. Sensitivity and specificity and positive predictive value of echocardiography findings in cardiac tamponade investigated in 50 patients with large pericardial effusions. Diagnosis of cardiac tamponade was established in 8/50 patients (16%) using clinical criteria and cardiac catheterization performed immediately before pericardiocentesis [41]. *RA* right atrium, *RV* right ventricle, *LA* left atrium, *IVS* interventricular septum, *VCI* inferior caval vein (Ristic et al. [41])

Fig. 3.11a,b. Doppler echocardiography demonstrating respiratory changes of flow velocities in cardiac tamponade. (a) On inspiration (Insp) (*arrowhead*), mitral E velocity decreases significantly and opposite changes occur on expiration (*Exp*) (*double arrowhead*). Reciprocal changes are identified on the bottom (b). Adapted with permission from Oh et al. (1993) [42]

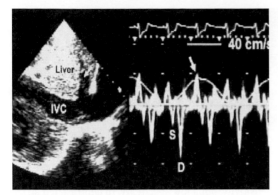

◻ Fig. 3.12. Congestion of inferior caval vein (*IVC*) in a patient with cardiac tamponade (two-dimensional echocardiography, subcostal view). Doppler echocardiography (*right*) revealed increased hepatic venous diastolic flow reversal. *S* systole, *D* diastole. Reproduced with permission from Tsang et al. (2000) [34]

and diastolic flows are reduced in systemic veins in expirium and reverse flow with atrial contraction is increased (Fig. 3.12).

Distinct respiratory variations of color M-mode Doppler flow propagation velocity (Vp) are also evident in the setting of cardiac tamponade [43]. Prior to pericardiocentesis, the Vp slope varies with respiration, with values ranging from 70 cm/s at end-inspiration to 100 cm/s at end-expiration.

After pericardiocentesis, this variation disappears, and Vp is constant at 60 cm/s. The increased flow propagation prior to pericardiocentesis is likely due to the accelerated LV relaxation that has been demonstrated in cardiac tamponade [44]. The positive and negative predictive values were high (82% and 88%, respectively) for abnormal right-sided venous flows (systolic predominance and expiratory diastolic reversals) but the latter could not be evaluated in more than one third of patients.

During cardiac tamponade, tricuspid and pulmonic valve flow velocities increase markedly with inspiration and mitral, aortic, and pulmonary vein flow velocities decrease compared with normal controls and with patients with asymptomatic effusions. However, associated conditions can both create (e.g., pleural effusions, chronic obstructive pulmonary disease, LV dysfunction) and obscure (e.g., RV hypertension) the echocardiographic signs of tamponade.

Computed Tomography and Magnetic Resonance Imaging

Computed tomography (CT) and magnetic resonance imaging (MRI) have high temporal and spatial resolution, large field of view, multiplanar capability, and offer possibility to image the entire pericardium as well as to evaluate the cardiac function during a single examination. Main indications are distinguishing focal pericardial thickening and small to moderate size pericardial effusions, detecting loculated pericardial effusion (Fig. 3.13), and establishing the diagnosis of constrictive pericarditis as well as the differential diagnosis to restrictive cardiomyopathy (Table 3.1). In patients with effusive-constrictive and constrictive pericarditis MRI can significantly contribute to the reduction of perioperative mortality by exclusion of patients with extensive myocardial fibrosis and/or atrophy.

Additional common indications are the visualization of pericardial masses and congenital anomalies and the evaluation of their relationship towards surrounding structures. Therefore, CT and MRI of the pericardium are important not only for establishing the diagnosis of pericardial diseases but also for the further clinical decision-making and the optimal choice of treatment in these patients.

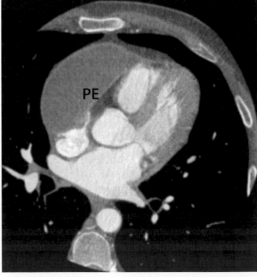

◻ Fig. 3.13. Localized pericardial effusion. CT-scan in a four chamber view. *PE* Pericardial effusion

Table 3.1. Pericardial changes in computed tomography and magnetic resonance imaging				
Pattern	Pathoanatomical basis	CT	MRI	Interpretation DD
Normal thickness	–	Thin line in front of the right atrium and right ventricle between mediastinum and subepicardial fat +++	Thin signal free line round the heart as long subepicardial and mediastinal fat present (for delineation) ++	No pathology
Thickened and smooth	Acute inflammatory process, effusion	CT-values for DD +++	MRI-signals for DD ++	Acute, subacute pericarditis, pericardial effusion, DD liquid, semiliquid, hemorrhagic, purulent, solid
Thickened irregular	Chronic inflammatory process	+++	+++	Chronic pericarditis, pericardial fibrosis, tumor, metastasis, post surgery
Thickened irregular, calcified	End-stage of inflammatory, traumatic or hemorrhagic process	High CT value +++	Poor signal ++	Pericarditis calcarea, calcified tumors

CT computed tomography, MRI magnetic resonance imaging, DD differential diagnosis, + visible, ++ good, +++ best visualization. Modified with permission from Maisch et al. (2004) [13].

Cardiac Catheterization and Invasive Hemodynamics

Patients in pericardial tamponade demonstrate at cardiac catheterization an elevated right atrial pressure, with a prominent x descent and a diminished or absent y descent (cardiac compression, which interrupts the venous return is maximal at end-diastole) (Fig. 3.14) [35]. In cardiac tamponade, the jugular pressure declines normally with inspiration (Kussmaul's sign absent), reflecting augmented systemic venous return. On the contrary, in constrictive or effusive-constrictive pericarditis, right heart failure, or severe tricuspid regurgitation, the mean central venous pressure does not decline during inspiration, and may even increase (Kussmaul's sign present).

The pulmonary capillary wedge pressure is elevated and nearly equal to the intrapericardial and right atrial pressure. Except in low-pressure tamponade, diastolic pressures in all heart chambers are usually 15–30 mmHg. These pressures are similar to pressures present in heart failure. However, cardiac tamponade does not cause alveolar pulmonary edema [46]. In contrast to constrictive pericarditis, ventricular diastolic pressure does not have

the dip and plateau configuration, but is elevated in early diastole and continues to rise throughout the diastole [47].

In contrast to constrictive pericarditis in cardiac tamponade, as in normal subjects, both the pulmonary wedge pressure and the central venous pressure

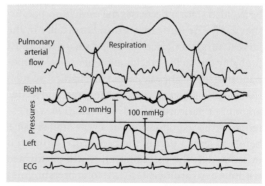

Fig. 3.14. Hemodynamic characteristics of cardiac tamponade. Marked elevation of diastolic pressures in the right ventricle, right atrium, and left ventricle and pericardial cavity. The right atrial pressure displays the loss of the y descent. Marked variations of the aortic and pulmonary artery pressures are consistent with pulsus paradoxus. *Right:* right atrial and ventricular pressures, *left:* aortic and left ventricular pressures. Reproduced with permission from Murgo et al. (1982) [45]

fall with inspiration. In constrictive pericarditis, the pulmonary wedge pressure is diminished in inspiration, but the central venous pressure is not. Equalization of the two venous pressures is often present only during inspiration. As pericardial fluid is drained, intrapericardial pressure falls below bi-atrial pressure. If this does not occur, the diagnosis of effusive constrictive disease should be considered [10].

Medical Management of Cardiac Tamponade

Cardiac tamponade is an absolute indication for urgent pericardial drainage [48]. Medical treatment is only a temporary measure until pericardiocentesis or surgical relief (e.g. in dissection of the aorta) can be performed. The benefit of inotropic support for hypotensive patients, with or without vasodilators (e.g. dobutamine) [49], is controversial [50]. Volume infusion, however, is useful for patients with hypovolemia [4]. Although we have never noticed such an event in our clinical practice, it was reported that intravenous administration of fluid can even precipitate tamponade in normovolemic or hypervolemic patients [51].

Although severely hypoxic patients or those inclining to respiratory arrest must be intubated and ventilated during the preparation for pericardiocentesis, prolonged, positive pressure ventilation should be avoided since it decreases the cardiac output further [52]. The initial procedural mortality in the largest surgical pericardioscopy series was most probably due to the precipitation of critical tamponade by general anesthesia and mechanical ventilation [53]. In patients with cardiac arrest and a large amount of pericardial fluid, resuscitation with external cardiac compression has a very limited value, before at least a part of the pericardial effusion is evacuated. If the resuscitation is still performed without pericardiocentesis, systolic pressure may even slightly rise, but diastolic pressure will fall and further reduce coronary perfusion pressure [51]. Intravenous administration of diuretics is contraindicated and could be fatal in patients on the edge of their compensatory mechanisms in tamponade [48]. Oliguria or anuria in patients with cardiac tamponade is not an indication for diuretics but for emergency pericardiocentesis. The diuresis will be very promptly resumed as soon as the pericardial effusion is evacuated and systemic pressure is normalized.

Future Perspectives and Recommendations

Pericardial effusion is from the clinical point of view one of the most important manifestations of pericardial diseases, ranging from undetectable or mild, to life-threatening cardiac tamponade. Prompt determination of its hemodynamic impact and etiology are essential. Some patients have only minor hemodynamic compromise and may be treated conservatively, or even on out-patient basis. Others, however, may have significantly compromised cardiac filling and require urgent hospitalization and pericardial drainage to avoid cardiac tamponade. The Guidelines of the European Society of Cardiology provide a simple decision-making algorithm in patients with pericardial effusion [48]. Importantly, the ability to treat the underlying cause, the long-term prognosis, and patient safety and comfort should be always considered in detail before selecting the diagnostic and treatment strategy.

References

1. Spodick DH. Pericardial diseases. In: Braunwald E, Zipes D, Libby P (eds) Heart disease: a textbook of cardiovascular medicine. Sixth Edition. WB Saunders, Philadelphia, 2001, pp 1823–1876
2. Sagrista-Sauleda J, Merce J, Permanyer-Miralda G, Soler-Soler J. Clinical clues to the causes of large pericardial effusions. Am J Med 2000; 109(2): 95–101
3. Soler-Soler J. Massive chronic pericardial effusion. In: Soler-Soler J, Permanyer-Miralda G, Sagrista-Sauleda J (eds) Pericardial diseases – old dilemmas and new insights. Kluwer, Amsterdam, 1990, pp 153–165
4. Spodick DH. Acute cardiac tamponade. N Engl J Med 2003; 349(7): 684–690
5. Imazio M, Demichelis B, Parrini I, et al. Day-hospital treatment of acute pericarditis: a management program for outpatient therapy. J Am Coll Cardiol 2004; 43(6): 1042–1046
6. Spodick DH. Physiology of cardiac tamponade. In: Spodick DH (ed) The pericardium: a comprehensive textbook. Marcel Dekker, New York, 1997, pp 180–190
7. Reddy PS, Curtiss EI, Uretsky BF. Spectrum of hemodynamic changes in cardiac tamponade. Am J Cardiol 1990; 66: 1487–1491

8. Delgado C, Barturen F. Atrial tamponade causing acute ischemic hepatic injury after cardiac surgery. Clin Cardiol 1999; 22(3): 242–244

9. Ramsaran EK, Benotti JR, Spodick DH. Exacerbated tamponade: Deterioration of cardiac function by lowering excessive arterial pressure in hypertensive cardiac tamponade. Cardiology 1995; 86: 77–79

10. Sagrista-Sauleda J, Angel J, Sanchez A, Permanyer-Miralda G, Soler-Soler J. Effusive-constrictive pericarditis. N Engl J Med 2004; 350(5): 469–475

11. Klopfenstein HS, Schuchard GH, Wann LS, et al. The relative merits of pulsus paradoxus and right ventricular diastolic collapse in the early detection of cardiac tamponade: an experimental echocardiographic study. Circulation 1985; 71: 829–833

12. Shabetai R. Pulsus paradoxus: definition, mechanisms, and clinical association. In: Seferovic PM, Spodick DH, Maisch B (eds) Pericardiology: contemporary answers to continuing challenges. Science, Belgrade, 2000, pp 53–62

13. Oliver C, Marin F, Pineda J, et al. Low QRS voltage in cardiac tamponade: a study of 70 cases. Int J Cardiol 2002; 83(1): 91–92

14. Gonzalez MS, Basnight MA, Appleton CP, Carucci M, Henry C, Olajos M. Experimental cardiac tamponade: a hemodynamic and Doppler echocardiographic reexamination of the relation of right and left heart ejection dynamics to the phase of respiration. J Am Coll Cardiol 1991; 18: 143–152

15. Toney JC, Kolmen SN. Cardiac tamponade: fluid and pressure effects on electrocardiographic changes. Proc Soc Biol Med 1966; 12: 642–648

16. Karatay CM, Fruehan CT, Lighty GW, Jr, Spear RM, Smulyan H. Acute epicardial distension in pigs: effect of fluid conductance on body surface electrocardiogram QRS size. Cardiovasc Res 1993; 27: 1033–1038

17. Brody DA. A theoretical analysis of intracavitary blood mass influence on the heart-lead relationship. Circ Res 1956; 4: 731– 738

18. Bruch C, Schmermund A, Dagres N, et al. Changes in QRS voltage in cardiac tamponade and pericardial effusion: reversibility after pericardiocentesis and after anti-inflammatory drug treatment. J Am Coll Cardiol 2001; 38(1): 219–226

19. Rushmer RF. Cardiovascular dynamics. WB Saunders, Philadelphia, PA, 1970, pp 76–81

20. Schlant RC, Hurst MD. Advances in electrocardiography. Grune and Stratton, New York, NY, 1976, pp 4–6

21. Friedman HS, Lajam F, Calderon J, Zaman Q, Marino ND, Gomes JA. Electrocardiographic features of experimental cardiac tamponade in closed-chest dogs. Eur J Cardiol 1977; 6: 311–322

22. Eisenberg MJ, Dunn MM, Kanth N, Gamsu G, Schiller NB. Diagnostic value of chest radiography for pericardial effusion. J Am Coll Cardiol 1993; 22: 588–593

23. Torrance DJ. Demonstration of subepicardial fat as an aid in the diagnosis of pericardial effusion or thickening. Am J Roentgenol 1955; 74: 850–855

24. Kremens V. Demonstration of the pericardial shadow on the routine chest roentgenogram: a new roentgen finding. Radiology 1955; 64: 72–80

25. Holt JF. Epicardial fat shadows in differential diagnosis. Radiology 1947; 48: 472–479

26. Lane EJ Jr, Carsky EW. Epicardial fat: Lateral plain film analysis in normals and in pericardial effusion. Radiology 1968; 91(1): 1–5

27. Carsky EW, Mauceri RA, Azimi F. The epicardial fat pad sign: analysis of frontal and lateral chest radiographs in patients with pericardial effusion. Radiology 1980; 137(2): 303–308

28. Woodring JH. The lateral chest radiograph in the detection of pericardial effusion: a reevaluation. J Ky Med Assoc 1998; 96(6): 218–224

29. Heinsimer JA, Collins GJ, Burkman MH, Roberts L Jr, Chen JT. Supine cross-table lateral chest roentgenogram for the detection of pericardial effusion. JAMA 1987; 257(23): 3266–3268

30. Spooner EW, Kuhns LR, Stern AM. Diagnosis of pericardial effusion in children: a new radiographic sign. Am J Roentgenol 1977; 128(1): 23–25

31. Tehranzadeh J, Kelley MJ. The differential density sign of pericardial effusion. Radiology 1979; 133(1): 23–30

32. Maisch B, Ristic AD. Tangential approach to small pericardial effusions under fluoroscopic guidance in the lateral view: The halo phenomenon [abstract]. Circulation 2001; 103(Suppl. A): II-730

33. Horowitz MDS, Schultz CS, Stinson EB, Harrison DC, Popp RL. Sensitivity and specificity of echocardiographic diagnosis of pericardial effusion. Circulation 1974; 50: 239–245

34. Tsang TS, Oh JK, Seward JB, Tajik AJ. Diagnostic value of echocardiography in cardiac tamponade. Herz 2000; 25(8): 734–740

35. Singh S, Wann LS, Schuchard GH, et al. Right ventricular and right atrial collapse in patients with cardiac tamponade – a combined echocardiographic and hemodynamic study. Circulation 1984; 70(6): 966–971

36. Merce J, Sagrista-Sauleda J, Permanyer-Miralda G, Evangelista A, Soler-Soler J. Correlation between clinical and Doppler echocardiographic findings in patients with moderate and large pericardial effusion: implications for the diagnosis of cardiac tamponade. Am Heart J 1999; 138 (4 Pt 1): 759–764

37. Ionescu A, Wilde P, Karsch KR. Localized pericardial tamponade: difficult echocardiographic diagnosis of a rare complication after cardiac surgery. J Am Soc Echocardiogr 2001; 14: 1220–1223

38. Joffe II, Jacobs LE, Kotler MN. Images in cardiovascular medicine. Pericardial tamponade. Circulation 1996; 94(10): 2667

39. Cikes I. Pericardial disease. In: Roelandt JRTC, Sutherland GR, Ilicento S, Linker DT (eds) Cardiac ultrasound. Livingstone, Edingburgh, 1993, pp 543–556

40. D´Cruz IA, Cohen HC, Prabhu R, Glick G. Diagnosis of cardiac tamponade by echocardiography. Changes in mitral valve motion and ventricular dimensions, with special reference to paradoxical pulse. Circulation 1975; 52: 460–465

41. Ristić AD, Kušić-Pajić A, Seferović PM, et al. Is two-dimensional echocardiography sensitive and specific enough to diagnose cardiac tamponade? Eur Heart J 2002; 23(Suppl.): 3307

42. Oh JK, Hatle LK, Mulvagh SL, Tajik AJ. Transient constrictive pericarditis: diagnosis by two-dimensional Doppler echocardiography. Mayo Clin Proc 1993; 68: 1158–1164

43. Togni M, Shabetai R, Blanchard D. Color M-mode Doppler flow propagation velocity in cardiac tamponade. J Am Coll Cardiol 2001; 37(1): 328–329

44. Nishikawa Y, Roberts JP, Talcott MR, Dysko RC, Tan P, Klopfenstein HS. Accelerated myocardial relaxation in conscious dogs during acute cardiac tamponade. Am J Phys 1994; 266(5 Pt 2): H1935–1943

45. Murgo JP, Uhl GS, Felter HG. Right and left heart ejection dynamics during pericardial tamponade in man. In: Reddy PS, Leon DF, Shaver JA (eds) Pericardial disease. Raven Press, New York, 1982, pp 189–201

46. Spodick DH. Low atrial natriuretic factor levels and absent pulmonary edema in pericardial compression of the heart. Am J Cardiol 1989; 63: 1271–1272

47. Shabetai R, Fowler NO, Guntheroth WG. The hemodynamics of cardiac tamponade and constrictive pericarditis. Am J Cardiol 1970; 26: 480–489

48. Maisch B, Seferovic PM, Ristic AD, et al. Task Force on the Diagnosis and Management of Pericardial Diseases of the European Society of Cardiology. Guidelines on the diagnosis and management of pericardial diseases. Executive summary. Eur Heart J 2004; 25(7): 587–610

49. Gascho JA, Martins JB, Marcus ML, Kerber RE. Effects of volume expansion and vasodilators in acute pericardial tamponade. Am J Physiol 1981; 240: H49–H53

50. Spodick DH. Medical treatment of cardiac tamponade. In: Caturelli G (ed) Cura intensiva cardiologica. TIPAR Poligrafica, Rome, 1991, pp 265–268

51. Hashim R, Frankel H, Tandon M, Rabinovici R. Fluid resuscitation-induced cardiac tamponade. Trauma 2002; 53: 1183–1184

52. Cooper JP, Oliver RM, Currie P, Walker JM, Swanton RH. How do the clinical findings in patients with pericardial effusions influence the success of aspiration? Br Heart J 1995; 73: 351–354

53. Nugue O, Millaire A, Porte H, et al. Pericardioscopy in the etiologic diagnosis of pericardial effusion in 141 consecutive patients. Circulation 1996; 94(7): 1635–1641

Pericardial Access and Drainage: Standard Techniques

Introduction

During more than 200 years of practice of pericardial drainage in the history of medicine physicians had to select either an open surgical approach or blind pericardiocentesis, mainly according to the personal preferences and training. In the absence of valid imaging the open approach was safer regarding the risk of puncturing the cardiac chambers instead of the effusion, the second approach had the lower risk for secondary infection.

With the wide availability of echocardiography and other imaging modalities an attempt to perform pericardial drainage without previous imaging would have to be regarded as "vitium artis". The precise determination of the size and distribution of the effusion by echocardiography enables the selection of the shortest route to the section of the pericardium where the effusion is the largest, and therefore significantly improves the feasibility and safety of the procedure.

However, even nowadays, the final selection if the surgical approach or pericardiocentesis guided by echocardiography only, or by fluoroscopy are selected depends not only upon the size and distribution of the effusion, but also upon the etiology of the disease, the personal experience of the operator, and the availability of the facilities and the equipment. The state-of-the art techniques for these three standard approaches to pericardial drainage will be reviewed in this chapter.

Indications for Pericardial Drainage

Pericardial drainage is indicated for clinical tamponade, suspicion of purulent, tuberculous, or neoplastic pericarditis, or for patients, who are symptomatic, despite one-week medical treatment [1]. Due to the high incidence of tamponade in the follow-up, drainage is also indicated in patients with effusions larger than 20 mm, measured in diastole in echocardiography (Fig. 4.1).

Pericardial drainage may not be necessary when the effusion is small and resolves spontaneously or under anti-inflammatory treatment (Table 4.1) [1]. In symptomatic patients with chronic moderately large effusions causing no hemodynamic compromise pericardiocentesis is indicated (level of evidence B, indication class IIa) if additional diagnostic procedures are available (e.g. pericardial fluid and tissue analyses, pericardioscopy, and epicardial/pericardial biopsy) to reveal the etiology of the disease and permit further causative therapy [2–15].

The decision to drain an effusion must take into account not only the echocardiography findings but

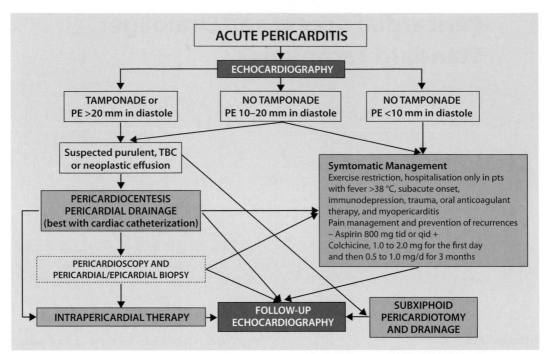

■ Fig. 4.1. Recommendations for the management of acute pericarditis and pericardial effusion. European Society of Cardiology Guidelines on diagnosis and management of pericardial diseases. Adapted with permission from Maisch et al. (2004) [1]

■ Table 4.1. Indications for pericardiocentesis according to the European Society of Cardiology Guidelines on diagnosis and management of pericardial diseases. Adapted with permission from Maisch et al. (2004) [1]

Class I indications

- Cardiac tamponade
- Effusions > 20 mm in echocardiography (diastole)
- Suspected purulent or tuberculous pericardial effusion (Fig. 4.2)

Class IIa indications

- Effusions 10–20 mm in echocardiography in diastole for diagnostic purposes other than purulent pericarditis or tuberculosis (pericardial fluid and tissue analyses, pericardioscopy, and epicardial/pericardial biopsy)
- Suspected neoplastic pericardial effusion

Class IIb Indications

- Effusions < 10 mm in echocardiography in diastole for diagnostic purposes other than purulent; neoplastic, or tuberculous pericarditis (pericardial fluid and tissue analyses, pericardioscopy, and epicardial/pericardial biopsy)

Class III – Contraindications

- Aortic dissection
- Relative contraindications: uncorrected coagulopathy, anticoagulant therapy, thrombocytopenia < 50000/mm3, small, posterior, and loculated effusions.
- Pericardiocentesis is not necessary when the diagnosis can be made otherwise or the effusions are small and resolving under anti-inflammatory treatment.

Class I: Conditions for which there is evidence and/or general agreement that a given procedure or treatment is useful and effective. *Class II:* Conditions for which there is conflicting evidence and/or a divergence of opinion about the usefulness/efficacy of a procedure or treatment. *Class IIa:* Weight of evidence/ opinion is in favor of usefulness/efficacy. *Class IIb:* Usefulness/efficacy is less well established by evidence/opinion but can (or should) be carried out if therapeutic consequences are to be expected.

also the clinical presentation and the risk-benefit ratio of the procedure. For example, large, chronic pericardial effusions affect intraocular pressure due to increased episcleral venous pressure [16]. Therefore, patients with glaucoma should undergo pericardiocentesis early, or if pericardiocentesis is not promptly feasible, patient should be referred for an ophthalmological examination with intraocular pressure measurement.

Aortic dissection is a major contraindication for pericardiocentesis [1, 17]. Relative contraindications include uncorrected coagulopathy, anticoagulant therapy, thrombocytopenia < 50.000/mm³, small, posterior, and loculated effusions. In acute traumatic hemopericardium and purulent pericarditis surgical drainage is more appropriate.

The decision to drain an effusion must take into account not only the echocardiographic findings but also the clinical presentation and the risk-benefit ratio of the procedure. For example, large, chronic pericardial effusions affect intraocular pressure due to increased episcleral venous pressure [16]. Therefore, patients with glaucoma should undergo pericardiocentesis, or if pericardiocentesis is not promptly feasible, referred for an ophthalmologic examination with intraocular pressure measurement.

Aortic dissection is a major contraindication for pericardiocentesis [1, 17]. Relative contraindications include uncorrected coagulopathy, anticoagulant therapy, thrombocytopenia < 50.000/mm³, small, posterior, and loculated effusions. In acute traumatic hemopericardium and purulent pericarditis surgical drainage is more appropriate.

Emergency Pericardiocentesis

Pericardiocentesis was performed for decades as a "blind" procedure, almost exclusively from the subxiphoid area, which has remained the most widely used approach (see Chapter 1) [18]. Currently, however, echocardiography is widely available and except in very rare urgent cases with clear diagnosis (e.g. complications of coronary interventions or endomyocardial biopsy) pericardiocentesis should not be attempted before seeing the current echocardiography findings. This is essential regardless of the technique selected for the further pericardial drainage.

If echocardiography is available in the emergency setting, urgent pericardiocentesis can be safely and successfully performed using the intercostal approach as described in the following section [19]. If the clinical status of the patient is rapidly deteriorating, diagnosis of the cardiac tamponade is certain but no echocardiography or fluoroscopic guidance can be immediately provided, pericardiocentesis should be performed with no further delay using the subxiphoid approach. A pigtail catheter should be inserted for drainage of the effusion, but if such a catheter is not available in the emergency setting a standard 7F central venous catheter can be used instead (Fig. 4.2).

Iatrogenic cardiac tamponade occurs most frequently in percutaneous mitral valvuloplasty, during or after transseptal puncture, particularly, if no biplane catheterization laboratory is available and a small left atrium is present. Whereas the puncture of the interatrial septum is asymptomatic, the passage of the free wall induces chest-pain immediately. If high-pressure containing structures are punctured, rapid deterioration will occur. However, if only the atrial wall is passed, the onset of symptoms and the tamponade may be delayed for 4 to 6 hours. Rescue pericardiocentesis is successful in 95–100% with a mortality of less than 1% [19]. Transsection or rupture of the coronary artery and acute or subacute cardiac tamponade may also occur during percutaneous coronary interventions [20, 21]. A breakthrough in the treatment of coronary perforation was achieved by introduction of membrane-covered graft stents [22]. Perforation of the coronary artery by a guide-wire is not infrequent but rarely causes a relevant pericardial hemorrhage.

During right ventricular endomyocardial biopsy, due to the low stiffness of the myocardium, perforation may occur, particularly, when the bioptome has not been opened before reaching the endocardial border. The rate of perforation is reported to be in the range of 0.3–5%, leading to tamponade and circulatory collapse in less than half of the cases [23–25]. The incidence of pericardial hemorrhage in left ventricular endomyocardial biopsy is lower (0.1–3.3%). Frank cardiac perforations seem to be accompanied by sudden bradycardia and hypotension [23]. Severe complications, leading to procedure related mortality were reported in only 0.05% in a

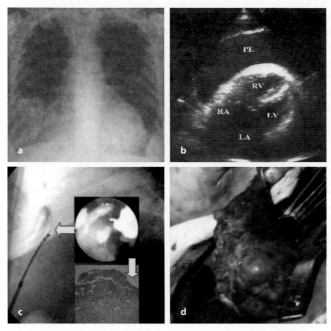

Fig. 4.2a–d. Large pericardial effusion in purulent pericarditis, a chest X-ray revealing an incapsulated pleural effusion in the basal left segment, **a** massive right-basal pneumonia and cardiomegaly (courtesy of Prof. K.J. Klose, MD, Marburg); **b** two-dimensional echocardiography (subxiphoid view) demonstrates a very large pericardial effusion (> 2 cm in diastole, PE). **c** Flexible percutaneous pericardioscopy (Storz AF1101B1, Tuttlingen) demonstrating purulent masses on the epicardial and parietal pericardial layers. Epicardial biopsy (horizontal arrow) revealed fibrino-purulent infiltration of the pericardium (vertical arrow); **d** surgical pericardiectomy via median sternotomy (courtesy of Prof. P. Petrović, MD, PhD, Belgrade). Reproduced with permission from Pankuweit et al. (2004) [14]

worldwide survey of more than 6000 cases [24] and in none of the 2537 patients from the registry of an experienced center [25].

Pacemaker leads penetrating the right ventricle or epicardial fixed electrodes may cause pericarditis with tamponade, adhesions, or constriction. A right bundle branch block instead of a usually induced left bundle branch block can be a first clue [26–29].

Hsu et al. [30] have described a technique of a life-saving transcardiac pericardial drainage using the transseptal puncture kit, after failure of conventional pericardiocentesis in a patient with radiofrequency catheter ablation-related acute tamponade. Although surgical repair for the perforation had to be performed subsequently, the patient survived without sequelae. The transcardiac approach may be an important and potentially life-saving adjunctive technique after failure of conventional pericardiocentesis in rapidly deteriorating or extremely unstable patients.

If the catheter is still in the pericardium when cardiac perforation and tamponade is recognized during catheterization or electrophysiology procedures, it can be used for a definitive aspiration and for the relief of tamponade. Fisher et al. [31] have reported two cases of cardiac perforation during radiofrequency ablation procedures for atrial fibrillation. In both cases tamponade was treated so that a long sheath was advanced over the ablating catheter that perforated into the pericardial space, before the ablating catheter was withdrawn. A 0.032-inch guidewire was advanced well into the pericardial space to stabilize and hold the position. Cardiac tamponade was resolved by aspiration through the sheath and surgical repair of the perforation was avoided by subsequent downsizing of the drainage catheters.

For the additional safety of pericardioscopy guided epicardial biopsy we recommend to use two guide wires, one for the eventual rescue procedures and another one for the advancement of the introducer set and for the endoscope. In the case of hemorrhage after epicardial biopsy the blood in the pericardial sac should be drawn and autotransfused, best through the femoral vein. This approach will stabilize the patient without a need for additional blood transfusion or surgical back-up.

If a perforation of cardiac chambers occurs during pericardiocentesis, the perforating catheter should be secured and kept in place. Percutaneous puncture and drainage can then be attempted again. Depending on the type, size, and location of the cardiac lesion, if percutaneous puncture and drainage are successful, the perforating catheter can be withdrawn and, surgery avoided by prompt drainage and autotransfusion of pericardial blood [32]. However, if the patient is still unstable, surgical repair should not be further postponed.

Even in medical emergencies strict aseptic and antiseptic conditions have to be respected during pericardiocentesis. The routine part of the preparation for the procedure should include, whenever possible, a chest X-ray and a basic laboratory evaluation, especially taking care of the coagulation status. In the presence of severe coagulation disorders pericardiocentesis has to be postponed until sufficient blood for transfusion, fresh frozen plasma platelets or coagulation factors are provided.

Echocardiography-Guided Pericardiocentesis

Evolution of Echo-Guided Pericardiocentesis

Pericardiocentesis is a life-saving percutaneous procedure for the management of cardiac tamponade or hemodynamically significant pericardial effusions. However, until two-dimensional (2D) echocardiography became available, pericardiocentesis was performed "blind". With the "blind" subxiphoid percutaneous approach to pericardiocentesis, serious complications were relatively common, and the procedures were associated with unacceptably high rates of effusion recurrence, morbidity and mortality [33, 34]. As a consequence, surgical decompression was commonly resorted to, and was advocated as a "safer" and more "definitive" procedure [35–38].

In an attempt to improve safety, pericardiocentesis had been performed under fluoroscopic guidance with or without electrocardiographic needle monitoring [39, 40]. Despite these additional measures, reported complications remained common, and included damage to the liver, myocardium, coronary arteries, and lungs [34].

Two-dimensional (2D) phased-array echocardiography was introduced into routine clinical use in late the 1970s [41]. This technology revolutionized visualization of cardiac anatomy and provided superior assessment of the location and distribution of pericardial fluid. Echocardiographically (echo)-guided pericardiocentesis was introduced at the

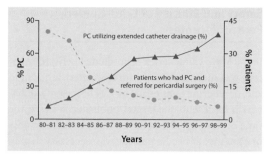

Fig. 4.3. Pericardiocentesis vs. surgical drainage of the pericardium in the Mayo clinic 1979–2000. PC pericardiocentesis. Reproduced with permission from Tsang et al. (2003) [46]

Mayo Clinic in 1979, and since that time, important procedural adaptations and modifications have been established that optimize safety and patient comfort, and minimize the recurrence of effusion. Echocardiographic guidance has substantially reduced the morbidity and mortality associated with pericardiocentesis. This technique has been modified and refined over the past two decades, and is currently widely used for the treatment of pericardial effusion (Fig. 4.3) [42–44]. The most important adaptation is the use of a pigtail catheter for extended drainage, which was associated with a significant decrease in the recurrence of pericardial effusions [44, 45].

The current state-of-the-art technique at the Mayo Clinic evolved from experience accumulated from 1127 consecutive procedures performed over 20 years [47]. A review of the Mayo experience with echo-guided pericardiocentesis revealed that the most common etiologies for the pericardial effusion were malignancy, post-cardiothoracic surgery, and cardiac perforation related to invasive percutaneous procedures [47].

Malignancy was formerly the most common etiology of an effusion for patients requiring pericardiocentesis. In more recent years, post-operative inflammation/bleeding following cardiothoracic surgery has surpassed it in numbers and is currently responsible for the largest number of pericardial effusions requiring treatment [47]. The other causes include infections, ischemic events (following myocardial infarction/rupture), connective tissue/inflammatory diseases, renal failure, anticoagulant use, drug-related, trauma, coagulopathies, post-irradiation, and some are "idiopathic".

Safety and Efficacy of Echo-Guided Pericardiocentesis

In the Mayo Clinic series, echo-guided pericardiocentesis was successful in with-drawing pericardial fluid and/or relieving tamponade in 97% of the procedures, which represents the largest published series at the time of writing [47]. In 89% of the procedures, only one attempt at needle passage was necessary to gain access into the pericardial space. Over the 21-year period of 1979–2000, 1127 echo-guided pericardiocentesis procedures were performed. There were a total of 14 major (1.2%) and 40 minor complications (3.5%) [47]. The major complications included the death of a 50-year-old woman with severe primary pulmonary hypertension, who did not survive an attempted surgical rescue following a right ventricular puncture that led to hemorrhagic tamponade. Non-fatal complications included chamber lacerations requiring surgery (5), injury to an intercostal vessel necessitating surgery (1), pneumothoraces requiring chest tube placement (5), ventricular tachycardia (1), and bacteriemia possibly related to pericardial catheter placement (1). Minor complications did not require specific treatment, except for monitoring and appropriate follow-up. These included transient chamber entries (11), small pneumothorax noted on radiographs (8), vasovagal response with transient fall in blood pressure (2), nonsustained supraventricular tachycardia (2), pericardial catheter occlusion (8), and probable pleuropericardial fistula (9). The safety and efficacy of echo-guided pericardiocentesis had been shown in various subgroups including pediatric patients [48], patients who were hemodynamically very unstable from cardiac perforation secondary to invasive percutaneous procedures [19], in postoperative patients [49], and in patients with malignancy [50] or connective tissue diseases [51].

Reduction of Effusion Recurrence with Catheter Drainage

The recurrence of pericardial effusion within 6 months of the initial procedure was 27% for patients who underwent simple pericardiocentesis, and 14% for those who had extended drainage using a pigtail catheter [47]. The frequency of effusion recurrence leading to repeat pericardiocentesis or surgery decreased significantly over time with the introduction and increased use of a pericardial pigtail catheter for more complete drainage [47], and safety of this adaptation has been established [45, 47]. Sclerotherapy, commonly used prior to 1993, was not found to be a significant predictor of recurrence. Corticosteroid use as concomitant therapy was more common in earlier years, and similar to nonsteroidals, was not predictive of recurrence in the Mayo clinic series. The lack of use of a pigtail catheter for extended drainage was the single most important predictor of effusion recurrence [47].

Technique of State-of-the-Art Echo-Guided Pericardiocentesis

Most 2D echocardiographic ultrasound machines are suitable for imaging and are portable to the bedside or procedure room. The necessary equipment and supplies are listed in Table 4.2. Special needles or catheters are generally not required, and a pericardiocentesis tray can be assembled from standard supplies.

The ideal site of needle entry is the point at which the largest fluid collection is closest to the body surface and from which a straight needle trajectory avoids vital structures. Since ultrasound does not penetrate air, it would not be difficult to avoid injury to the lungs. Based on the Mayo clinic series, the left chest wall was the preferred location for entry under echocardiographic site selection [47]. The subcostal route is not commonly used. It involves a longer path to reach the fluid, passes anterior to the liver capsule, and is directed toward the right heart chambers. The specific direction of the ultrasound beam, which best avoids all vital structures is the needle trajectory of choice. The intended needle trajectory should be evaluated by echocardiography multiple times to confirm the optimal direction and depth the needle will be advanced. The use of a 16-gauge polytef-sheathed intravenous needle for entry has eliminated the need for electrocardiographic monitoring of a steel needle. Once the fluid space is entered, only the polytef sheath is advanced. The steel core is immediately withdrawn. This latter step ensures safe manipulation after entry into the fluid-filled space

■ **Table 4.2.** Equipment and supplies for echo-guided pericardiocentesis [44]

Pericardiocentesis tray

1.	Povidone-iodine solution (skin antiseptic)
2.	Sterile transparent plastic drape (1030 Drape, Baxter)
3.	One 20- to 25-gauge needle for local anesthetic infiltration
4.	1% to 2% lidocaine (local anesthetic)
5.	Multiple 16- to 18-gauge (5.1- to 8.3-cm) polytef-sheathed venous "intracath" needles (Deseret)
6.	Syringes (10 to 20 ml) and one large syringe (60 ml)
7.	Specimen-collecting tubes for fluid analyses and cultures
8.	Plastic tubing (30 cm long) and three-way stopcock
9.	Scalpel (No. 11 blade)
10.	4 by 4 gauze dressing

Other supplies

1.	Sheath introducer set (Cordis): a) Fine-gauge (0.035-mm) polytef-coated, floppy-tipped guide wire b) A dilator and introducer sheath (6F to 8F)
2.	A 65-cm standard pigtail angiocatheter (6F to 8F) with multiple side holes (Cordis)
3.	Fluid receptacle (1 l vacuum bottle)
4.	Manometer (for pericardial pressure measurement)
5.	Dressings and antiseptic ointment
6.	Sterile isotonic saline (for flushing catheter)
7.	Sterile gloves, mask, and gown

and avoids the potential for sharp needle injury to a vital structure. Critical aspects of the procedure are:

1. Determination of the ideal entry site and needle trajectory,
2. Use of a polytef-sheathed needle, and
3. Advancement of the needle in a straight line without side-to-side manipulation during needle entry.

Confirmation of the polytef sheath position any time during the procedure can be achieved by echocardiographic imaging from a remote window while agitated saline (echo-contrast) is injected. Pericardial pressure can be measured, if desired, using a simple manometer attached to the introducing polytef sheath.

Introduction of a pigtail catheter into the pericardial sac provides better control of fluid withdrawal and assures continued access to the pericardial space for extended fluid drainage. The increasing use of a pericardial catheter has been associated with reduced recurrence of effusion and decreased the utilization of pericardial surgery [47, 50].

Initially, the effusion is completely drained via the catheter. Any additional fluid that accumulates is aspirated intermittently as opposed to continuously. Continuous catheter drainage was associated with a high incidence of catheter obstruction by proteinaceous components of the pericardial fluid. This problem can be avoided with intermittent drainage, typically every 4 to 6 hours or as clinically indicated. The catheter should be flushed with sterile saline after each withdrawal to maintain patency. The catheter is left in the pericardial space until net fluid output is less than 25 ml per 24 hours. Standard indwelling catheter care, with a complete change of dressing every 72 hours, is recommended. The patient can generally be ambulatory shortly after the procedure.

The contraindications to echo-guided pericardiocentesis are few. Theoretically, pericardiocentesis is contraindicated in the setting of myocardial rupture or aortic dissection because of the risk of extending the rupture or dissection with decompression [51]. The following is a step-by-step guide to echo-guided pericardiocentesis.

Echocardiography to Assess Location, Size, and Hemodynamic Impact of Effusion

If the clinical presentation permits, both 2D and Doppler studies are performed to assess the size, distribution, and hemodynamic impact of the effusion. In an emergency situation, an abbreviated 2D examination to localize the effusion and identify the ideal entry site and needle trajectory for pericardiocentesis is usually performed (Figs. 4.4 and 4.5).

Selection of the Ideal Entry Site

This is the point on the body surface where the effusion is closest to the transducer and the fluid collection is maximal. The distance from the skin to the

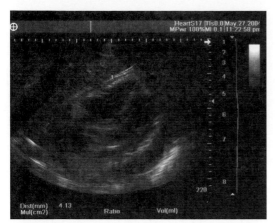

■ Fig. 4.4. Two-dimensional echocardiography – subxiphoid view showing a large pericardial effusion with only 4 mm diastolic separation of the pericardial layers in front of the right ventricle and ~2 cm separation in front of the left ventricle. The subxiphoid approach for pericardiocentesis would be inconvenient and risky in this patient (the same patient, studied at the same time as in Fig. 4.5). Courtesy of Arsen D. Ristić, MD (Belgrade)

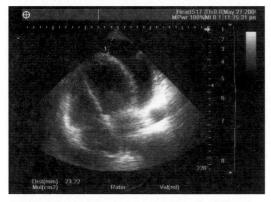

■ Fig. 4.5. Two-dimensional echocardiography – apical four chamber view showing a large pericardial effusion with a 23 mm diastolic separation in front of the apical segment of the left ventricle. Apical intercostal approach is the procedure of choice for pericardiocentesis in this patient (the same patient, studied at the same time as in Fig. 4.4). Courtesy of Arsen D. Ristic, MD (Belgrade)

pericardial space is assessed. The needle trajectory is defined by the angulation of the hand-held transducer. A straight trajectory that best avoids vital structures, including the liver, myocardium, and lung, is identified. Since ultrasound does not penetrate air-filled spaces, the lungs are effectively avoided. The operator

should select a site that avoids the internal mammary artery (3 to 5 cm from the parasternal border) and the vascular bundle at the inferior margin of each rib. The intended point of entry is marked on the skin with an indelible pen, and the direction of the ultrasound beam is carefully and repeatedly noted. This optimal needle trajectory should be transfixed in the operator's mind. Any repositioning of the patient should prompt reassessment of entry site and trajectory.

Sterile Preparation, Local Anesthetic Administration

Povidone-iodine is used as skin antiseptic. A transparent plastic sheet (1030 Drape, Baxter) allows both visualization of the sterile field and echocardiographic imaging, if needed. A 20- to 25-gauge needle is used to deliver lidocaine (1% to 2%) at the selected site. On the chest wall, the superior margin of a rib is used as a landmark. Generally, sedatives or anxiolytics are not necessary, but can be given if the situation warrants.

Insertion of the Polytef-Sheathed Needle

The polytef-sheathed "intracath" (16- to 18-gauge, 5.1- to 8.3-cm) Deseret needle with an attached saline-filled syringe is positioned at the predetermined entry site and angulation. In the predefined trajectory and with gentle aspiration, the sheathed needle is advanced in the direction of the fluid space. On entering the fluid, the needle is advanced approximately 2 mm further. The polytef sheath is then advanced over the needle, and the steel core is withdrawn. Only the polytef sheath remains in the fluid space.

Saline Echo-Contrast for Confirmation of Position

The position of the sheath can be confirmed by injecting 5 ml of agitated saline through the sheath. This should be performed particularly if bloody fluid has been aspirated or if there is any question of the sheath position. The echo-contrast effect is monitored by 2D echocardiography from a position outside the sterile field or through the underside of the transparent sheet. Saline echo-contrast medium is prepared with two syringes (one containing 5 ml of saline, the other empty), each connected to a three-way stopcock. The saline is agitated by rapidly injecting it back and forth between the two syringes. The agitated saline (echo-contrast) is then quickly injected into the polytef sheath, and the contrast effect is observed by 2D echocardiography. If contrast appears in the pericardial sac, the procedure can continue. If the sheath is not in the pericardial space, it should be repositioned by withdrawal or another needle passage should be attempted.

Diagnostic Tap

Fluid is aspirated directly into a syringe or via a three-way stopcock with extended flexible tubing. The fluid is sent for diagnostic tests.

Catheter Drainage

a) A guide wire is advanced through the polytef sheath before any appreciable amount of pericardial fluid is withdrawn. The polytef sheath is removed over the guide wire.
b) A small stab incision of the skin is made at the entry site, followed by introduction of a dilator (6–8 F, Cordis) over the guide wire. Predilatation of the chest wall passage facilitates subsequent insertion of the introducer sheath-dilator (6–8 F, Cordis) and minimizes burring of the sheath tip.
c) The guide wire and dilator are removed, leaving only the sheath in the pericardial sac. (The introducer sheath technique is used rather than direct catheter passage over the guide wire because the catheter tip occasionally pulls the wire out of the pericardial sac. The sheath is particularly helpful for traversing longer distances or passing through a sclerotic pericardial sac.)
d) The pigtail angiocatheter (65 cm, Cordis) is inserted through the introducer sheath, and fluid is aspirated to ensure good return.

e) After insertion of the pigtail catheter, the introducer sheath is removed, leaving only the smooth-walled pigtail catheter in the pericardial space. The potential complication caused by a frayed sheath tip can be eliminated by withdrawing the sheath after the pigtail catheter is secured in the pericardial sac.
f) Agitated saline echo-contrast injection is repeated as necessary to confirm the position of the catheter or sheath.
g) The pericardial fluid is drained completely by syringe suction, with echocardiographic assessment of residual fluid and Doppler hemodynamics as needed. Manual syringe aspiration is preferred to vacuum suction because the former provides better control and collapse of the tubing is effectively avoided.

Dressing

The pericardial catheter is secured to the chest wall by suture or appropriate dressing or both. Antiseptic ointment is applied to the entry site, and aseptic dressings are applied.

Intermittent Catheter Drainage and Maintenance

Education for nursing staff is crucial to ensure appropriate care and maintenance of the pericardial catheter.
a) Pericardial fluid is aspirated intermittently via a three-way stopcock with aseptic technique (usually every 4 to 6 hours, or as clinically indicated). To avoid catheter plugging, continuous drainage is not used.
b) At the end of each fluid withdrawal, the catheter is flushed with sterile isotonic saline to maintain patency. Aspirations and flushing inputs are charted and net volumes recorded.
c) The site should be redressed periodically (usually every 72 hours), and guidelines for proper care of the site should be analogous to those for any central line.
d) The attending physician should be notified if there is (1) a sudden increase in the volume of aspirated fluid, (2) a change in the appearance of

the fluid, especially if the fluid becomes bloody or purulent, (3) acute chest pain, or (4) a change in vital signs, for example, development of tachycardia, hypotension, tachypnea, or a fever.

e) The catheter is removed once the drainage has decreased to less than 25 ml in 24 hours and follow-up echocardiography reveals no significant residual pericardial effusion. While the pericardial catheter is in place, the patient may be ambulatory as tolerated without restriction of upper body movement. Continuous electrocardiographic monitoring has not been found necessary. Minor discomfort can be managed with simple analgesics. Underlying conditions should be treated as clinically indicated [52].

In summary, echo-guided pericardiocentesis has an excellent profile in simplicity, safety, and efficacy. The use of a pericardial pigtail catheter reduces the recurrence of effusion. The technology is widely accessible without requirement for specialized facilities and personnel. Echo-guided pericardiocentesis

with extended catheter drainage can now supplant more invasive procedures as the initial strategy for the management of hemodynamically significant pericardial effusions. In the majority of the cases, it is the definitive procedure and surgical management is usually not necessary.

Pericardiocentesis Guided by Fluoroscopy

Unless the situation is immediately life threatening, experienced staff should perform pericardiocentesis in a facility equipped for radiographic, echocardiographic, and hemodynamic monitoring to optimize the success and safety of the procedure. Elective pericardiocentesis should always be carried out or supervised by an experienced operator. Intravenous saline solution should be given to hypovolemic patients with cardiac tamponade awaiting pericardial drainage in an effort to expand the intravascular volume. Dobutamine or nitroprusside may be used to stabilize cardiac output after the blood

Table 4.3. Sets for pericardiocentesis available on the international market. Utilization of any combination of standard angiographic components including any needle large enough for a 0,038" J-tip guidewire, introducer set and a pig-tail catheter is also possible. Widely available central venous catheters are especially suitable for emergency procedures

Sets for Pericardiocentesis	Type/Description
ARROW Intl. Inc.	— AK-00376 8F Set
Boston Scientific	— Meadox kit, PeriVac pericardiocentesis kit (F8 pig-tail catheter with a J-tip 0,038" guidewire)
B-Braun, Melsungen	— Cordican drainage kit with beveled end (braunula technique with a beveled steel stylet), F5 size — Cordican Seldinger drainage kit, F5 and F8, with a J-tip 0,038" guidewire
William Cook Europe	— C-PCS-500-TTL (Teitel pediatric pericardiocentesis set including ECG cable and 30 cm 5-F pig-tail catheter with 6 side-ports and a J-tip 0,028" guidewire) — C-PCS-830-LOCK (Lock's pericardiocentesis set including a 40 cm 8,3-F pig-tail catheter with 6 side-ports and a J-tip 0,028" guidewire) — C-PCS-850 (8.5 F, 22 cm long, straight-tip catheter with 4 side-ports, J-tip 0,038" guidewire, and a ECG cable) — C-PCSY-1000-SPAC (emergency pericardiocentesis and tray including ECG cable, coaxial catheter/needle set, and a 19 cm long, 10F straight-tip catheter with 2 side-ports) — C-PCSY-830-AT (Tilkian's pericardiocentesis set including ECG cable, a 40 cm 8,3-F pig-tail catheter with 6 side-ports and a J-tip 0,038" guidewire) — C-PPD-850 (Fuhrman's pleral/pneumopericardial drainage set, including a 15 cm 8.5-F pig-tail catheter with 6 side-ports and J-tip 0,028" guidewire) — C-PPD-500-Wood and C-PPD-600-Wood (pleral/pneumopericardial drainage set for neonates including a 8 cm 5F or 6F pig-tail catheter with 10 side-ports and peal-away straightener – no guidewire is needed)

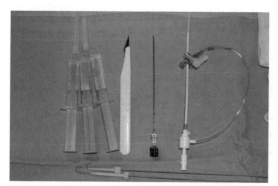

◘ Fig. 4.6. Pericardiocentesis set comprising a 10 cm Tuohy needle with a mandrel, standard vascular 7F introducer set, 3x 5 ml syringes for local anesthesia (lidocain 1–2% or mepivacain 1%), a scalpel (small incision of the skin to facilitate the entrance of the needle and introducer set through the subcutaneous tissue), and two J-tip, 0.038″ exchange guidewires

volume has been expanded, but only as a temporary measure and with careful hemodynamic monitoring.

Unless the procedure is considered extremely urgent, a clotting profile and chest X-ray should be obtained before pericardiocentesis. Although complications requiring blood transfusion are very rare nowadays, it is prudent to obtain 2–3 units of cross-tested blood before beginning the procedure.

Various specialized sets for pericardiocentesis are available on the market (Table 4.3), but standard vascular introducer sets, guidewires, and pigtail angiography catheters can be successfully applied as well (Fig. 4.6).

Pericardiocentesis guided by fluoroscopy is performed in the cardiac catheterization laboratory with ECG and systemic blood pressure monitoring. Aseptic conditions are again essential. Resuscitation equipment and medications should be available. Direct ECG monitoring from the puncturing needle is not an adequate safeguard and should not be applied [1, 53]. The subxiphoid approach has been used most commonly, with a long needle with a mandrel (Tuohy or thin-walled 18-gauge; Figs. 4.7, 4.8) directed towards the left shoulder at a 30° angle to the skin.

This route is extrapleural and avoids the coronary, pericardial, and internal mammary arteries. The operator intermittently attempts to aspirate fluid and injects small amounts of diluted contrast media. The lateral angiographic view provides the best visualization of the puncturing needle and its relation to the diaphragm and the pericardium (Fig. 4.8). If hemorrhagic fluid is freely aspirated a few milliliters of the contrast medium may be injected under fluoroscopic observation (Fig. 4.8b). The appearance of a sluggish layering of the contrast medium inferiorly indicates that the needle is correctly positioned. A soft J-tip guidewire is introduced and after dilatation exchanged for a multi-holed pigtail catheter (Figs. 4.9 and 4.10).

It is essential to check the position of the guidewire in at least two angiographic projections (lateral view and antero-posterior angiographic view). If the guidewire was erroneously placed intracardially, this should be recognized before insertion of the dilator and drainage catheter. If, despite the caution, the introducer set or the catheter have perforated the heart and are laying intracardially, the catheter should be very carefully secured and the patient promptly transferred to the cardiac surgery. Alternatively, a second puncture can be attempted. If successful, surgery may be avoided using autotransfusion of pericardial blood to the femoral vein after retraction of the falsely positioned first catheter.

Before and at the end of drainage, intrapericardial pressure should be registered (Fig. 4.11). It is prudent to drain the pericardial fluid in steps of less than 1 l at a time to avoid the acute right-ventricular dilatation ("sudden decompression syndrome") [54]. After the procedure, patients should be monitored (vital signs, serial echocardiograms) for recurrent tamponade, particularly those with hemorrhagic effusions, which may occur despite the presence of an intrapericardial catheter (best for 24 hours in an intensive or semi-intensive care unit). Diluted fibrinolytics may be instilled in the catheter to prevent fibrin deposition.

Pericardial drainage is a final treatment for nearly one half of patients with "idiopathic" chronic pericardial effusion. In addition, the significant incidence of unforeseen cardiac tamponade is eliminated [55]. Intrapericardial instillation of triamcinolone can prevent recurrences in up to 90% of patients with autoreactive pericarditis [8]. However, subxiphoid pericardiotomy, percutaneous balloon pericardiotomy or the surgical creation of a pleuropericardial or a peritoneal-pericardial window may be required in severely symptomatic and/or frequently relapsing pericardial effusions.

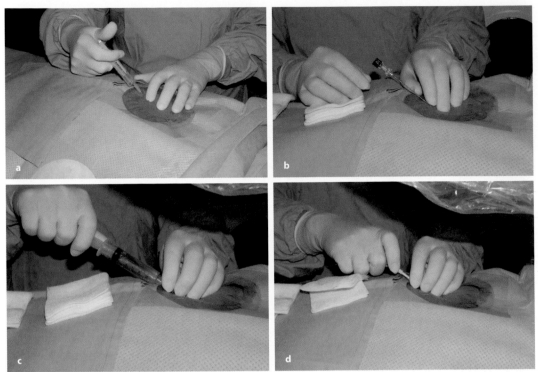

▣ **Fig. 4.7a–d.** Pericardiocentesis guided by fluoroscopy – step I. **a** Palpation of the subxiphoid position appropriate for puncture (1–2 cm between the xiphoid processus and the left costal arch and application of the local anesthetic (lidocain 1–2% or mepivacain 1%). **b** Puncture using the Tuohy needle with a mandrel [mandrel (*red cap*) will be removed when the subcutaneous tissue and the diaphragm are passed]. **c** Under intermittent aspiration and injections of the small amounts of the angiographic contrast, the needle is slowly approaching the pericardium, approximately tangentially to the epicardial halo phenomenon, until the effusion is aspirated. **d** 0,038″ J-guide wire is inserted in the pericardium

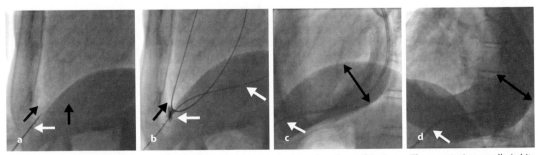

▣ **Fig. 4.8a–d.** Pericardiocentesis guided by fluoroscopy – step 1 – lateral angiographic view. **a** The puncturing needle (*white arrow*) is slowly approaching the heart shadow and the epicardial halo phenomenon (*black arrows*). **b** The needle was exchanged for a 0,038″ J-tip guide wire. **c** Lateral view – guidewire was exchanged for a 7F drainage catheter and after taking the 100 ml effusion samples for laboratory analyses the position of the catheter, size and distribution of the effusion was confirmed by intrapericardial injection of 40–50 ml of the contrast media. **d** Antero-posterior view – pericardial drainage catheter is in a proper position, injection of the contrast media demonstrates a large, circular pericardial effusion

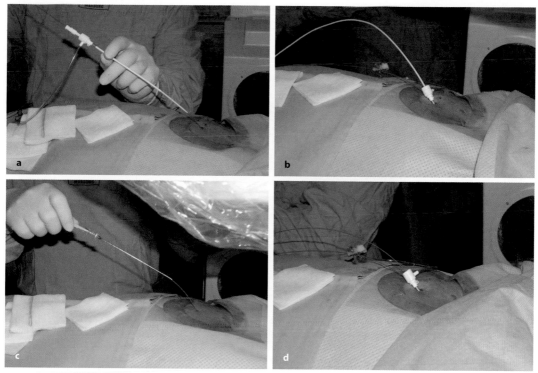

Fig. 4.9a–d. Pericardiocentesis guided by fluoroscopy – step II. **a** Withdrawal of the Tuohy needle, while keeping the J-tip guide wire in the pericardium. **b** Insertion of the 7F introducer-set into the pericardium (dilator + sheat) over the guidewire. **c** Dilator is withdrawn and the J-tip guide-wire remains intrapericardially. **d** Introduction of the 7F pigtail catheter over the guide-wire (in serous effusions 5F catheter is sufficient for drainage)

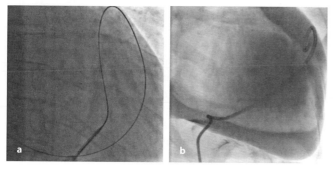

Fig. 4.10a,b. Another example of pericardio-centesis guided by fluoroscopy – step II – antero-posterior angiographic view. **a** Insertion of the dilator over the 0.038-inch J-tip guidewire. **b** Pigtail drainage catheter in "loop position" around the heart, from the frontal to the lateral and posterior side (most favorable position)

Feasibility of Fluoroscopy-Guided Pericardiocentesis

The likelihood of procedural success of pericardio-centesis is high in patients with anterior effusion and in those with an echocardiographically measured pericardial free space of 10 mm or more in diastole, either from the subxiphoidal view or from the apical view. This was confirmed by Krikorian and Hancock's study of 123 patients [33]: The procedure was successful in 93% of cases if the effusion was large and of both anterior and posterior location, whereas the rate of success was only 58% with small and posteriorly located effusions. Analyzing the predictors

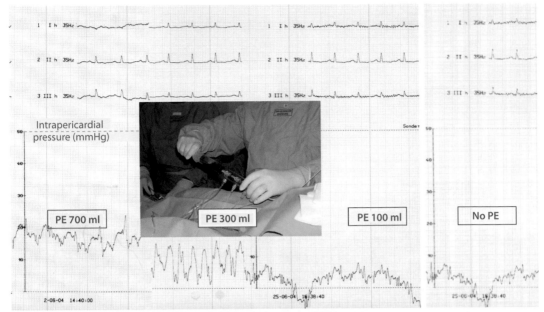

◘ Fig. 4.11. Pericardiocentesis guided by fluoroscopy – step III. Connection of the catheter to the manifold system, registration of the intrapericardial pressure and manual aspiration of the pericardial effusion. Other lines attached to the manifold are 1) pressure transducer (mmHg), 2) normal saline, and 3) angiographic contrast media. Additional 3-way connector was attached to the distal part to enable intermittent aspiration (60 cc syringe) and collection of the effusion in a standard 2 l urine collection bag. Note that intrapericardial pressure is falling from the mean value of 18 mmHg to the mean of 10 mmHg after drainage of 400 ml of effusion, further to the mean pressure of 3 mmHg after drainage of 600 ml, and will finally slightly below zero after drainage of the entire 700 ml of pericardial effusion (pressure curves from left to the right)

of failure in echocardiography-guided pericardiocentesis Cooper et al. [56] observed that the only parameter associated with unsuccessful aspiration was loculation of pericardial effusion, particularly after cardiac surgery.

However, in a recent large series of patients from the Mayo Clinic pericardiocentesis of loculated pericardial effusion after cardiac surgery, reached with echocardiographic guidance an efficacy of 96% with only 2% of major complications [49]. A rescue pericardiocentesis after cardiac perforation, guided by echocardiography, successfully relieved tamponade in 99% of 88 patients, and was the only and definitive therapy in 82% of the cases.

In the pericardiocentesis study conducted in Belgrade [4, 57] both fluoroscopic control and hemodynamic monitoring contributed to a better feasibility of the procedure (93.1% vs. 73.3%) in comparison to emergency pericardial puncture with no imaging control. The Marburg Registry with procedures involving pericardiocentesis and pericardioscopy under fluoroscopic control by using the "halo phenomenon" as guidance pericardioscopy even of small effusions was successful in 93.3% of cases. The 6.7% of cases with failure to access the pericardial sac were due to loculated effusions.

The Role of Cardiac Catheterization During Pericardiocentesis

Right-heart catheterization can be performed simultaneously with pericardiocentesis, providing the information about the hemodynamic status of the patient and the possibility to monitor the improvement as the effusion is drained. Importantly, this approach would enable prompt diagnosis of effusive-constrictive pericarditis immediately after the drainage of pericardial effusion is completed. Invasive hemodynamics and measurement of pericardial pressures are also use-

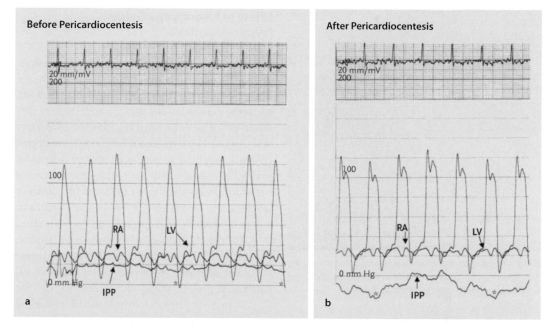

□ **Fig. 4.12a,b.** The role of cardiac catheterization in diagnosis of effusive-constrictive pericarditis. Before pericardiocentesis (**a**), the intrapericardial pressure (*IPP*), right atrial (*RA*) pressure, and end-diastolic left ventricular (*LV*) pressure were elevated. After pericardiocentesis (**b**), the intrapericardial pressure drops below 0 mmHg, whereas the right atrial and left ventricular pressures remained unchanged and a dip-plateau morphology of left intraventricular pressure is apparent. *Asterisks* indicate the end of the inspiratory phase. Adapted with permission from Sagrista-Sauleda et al. (2004) [60]

ful for the diagnosis and guidance of the procedure, particularly in questionable cases (see Chapter 3) [58].

Angiography may show atrial collapse and small hyperactive ventricular chambers. Coronary angiography sometimes demonstrates ouvert coronary compression in diastole and may expose associated coronary artery disease [59].

After successful pericardiocentesis, if intrapericardial pressure falls to zero or becomes negative, while right atrial pressure remains elevated, various diagnostic alternatives should be considered. The differential diagnosis includes effusive-constrictive pericarditis (Fig. 4.12) (especially in patients with tuberculosis or prior irradiation for neoplastic disease), preexisting left ventricular dysfunction, tricuspid valve disease, and restrictive cardiomyopathy.

In the study or Sagrista-Sauleda et al. [60] 15 patients with effusive-constrictive pericarditis were identified out of 190 individuals, who underwent combined pericardiocentesis and catheterization.

Before catheterization, concomitant constriction was recognized in only seven patients. Therefore, without cardiac catheterization the diagnosis would have been missed in 8/15 patients (53.3%). At catheterization, all patients had elevated intrapericardial pressure (median, 12 mmHg; interquartile range, 7 to 18) and elevated right atrial and end-diastolic right and left ventricular pressures. After pericardiocentesis, the intrapericardial pressure decreased (median value, –5 mmHg; interquartile range, –5 to 0), whereas right atrial and end-diastolic right and left ventricular pressures, although slightly reduced, remained elevated, with a dip-plateau morphology (Fig. 4.12).

Simultaneous right ventricular and puncturing needle contrast injections enables opacification of the right ventricle and the path of the pericardiocentesis needle and may additionally improve the safety of pericardiocentesis by establishing the position of the pericardium between the endocardium and epicardium of the diaphragmatic wall of the right ventricle (Fig. 4.13) [57]. The procedure was investigated in 59

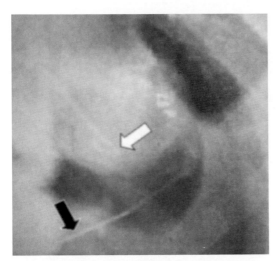

Fig. 4.13. Pericardiocentesis under fluoroscopic control using right ventricular angiography (*white arrow*) and puncturing needle contrast injection (*black arrow*) [57]

patients undergoing subxiphoid pericardiocentesis divided in two groups. Group 1 included 30 patients (43.3% males, mean age 51.8 ± 13.2 years) who had to undergo emergency subxiphoid pericardiocentesis with no imaging control. Group 2 comprised 29 patients (58.6% males, mean age 54.2 ± 9.6 years) who underwent pericardiocentesis guided by simultaneous right ventricular and puncturing needle contrast injections. In Group 2, right heart catheterization and right ventriculography were performed immediately before pericardiocentesis, outlining the inferior right ventricular border. Pericardium was accessed subxiphoidally using a Tuohy needle on a syringe with 50% radiography contrast. The needle was advanced under radiographic control (PA position), with frequent contrast injections, until pericardial fluid was aspirated. Simultaneously, manual contrast injections from the RV pigtail catheter were performed in order to improve orientation and safety. After obtaining pericardial fluid, a J guide wire was introduced, its position checked in lateral and RAO view, and exchanged for 8-F pigtail catheter. The procedure was successful in 22/30 patients (73.4%) from Group 1 and in 27/29 patients (93.1%) from Group 2 (Chi^2=4.1; p<0.05). In two patients from Group 2, in whom the procedure was not feasible, pericardial infiltration was misdiagnosed as effusion by echocardiography.

Safety of Fluoroscopy-Guided Pericardiocentesis

Although pericardiocentesis is usually well-tolerated, pulmonary edema, circulatory collapse, and acute RV and LV dysfunction have been reported after drainage of the pericardial effusion [61, 62]. We have also observed an extreme vagal reaction in one patient with consecutive sinus bradycardia and 2nd degree AV block requiring atropine and transient ventricular pacing. Too rapid drainage of the large volume of pericardial effusion can be followed by transient severe acute LV systolic failure in the absence of any prior history of left ventricular dysfunction [63]. Therefore, drainage of more than 1 l effusion should be avoided and prolonged catheter drainage should be provided for the remaining effusion. All patients, especially those with underlying cardiac disease, including myocarditis, should be monitored for postdrainage decompensation [64].

The most serious complications of pericardiocentesis are: laceration and perforation of the myocardium and the coronary vessels. Rarely patients can experience air embolism, pneumothorax, arrhythmias (usually vasovagal bradycardia), and puncture of the peritoneal cavity (Fig. 4.14) or abdominal viscera [4, 65]. Internal mammary artery fistulas, acute pulmonary edema, and purulent pericarditis were also reported [66].

Although the major complications are rare, blood transfusion (400–600 ml) should be provided and cross-matched before the pericardiocentesis, to allow time for treatment of potential major complications. Vagal reaction complicating tamponade or pericardiocentesis should be treated with atropine. Positive pressure breathing should be avoided before pericardial drainage is begun [11].

In a series of 352 fluoroscopy-guided percutaneous pericardiocenteses procedures [67] only 13 major complications occurred: three cardiac perforations (0.9%), two cardiac arrhythmias (0.6%), four cases of arterial bleeding (1.1%), two cases of pneumothorax (0.6%), one infection (0.3%), and one major vagal reaction (0.3%). No significant difference in complications was found between pericardiocenteses for pericardial effusions after cardiac surgery (208 patients) and those for effusions of non-surgical (144 patients) origin. In the Marburg experience with

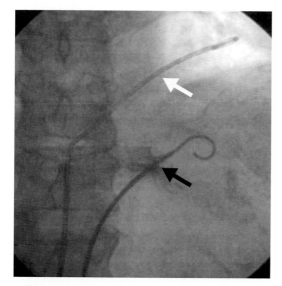

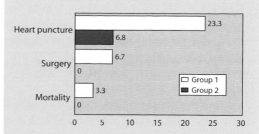

■ **Fig. 4.15.** Safety of pericardiocentesis guided by fluoroscopy and simultaneous right ventricular and puncturing needle contrast injections. Group 1 – 30 patients (43.3% males, mean age 51.8 ± 13.2 years) undergoing emergency subxiphoid pericardiocentesis with no imaging control. Group 2 – 29 patients (58.6% males, mean age 54.2 ± 9.6 years) that underwent pericardiocentesis guided by simultaneous right ventricular and puncturing needle contrast injections

■ **Fig. 4.14.** Complication of subxiphoid pericardiocentesis under fluoroscopic guidance. Anteroposterior fluoroscopic view. Pigtail catheter (*black arrow*) was erroneously placed intraperitonealy. The patient complained on abdominal pain and had a vagal reaction. Pericardiocentesis was repeated and another pigtail catheter (*white arrow*) was placed intrapericardially. The first catheter could be withdrawn without further complication or need for surgical intervention

fluoroscopic control of pericardiocentesis (n = 234 patients) there was no mortality and the incidence of major complications was significantly reduced by utilizing the epicardial halo phenomenon and the tangential approach in the lateral view. Major complications included 3 cases (1.3%) of cardiac perforation or arterial bleeding (none requiring surgery but all could be solved by autotransfusion), one major vagal reaction (0.4%), but no pneumothoraces.

In an early study of fluoroscopic guidance of pericardiocentesis and simultaneous right ventricular and puncturing needle contrast injection in the Belgrade Center, major complications in Group 1 included eight punctures of the heart chambers, 2/8 patients needed surgery, and one patient died before reaching the operating room (mortality 3.3%, major complications 23.3%) (Fig. 4.15).

In Group 2, incidental RV puncture occurred in two pts. (6.8%). However, further complications were prevented by a proper recognition of the guide-wire position. In both patients the procedure was successfully completed, after the removal and repositioning

of the guide wire (Group 1 vs. 2, $Chi^2 = 4.0$; $p < 0.05$). The procedure was especially useful in preventing major complications during pericardiocentesis in patients with neoplastic infiltrations of the pericardium.

Surgical Drainage of the Pericardium

If the heart cannot be reached by a needle or catheter, surgical drainage is required, usually through a subcostal incision. Furthermore, surgical drainage is desirable in patients with intrapericardial bleeding and in those with clotted hemopericardium or thoracic conditions that make pericardiocentesis difficult or ineffective [13]. Open surgical drainage has the potential benefit of resecting a portion of the anterior central diaphragm and creating a chronically open channel between the pericardium and peritoneum. The open approach also allows the surgeon to break up adhesions and loculations with a finger or a suction device and place a large drainage tube, which is especially important in purulent pericarditis.

McDonald et al. [68] compared outcomes of patients treated with percutaneous pericardial catheter drainage (n = 96) with outcomes after open subxiphoid pericardial drainage (n = 150) performed over 5-years time in a single institution. The duration of drainage, total drained volume, and mean follow-up (2.6 years) were similar in both groups. Effusions were malignant in 79 (32%) patients and benign in 167

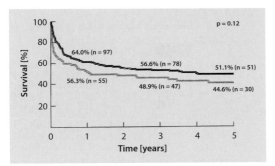

□ **Fig. 4.16.** Actuarial survival plot of treatment groups by the Kaplan-Meier method. Numeric percentages on the curve represent survival at 1, 3, and 5 years. Open drainage (*black line*; n = 150) = subxiphoid pericardiotomy; catheter drainage (*gray line*; n = 96) = percutaneous pericardial catheter drainage, p > 0.05 by Mantel. Reproduced with permission from McDonald et al. (2003) [68]

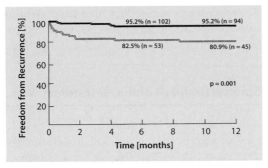

□ **Fig. 4.17.** Freedom from reintervention for recurrent pericardial effusion by the Kaplan-Meier method. Numeric percentages on the curve represent 6 and 12 months. Open drainage (*black line*; n = 150) = subxiphoid pericardiotomy; catheter drainage (*gray line*; n = 96) = percutaneous pericardial catheter drainage, p < 0.01 by Mantel. Reproduced with permission from McDonald et al. (2003) [68]

(68%) patients. No direct procedural mortality occurred, but the inhospital mortality was significantly higher in the percutaneous in comparison to the open surgical group (22.9% vs. 10.7%; p = 0.01). The 5-year survival was 51% in the open surgical group versus 45% in the percutaneous group (Fig. 4.16). This result was achieved despite a greater proportion of patients with malignant disease in the the open-surgery group (35% vs. 28%).

Recurrences were seen in 16.5% of patients in the percutaneous group compared with 4.6% in the open group (p = 0.002; Fig. 4.17). Malignancy was confirmed in 16/27 (59%) of percutaneous procedures performed on patients with known malignancy. In the open group, cytological and pathologic evaluation of the pericardial specimens revealed malignancy in 32/52 (62%) of patients with previously known malignancy [68].

Similarly, Allen and coworkers [69], have found a 30% recurrence rate for percutaneous drainage and 1.1% for subxiphoid pericardiostomy (retrospective study). Percutaneous catheter drainage in other reported series resulted in a recurrence rate of 0–30%, mean 16.2% [69–74]. Open subxiphoid drainage in published reports resulted in a recurrence rate of 0–9.1%, mean 3.2% [69, 70, 75–85]. However, these series included neither comprehensive evaluation of the etiology of the disease nor specific systemic or intrapericardial treatment that significantly diminishes recurrence rates after pericardiocentesis [8, 9].

In the study of McDonald et al. [68] the choice of the procedure was determined by the cardiologist performing the echocardiogram. If the echocardiogram suggested that the effusion was loculated or mostly posterior and inferior without a clear percutaneous trajectory for catheter drainage, the patient

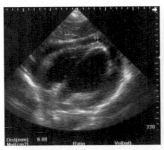
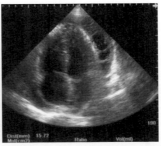

□ **Fig. 4.18.** Large pericardial effusion with massive pericardial adhesions indicated for surgical drainage

was referred for open drainage. An example of an echocardiographical finding that would be an indication for surgical drainage of pericardial effusion can be appreciated at the Fig. 4.18.

The disadvantages of the open surgical procedures remain general anesthesia (risk of sudden hypotension in patients with large effusions/cardiac tamponade), a need to perform a 6- to 8-cm vertical incision in the upper abdomen as well as to resect the xiphoid process in some cases.

The advantage of the open surgical procedure over pericardiocentesis in enabling large pericardial samples for pathohistological examination is currently compensated with the introduction of flexible percutaneous pericardioscopy and aimed pericardial and epicardial biopsy (Fig. 4.2, down-left) [3, 8, 9].

Future Perspectives and Recommendations

The risk of serious damage to the heart or a coronary artery during pericardiocentesis was notably diminished in the last two decades due to the echocardiography and fluoroscopy guidance, but is certainly not reduced to zero. Although less frequently, open techniques may also result in complications. In critical tamponade the choice of the procedure has to be based on the risk/benefit assessment for each specific case and on the availability of trained personnel and facilities for either of the two procedures.

References

1. Maisch B, Seferovic PM, Ristic AD, et al. Task Force on the Diagnosis and Management of Pricardial Diseases of the European Society of Cardiology. Guidelines on the diagnosis and management of pericardial diseases. Executive summary. Eur Heart J 2004; 25(7): 587–610
2. Zayas R, Anguita M, Torres F, et al. Incidence of specific etiology and role of methods for specific etiologic diagnosis of primary acute pericarditis. Am J Cardiol 1995; 75: 378–382
3. Seferovic PM, Ristic AD, Maksimovic R, Tatic V, Ostojic M, Kanjuh V. Diagnostic value of pericardial biopsy: improvement with extensive sampling enabled by pericardioscopy. Circulation 2003; 107: 978–983
4. Seferovic PM, Ristic AD, Maksimovic R, Mitrovic V. Therapeutic pericardiocentesis: Up-to-date review of indications, efficacy, and risks. In: Seferović PM, Spodick DH, Maisch B (eds) Pericardiology: contemporary answers to continuing challenges. Science, Belgrade, 2000, pp 417–426
5. Meyers DG, Meyers RE, Prendergast TW. The usefulness of diagnostic tests on pericardial fluid. Chest 1997; 111(5): 1213–1221
6. Maisch B, Bethge C, Drude L, Hufnagel G, Herzum M, Schönian U. Pericardioscopy and epicardial biopsy: new diagnostic tools in pericardial and perimyocardial diseases. Eur Heart J 1994; 15(Suppl. C): 68–73
7. Maisch B, Pankuweit S, Brilla C, et al. Intrapericardial treatment of inflammatory and neoplastic pericarditis guided by pericardioscopy and epicardial biopsy – results from a pilot study. Clin Cardiol 1999; 22(Suppl 1): I17–22
8. Maisch B, Ristić AD, Pankuweit S. Intrapericardial treatment of autoreactive pericardial effusion with triamcinolone: the way to avoid side effects of systemic corticosteroid therapy. Eur Heart J 2002; 23: 1503–1508
9. Maisch B, Ristić AD, Pankuweit S, Neubauer A, Moll R. Neoplastic pericardial effusion: efficacy and safety of intrapericardial treatment with cisplatin. Eur Heart J 2002; 23: 1625–1631
10. Millaire A, Wurtz A, de Groote P, Saudemont A, Chambon A, Ducloux G. Malignant pericardial effusions: usefulness of pericardioscopy. Am Heart J 1992; 124(4): 1030–1034
11. Nugue O, Millaire A, Porte H, et al. Pericardioscopy in the etiologic diagnosis of pericardial effusion in 141 consecutive patients. Circulation 1996; 94(7): 1635–1641
12. Porte HL, Janecki-Delebecq TJ, Finzi L, Metois DG, Millaire A, Wurtz AJ. Pericardioscopy for primary management of pericardial effusion in cancer patients. Eur J Cardiothorac Surg 1999; 16(3): 287–291
13. Merce J, Sagrista-Sauleda J, Permanyer-Miralda G, Soler-Soler J. Should pericardial drainage be performed routinely in patients who have a large pericardial effusion without tamponade? Am J Med 1998; 105: 106–109
14. Pankuweit S, Ristić AD, Seferović PM, Maisch B. Bacterial pericarditis: diagnosis and management. Am J Cardiovasc Drugs 2005; 5(2): 103–112
15. Maisch B, Karatolios K. New possibilities of diagnostics and therapy of pericarditis. Internist (Berl) 2008; 49(1): 17–26
16. Erdol C, Erdol H, Celik S, Baykan M, Gokce M. Idiopathic chronic pericarditis associated with ocular hypertension: probably an unknown combination. Int J Cardiol 2003; 87(2–3): 293–295
17. Erbel R, Alfonso F, Boileau C, et al. Task Force on Aortic Dissection, European Society of Cardiology. Diagnosis and management of aortic dissection. Eur Heart J 2001; 22(18): 1642–1681
18. Fagan SM, Chan KI. Pericardiocentesis. Blind no more! Chest 1999; 116: 275–276
19. Tsang TS, Freeman WK, Barnes ME, Reeder G, Packer D, Seward J. Rescue echocardiographically guided pericardiocentesis for cardiac perforation complicating catheter-based procedures. The Mayo Clinic experience. J Am Coll Cardiol 1998; 32(5): 1345–1350

20. Jungbluth A, Düber C, Rumpelt HJ, Erbel R, Meyer J. Koronararterienmorphologie nach perkutaner transluminaler Koronarangioplasatie (PTCA) mit Hämoperikard [Morphology of the coronary arteries following percutaneous transluminal coronary angioplasty with hemopericardium]. Z Kardiol 1988; 77: 125–129

21. Liu F, Erbel R, Haude M, Ge J. Coronary arterial perforation: prediction, diagnosis, management, and prevention. In: Ellis SG, Holmes DR (eds) Strategic approaches in coronary intervention. 2nd edn. Lippincott, Philadelphia, 2000, pp 501–514

22. von Birgelen C, Haude M, Herrmann J, et al. Early clinical experience with the implantation of a novel synthetic coronary stent graft. Cathet Cardiovasc Interv 1999; 47: 496–503

23. Levine MJ, Baim DS. Endomyocardial biopsy. In: Grossmann W, Baim DS (eds) Cardiac catheterization, angiography and interventions. Lea & Febiger, Philadelphia, 1991, pp 383–395

24. Sekiguchi M, Take M. World survey of catheter biopsy of the heart. In: Sekiguchi M, Olsen EGJ (eds) Cardiomyopathy. Clinical, pathological, and theoretical aspects. University Park Press, Baltimore, 1980, pp 217–225

25. Maisch B. Myokardbiopsien und Perikardioskopien. In: Hess OM, Simon RWR (eds) Herzkatheter: Einzatz in Diagnostik und Therapie. Springer, Berlin, 2000, pp 302–349

26. Kiviniemi MS, Pirnes MA, Eranen HJ, Kettunen RV, Hartikainen JE. Complications related to permanent pacemaker therapy. Pacing Clin Electrophysiol 1999; 22(5): 711–720

27. Matsuura Y, Yamashina H, Higo M, Fujii T. Analysis of complications of permanent transvenous implantable cardiac pacemaker related to operative and postoperative management in 717 consecutive patients. Hiroshima J Med Sci 1990; 39(4): 131–137

28. Spindler M, Burrows G, Kowallik P, Ertl G, Voelker W. Postpericardiotomy syndrome and cardiac tamponade as a late complication after pacemaker implantation. Pacing Clin Electrophysiol 2001; 24(9 Pt 1): 1433–1434

29. Elinav E, Leibowitz D. Constrictive pericarditis complicating endovascular pacemaker implantation. Pacing Clin Electrophysiol 2002; 25(3): 376–377

30. Hsu LF, Scavée C, Jaïs P, Hocini M, Haïssaguerre M. Transcardiac pericardiocentesis: an emergency life-saving technique for cardiac tamponade. J Cardiovasc Electrophysiol 2003; 14(9): 1001–1003

31. Fisher JD, Kim SG, Ferrick KJ, Gross JN, Goldberger MH, Nanna M. Internal transcardiac pericardiocentesis for acute tamponade. Am J Cardiol 2000; 86(12): 1388–1389

32. Maisch B, Ristić AD, Herzum M, Funck R, Moosdorf R. Feasibility of rescue pericardiocentesis under fluoroscopic guidance [abstract]. Eur Heart J 2003; 24(Suppl.): P2902

33. Krikorian JG, Hancock EW. Pericardiocentesis. Am J Med 1978; 65: 808–814

34. Wong B, Murphy J, Chang DJ, Hassenein K, Dunn M. The risks of pericardiocentesis. Am J Cardiol 1979; 44: 1110–1114

35. Fontenelle LJ, Cuello L, Dooley BN. Subxiphoid pericardial window: a simple and safe method for diagnosing and treating acute and chronic pericardial effusions. J Thorac Cardiovasc Surg 1971; 62: 95–97

36. Alcan KE, Zabetakis PM, Marino ND, Franzone AJ, Michelis MF, Bruno MS. Management of acute cardiac tamponade by subxiphoid pericardiotomy. JAMA 1982; 247: 1143–1148

37. Piehler JM, Pluth JR, Schaff HV, Danielson GK, Orszulak TA, Puga FJ. Surgical management of effusive pericardial disease. Influence of extent of pericardial resection on clinical course. J Thorac Cardiovasc Surg 1985; 90: 506–516

38. Ghosh S, Larrieu A, Ablaza S, Grana V. Clinical experience with subxyphoid pericardial decompression. Intern Surg 1985; 70: 5–7

39. Bishop LHJ, Estes EHJ, McIntosh HD. The electrocardiogram as a safeguard in pericardiocentesis. JAMA 1956; 162: 264–265

40. Duvernoy O, Borowiec J, Helmius G, Erikson U. Complications of percutaneous pericardiocentesis under fluoroscopic guidance. Acta Radiol 1992; 33: 309–313

41. Tajik AJ. Echocardiography in pericardial effusion. Am J Med 1977; 63: 29–40

42. Cikes I. New echocardiographic possibilities in the etiological diagnosis and therapy of pericardial diseases. In: Hanrath P, Bleifeld W, Souqquet J (eds) Cardiovascular diagnosis by ultrasound: transesophageal, computerized, contrast, doppler echocardiography. Vol. 22. Martinus Nijhoff, The Hague, 1982, pp 188–201

43. Taavitsainen M, Bondestam S, Mankinen P, Pitkaranta P, Tierala E. Ultrasound guidance for pericardiocentesis. Acta Radiol 1990; 32: 9–11

44. Tsang T, Freeman W, Sinak L, Seward J. Echocardiographically guided pericardiocentesis: evolution and state-of-the-art technique. Mayo Clin Proc 1998; 73: 647–652

45. Kopecky SL, Callahan JA, Tajik AJ, Seward JB. Percutaneous pericardial catheter drainage: report of 42 consecutive cases. Am J Cardiol 1986; 58: 633–635

46. Tsang TSM, Barnes ME, Gersh BJ, Bailey KR, Seward JB. Outcomes of clinically significant idiopathic pericardial effusion requiring intervention. Am J Cardiol 2003; 91: 704–707

47. Tsang T, Enriquez-Sarano M, Freeman W, et al. Consecutive 1127 therapeutic echocardiographically guided pericardiocenteses: clinical profile, practice patterns, and outcomes spanning 21 years. Mayo Clin Proc 2002; 77: 429–436

48. Tsang T, El-Najdawi E, Freeman W, Hagler D, Seward J, O'Leary P. Percutaneous echocardiographically guided pericardiocentesis in pediatric patients: evaluation of safety and efficacy. J Am Soc Echocardiogr 1998; 11: 1072–1077

49. Tsang T, Barnes M, Hayes S, et al. Clinical and echocardiographic characteristics of significant pericardial effusions following cardiothoracic surgery and outcomes of echoguided pericardiocentesis for management – Mayo clinic experience, 1979–1998. Chest 1999; 116: 322–331

50. Tsang T, Seward J, Barnes M, et al. Outcomes of primary and secondary treatment of pericardial effusion in patients with malignancy. Mayo Clin Proc 2000; 75: 248–253

51. Isselbacher EM, Cigarroa JE, Eagle KA. Cardiac tamponade complicating proximal aortic dissection. Is pericardiocentesis harmful? Circulation 1994; 90: 2375–2378

52. Cauduro S, Moder K, Tsang T, Seward J. Clinical and echo-cardiographic characteristics of hemodynamically significant pericardial effusions in patients with systemic lupus erythematosus. Am J Cardiol 2003; 92: 1370–1372

53. Tweddell JS, Zimmerman AN, Stone CM, et al. Pericardiocentesis guided by a pulse generator. J Am Coll Cardiol 1989; 14(4): 1074–1083

54. Armstrong WF, Feigenbaum H, Dillon JC. Acute right ventricular dilation and echocardiographic volume overload following pericardiocentesis for relief of cardiac tamponade. Am Heart J 1984; 107: 1266–1270

55. Sagrista-Sauleda J, Angel J, Permanyer-Miralda G, Soler-Soler J. Long-term follow-up of idiopathic chronic pericardial effusion. N Engl J Med 1999; 341: 2054–2059

56. Cooper JP, Oliver RM, Currie P, Walker JM, Swanton RH. How do the clinical findings in patients with pericardial effusions influence the success of aspiration? Br Heart J 1995; 73: 351–354

57. Ristic AD, Seferovic PM, Petrovic P, et al. Pericardiocentesis feasibility and safety revisited: improvement with simultaneous right ventricular and puncturing needle contrast injections [abstract]. J Am Coll Cardiol 1999; 32(Suppl. A): 516A

58. Hoit BD. Management of effusive and constrictive pericardial heart disease. Circulation 2002; 105: 2939–2942

59. O'Rourke RA, Fischer DP, Escobar EE, Bishop VS, Rapaport E. Effect of acute pericardial tamponade on coronary blood flow. Am J Physiol 1967; 212(3): 549–552

60. Sagrista-Sauleda J, Angel J, Sanchez A, Permanyer-Miralda G, Soler-Soler J. Effusive-constrictive pericarditis. N Engl J Med 2004; 350(5): 469–475

61. Wolfe MW, Edelman ER. Transient systolic dysfunction after relief of cardiac tamponade. Ann Intern Med 1993; 119: 42–44

62. Hamaya Y, Dohi S, Ueda N, et al. Severe circulatory collapse immediately after pericardiocentesis in a patient with chronic cardiac tamponade. Anesth Analg 1993; 77: 1278–1281

63. Chamoun A, Cenz R, Mager A, et al. Acute left ventricular failure after large volume pericardiocentesis. Clin Cardiol 2003; 26(12): 588–590

64. Spodick DH. Pericardial effusion and hydropericardium without tamponade. In: Spodick DH (ed) The pericardium: a comprehensive textbook. Marcel Dekker, New York, 1997, pp 126–152

65. Bender F. Hemoperitoneum after pericardiocentesis in a CAPD patient. Perit Dial Int 1996; 16(3): 330–334

66. Evron E, Goland S, Somin M, Sthoeger ZM. Purulent pericarditis. Harefuah 1996; 130(9): 602–603

67. Duvernoy O, Borowiec J, Helmius G, Erikson U. Complications of percutaneous pericardiocentesis under fluoroscopic guidance. Acta Radiol 1992; 33(4): 309–313

68. McDonald JM, Meyers BF, Guthrie TJ, Battafarano RJ, Cooper JD, Patterson GA. Comparison of open subxiphoid pericardial drainage with percutaneous catheter drainage for symptomatic pericardial effusion. Ann Thorac Surg 2003; 76: 811–816

69. Allen KB, Faber LP, Warren WH, Shaar CJ. Pericardial effusion: subxiphoid pericardiostomy versus percutaneous catheter drainage. Ann Thorac Surg 1999; 67: 437–440

70. Girardi LN, Ginsburg RJ, Burt ME. Pericardiocentesis and intrapericardial sclerosis: effective therapy for malignant pericardial effusions. Ann Thorac Surg 1997; 64: 1422–1428

71. Celermajer DS, Boyer MJ, Bailey BP, Tattersall MHN. Pericardiocentesis for symptomatic malignant pericardial effusion: a study of 36 patients. Med J Aust 1991; 154: 19–22

72. Kopecky SL, Callahan JA, Tajik J, Seward JB. Percutaneous pericardial catheter drainage: report of 42 consecutive cases. Am J Cardiol 1986; 58: 633–635

73. Shepherd FA, Morgan C, Evans WK, Ginsberg JF, Watt D, Murphy K. Medical management of malignant pericardial effusion by tetracycline sclerosis. Am J Cardiol 1987; 60: 1161–1166

74. Davis S, Rambotti P, Grignani F. Intrapericardial tetracycline sclerosis in the management of malignant pericardial effusion: an analysis of thirty-three cases. J Clin Oncol 1984; 2(6): 631–636

75. Santos GH, Frater RWN. The subxiphoid approach in the treatment of pericardial effusion. Ann Thorac Surg 1977; 23: 467–470

76. Prager RL, Wilson CH, Bender HW. The subxiphoid approach to pericardial disease. Ann Thorac Surg 1982; 34: 6–9

77. Levin BH, Aaron BL. The subxiphoid pericardial window. Surg Gynecol Obstet 1982; 155: 804–806

78. Ghosh SC, Larrieu AJ, Ablaza SGG, Grana VP. Clinical experience with subxiphoid pericardial decompression. Int Surg 1985; 70: 5 7

79. Reitknecht F, Regal AM, Antkowiak JG, Takita H. Management of cardiac tamponade in patients with malignancy. J Surg Oncol 1985; 30: 19–22

80. Palatianos GM, Thurer RJ, Pompeo MQ, Kaiser GA. Clinical experience with subxiphoid drainage of pericardial effusion. Ann Thorac Surg 1989; 48: 381–385

81. Sugimoto JT, Little AG, Ferguson MK, et al. Pericardial window: mechanism of efficacy. Ann Thorac Surg 1990; 50: 442–445

82. Park JS, Rentschler R, Wilbur D. Surgical management of pericardial effusion in patients with malignancies. Cancer 1991; 67: 76–80

83. Chan A, Rischin D, Clark CP, Woodruff RK. Subxiphoid partial pericardiectomy with or without sclerosant instillation in the treatment of symptomatic pericardial effusions in patients with malignancy. Cancer 1991; 68(5): 1021–1025

84. Okamoto H, Shinkae T, Tamakido M, Saijo N. Cardiac tamponade caused by primary lung cancer and the management of pericardial effusion. Cancer 1993; 71: 93–98

85. Moores DWO, Allen KB, Gillman DJ, et al. Subxiphoid pericardial drainage for pericardial tamponade. J Thorac Surg 1995; 109: 546–552

Alternative Techniques for Pericardiocentesis

Introduction

Pericardiocentesis of moderate, small or loculated pericardial effusions is a controversial issue. It should not be routinely performed if the patient is not symptomatic and effusion is spontaneously resolving and unless further diagnostic and/or therapeutic options are available (e.g. pericardioscopy, epicardial or pericardial biopsy, application of intrapericardial treatment). In addition, access to the small or moderated effusions requires a learning curve. Several experimental and few clinical concepts have been developed for access of a small pericardial effusion or normal pericardium. These procedures will be reviewed in the following sections.

Pericardiocentesis Guided by Epicardial Halo Phenomenon

For the diagnosis of pericardial effusion in the pre-echocardiography era the radiological findings were of greatest importance. One of the most valuable tools was the evaluation of the epicardial halo phenomenon. However, the correlation of this phenomenon with the presence of and/or the size of pericardial effusion was never resolved. In an effort to improve feasibility and safety of pericardiocentesis for small

pericardial effusions we have noted the applicability of the sign for fluoroscopic guidance of the procedure.

In most of the patients with pericardial effusion there is a clear fluoroscopic distinction between the epicardial surface of the heart and the surroundings, which can be appreciated best in the left lateral view (90 degrees) in the cine fluoroscopy (Fig. 5.1, Video 1.3). In the pre-echocardiography era this sign was utilized for the follow-up of pericardial effusions [1–3]. The halo phenomenon, however, has not been previously applied to guide pericardiocentesis.

In our own experience the sensitivity of the epicardial halo sign for the detection of pericardial effusion was 84.1% and 92.0% in anterior-posterior (PA) and lateral angiographic view respectively [4]. As expected, the specificity of the sign for the detection of pericardial effusion was lower: 57.2% and 44.9% (PA vs. lateral view) revealing a likelihood ratio to establish the effusion of 1.5 and 1.7 in PA angiographic view and lateral angiographic view respectively.

Eisenberg et al. [5] demonstrated 94% specificity, but only 12% sensitivity of the epicardial halo sign in 83 patients with pericardial effusion and in 17 controls with no effusion. The results were better for large and moderate effusions with 92% specificity and 22% sensitivity. These findings confirm that the epicardial halo sign is sensitive enough that it could

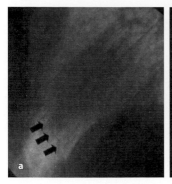
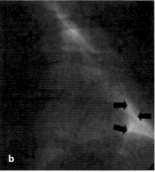

Fig. 5.1a,b. The epicardial halo phenomenon in lateral angiographic view (**a**) and in the anterior-posterior angiographic view (**b**)

be used for guidance of pericardiocentesis in the large majority of patients. The low specificity of the sign is not a limitation for guidance of pericardiocentesis since all patients undergoing the procedure will certainly have to undergo echocardiography before establishing the indication for the drainage of pericardial effusion. Of note, the intensity of the epicardial halo sign may depend on the size of the pericardial effusion, the body-mass index, the technical features of the radiology equipment, as well as the age of the patient and the heart rate and there is therefore a small subpopulation of patients in which it cannot be applied for guidance of pericardiocentesis [4].

Physical Origin of the Sign

Regarding the origin of the epicardial halo phenomenon two main hypotheses have been discussed in the literature. The first explains the epicardial halo as a radiological projection of the subepicardial fat layer [1, 6, 7]. Other experimental and clinical studies, however, have shown that the intensity of the sign correlated with the size of pericardial effusion [8]. In an attempt to explain the origin of the sign Tehranzadeh and Kelly [8] constructed an original model demonstrating that the difference between the X-ray absorption coefficient of the blood in the cardiac chambers and of the transudate in the pericardial space is the most important contributing factor for the appreciation of the halo phenomenon.

Our findings partially support this view, since in our experience, the intensity of the sign was reduced after evacuation of pericardial effusion. However,

there is still no good explanation for the origin of the sign in patients with coronary artery disease who had no pericardial effusion on echocardiography, except probably the presence of epicardial fat [9].

Tangential Approach to the Pericardial Surface

The epicardial halo delineates the epicardial surface of the heart and is used to guide the pericardiocentesis as a line or a border that the needle tip should not cross during the procedure (Fig. 5.2). For the guidance of pericardiocentesis the sign is considered positive, when a halo is visualized in the 90 degrees lateral projection on fluoroscopy, as an anterior demarcation line of higher radiographic density than both the pericardial effusion and the heart shadow, thicker than 2 mm (see Fig. 5.1a). A positive epicardial halo sign may also be noticed, although less frequently, in the frontal projection (see Fig. 5.1b) as an elliptical stripe paralleling the lower left heart border [2, 10].

The procedure is performed in the cardiac catheterization laboratory, using the Tuohy-17, blunt-tip introducer needle, subxiphoid route and local anesthesia. The tangential approach assumed that the puncturing needle is directed posteriorly until the tip passes the bony cage, then the hub of the needle is pressed toward the diaphragm and the needle is advanced tangentially to the epicardial halo. In this way, the needle is directed to the area where the accumulation of the effusion is certainly larger than in the frontal region of the pericardium, assuming that

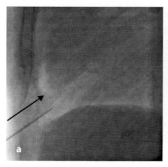 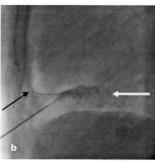

Fig. 5.2a,b. Fluoroscopic guidance of pericardiocentesis using the epicardial halo phenomenon in the lateral angiographic view. *Black arrows* are pointing to the halo phenomenon. *Horizontal black arrow* shows puncture needle approximately tangential to the heart shadow. The *horizontal white arrow* is depicting angiographic contrast in the pericardial space after successful puncture. The left-sided image (**a**) is showing the puncturing needle approaching the pericardium, the right-sided image (**b**) is demonstrating the successful pericardial puncture

the patient is lying on his back in the steady supine position. The mandrel is then removed and the needle is attached to a syringe containing 1% lidocaine or angiography contrast medium.

The operator intermittently attempts to aspirate fluid and injects a small amount of lidocaine or contrast medium. After aspiration of pericardial fluid, a J-tip guidewire is introduced and after dilatation exchanged for a pigtail catheter in order to drain the effusion safely.

Feasibility and Safety of Pericardiocentesis Guided by the Epicardial Halo Phenomenon

In our experience, the application of the halo phenomenon for the guidance of pericardiocentesis in patients with small/moderate effusions resulted in an improved procedural feasibility independent from the size of the effusion (Table 5.1). When the epicardial halo phenomenon was not used for the guidance of pericardiocentesis the success rate was significantly lower for very small effusions (< 200 ml) in comparison to the large effusions (> 300 ml; 76.7% vs. 93.3%, p < 0.01). There were no significant differences regarding the patients' characteristics (Table 5.1) and the etiologies of pericardial effusion of the patients selected for either group [4].

Furthermore, the diagnostic value of pericardiocentesis and of further analyses of the pericardial fluid and tissue obtained by pericardioscopically guided epicardial biopsy was consistently high regardless of the size of the pericardial effusion with a low proportion of false negative findings.

There was no mortality in either group and the incidence of complications was low in all patients who underwent pericardiocentesis. Remarkably, significant complications occurred only in patients who underwent pericardiocentesis before the epicardial halo phenomenon was applied to guide the procedure (0% vs. 3.8%; p < 0.05).

Table 5.1. Patients' age and sex distribution, and procedural feasibility obtained by two different approaches (group 1 – tangential approach using the epicardial halo phenomenon for guidance in 90 degrees lateral angiographic view; group 2 – standard orthogonal approach with frontal view fluoroscopic control and no halo guidance) [4]

	n	Males [%]	Age [years]	Total feasibility	Feasibility in patients with PE > 300 ml	Feasibility in patients with PE 200–300 ml	Feasibility in patients with PE < 200 ml
Group 1 (halo guidance)	76	53.9	55.8±13.7	70/76 (92.1%)	20/21 (95.2%)	25/27 (92.6%)	25/28 (89.3%)
Group 2 (no halo guidance)	158	58.2	50.4±15.2	138/158 (87.3%)	70/75 (93.3%)	45/53 (84.9%)*	23/30 (76.7%)*†

PE: pericardial effusion; * Group 1 vs. Group 2: p < 0.05; † - Feasibility in patients with PE > 300 ml vs. PE < 200 ml in Group 2: p < 0.05

Clinical Implications of the Epicardial Halo Phenomenon

In our experience the halo sign reliably detected the "epicardial border zone" thus enabling a safe access to small pericardial effusions. The sensitivity of the sign was determined by the size of pericardial effusion [1], the body-mass index and by technical factors. Fluoroscopy with short exposure time [6] and low imaging energy increase the probability of detecting the halo phenomenon [2, 12].

In previous studies analyzing plain chest radiographs the sign was noted in 52–68% [2, 8, 13] in patients with pericardial effusion. Most of the studies reported a better appreciation of the sign on the lateral than on the frontal projection (41% vs. 23%) [2, 5, 13]. However, there were also some opposite findings (frontal radiographs 62% vs. lateral films 41%) [8]. In 12% [2] and 30% [8] of the patients the sign is present on both frontal and lateral radiographs. Jorgens et al. [14] described the cinefluoroscopic approach, which was considerably more reliable in diagnosing effusions. The same was confirmed in the study of Botsch [1] revealing a positive epicardial halo in 29/33 (87.9%) patients with moderate or large pericardial effusions.

An additional advantage could be the supine position of the patient [3]. In 35 patients with pericardial effusion, the "epicardial fat stripe" sign was positive in 51% of the patients using the supine cross-table lateral chest roentgenograms in contrast to 31% of positive conventional lateral roentgenograms. The sign was positive using the supine lateral roentgenograms in 20%, 36%, and 86% of patients with small, moderate, and large effusions, respectively. In conventional lateral roentgenograms the sign was present in 17% of patients without pericardial effusion, and in 30%, 27%, and 36% of patients with small, moderate, and large effusions, respectively.

Despite significant advances introduced by fluoroscopic and echocardiographic guidance, pericardiocentesis of pericardial effusion smaller than 300 ml remains difficult and controversial. Pericardiocentesis guided by the epicardial halo phenomenon offers a simple alternative and enables safe drainage of pericardial effusions that would not be accessible or even attempted with the standard approach [4, 15].

The safety of pericardiocentesis has significantly improved with the introduction of echocardiographic or fluoroscopic guidance. Procedure-related mortality was up to 18% in the 1970s [16] and 2-4% [17] in the 1980s. However, the recent large echocardiographic series (1127 therapeutic echo-guided pericardiocenteses in 977 patients) reported 1.2% major complications and 3.5% minor complications [18]. In our experience with fluoroscopic control of pericardiocentesis there was no mortality and the incidence of major complications was significantly reduced by utilizing the epicardial halo phenomenon and the tangential approach in the lateral view [4].

Pericardial Effusion Access Using PerDUCER® Device

The concept of pericardiocentesis with the PerDUCER® device includes a combination of vacuum suction and tangential puncture of the parietal pericardium [19, 20]. It contains a 21-gauge introducer needle located inside of a stainless steel sheath. The sheath ends with a plastic view tube and a hemispheric side-hole cavity, where the pericardium is captured by vacuum and tangentially punctured by an introducer needle. The size of the side-hole determines the maximum thickness of the pericardium that can be captured (2 mm). The device has a patent in the USA and is approved for experimental and clinical application in Europe, but not yet approved by the Food and Drug Administration in the USA.

The procedure includes two major steps:
1. subxiphoid access to the anterior mediastinum (Fig. 5.3); and
2. pericardial capture, puncture, insertion of the guidewire, and catheter for sampling of pericardial fluid or delivery of intrapericardial treatment (Fig. 5.4; CD-ROM – Video 5).

This concept has offered a potentially promising technique to access the pericardium in the absence of effusion and deliver intrapericardial treatment for the various diseases of the heart. The pericardial access with the PerDUCER® device in the absence of effusion is reviewed separately in this book (see

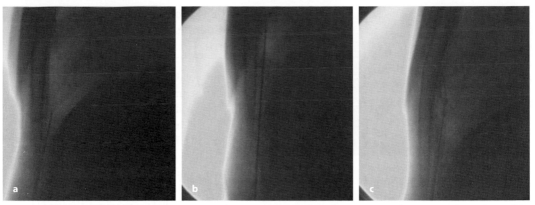

◻ Fig. 5.3a–c. Subxiphoid access to the anterior mediastinum (left lateral view) in **a** patient with autoreactive perimyocarditis: a puncture with a blunt cannula; **b** insertion of the 0.038-inch J-tip guidewire, and **c** 19F introducer set (16.5 F also applicable). Adapted with permission from Maisch et al. (2001) [21]

Chapter 6). In this section we will discuss only the clinical experience in pericardiocentesis with Per-DUCER® in patients with pericardial effusion.

Endoscopic Guidance in Patients with Perimyocarditis

To evaluate the feasibility of the procedure in humans and the contribution of endoscopic guidance during pericardiocentesis with the PerDUCER®, we applied this approach in six patients with myopericarditis participating in the study of intrapericardial treatment with triamcinolone (3 men, mean age 43 ± 13 years, with acute, virus-negative (n = 4) or recurrent autoreactive myopericarditis (n = 2), pericardial effusion in all < 180 ml) (Table 5.4). Only symptomatic patients with small pericardial effusions and negative polymerase chain reaction findings in endomyocardial biopsies for cardiotropic microbial agents (influenza A/B, cytomegalovirus, enterovirus, adenovirus, herpes simplex virus, Ebstein-Barr virus, Borrelia burgdorferi, Parvo B19, Chlamydia pneumoniae, and Mycobacterium tuberculosis, were included in the study.

◻ Table 5.2. Patients with autoreactive myopericarditis who underwent PerDUCER® procedure in order to obtain intrapericardial treatment with triamcinolone. Adapted with permission from Maisch et al. (2001) [21]

	Sex	Age	Duration of the disease	LVEDD [cm]	LVEF [%] (echo)	PE volume (drainage or echo)	PerDUCER® procedure successful
Group 1							
Case 1	M	26	1	5.6	59	110	Yes
Case 2	F	59	20	4.6	65	50	Yes
Case 3	F	45	3	5.8	45	160	No
Group 2							
Case 1	M	32	1	5.2	65	180	No
Case 2	M	38	2	4.9	60	170	No
Case 3	F	57	16	6.0	40	120	No

Group 1 – patients undergoing pericardiocentesis with the PerDUCER® device guided by pericardioscopy; Group 2 – patients undergoing pericardiocentesis with PerDUCER® device with no pericardioscopy guidance; *LVEDD* left ventricular end-diastolic diameter; *LVEF* left ventricular ejection fraction; *PE* pericardial effusion; echo echocardiography.

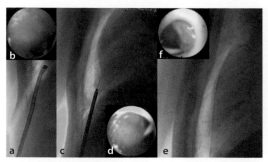

◨ **Fig. 5.4a–f.** Key steps in the application of the PerDUCER® device (left lateral view): **a** advancement of the flexible endoscope; **b** selection of the portion of the pericardium with no adhesion and fat deposition; **c** insertion of the PerDUCER® device, manual vacuum suction, capture and puncture of the parietal pericardium in the distal view tube of the instrument, and introduction of the intrapericardial 0.018-inch J-tip guidewire; **d** verification of the guidewire position by pericardioscopy; **e** dilatation and insertion of the 5.4 F intrapericardial catheter; **f** endoscopic verification of the intrapericardial position of the catheter. Adapted with permission from Maisch et al. (2001) [21]

All procedures were performed in the cardiac catheterization laboratory with the patient under local anesthesia. The selection of the pericardial site for the application of the PerDUCER® was guided by flexible endoscopy (AF 1101 Bl, Karl Storz, Tuttlingen, Germany; Fig. 5.4). An intrapericardial catheter was left for 48 hours. Before its removal all residual fluid was evacuated.

In 3 patients from group 1, after access to the mediastinal space, it was possible to identify the pericardial surface endoscopically, and in 2 patients, it was possible to find an area free of adipose tissue and adhesions to successfully apply the PerDUCER (Figs. 5.4a,b). In the third patient, the procedure failed due to pericardial adhesions and fibrosis, previously not detected by computed tomography, but revealed by pericardioscopy. In group 2, although access to the mediastinal space and contact to the pericardial surface were achieved, it was not possible to enter the pericardium. These patients were further treated with oral medications. In 2 of 4 patients, the amount of pericardial effusion increased two and four weeks after the initial, unsuccessful PerDUCER® procedure, and standard, fluoroscopically guided pericardiocentesis and intrapericardial instillation of triamcinolone were performed. There were no acute or late complications in any of the procedures.

PerDUCER® Procedure in Patients with Moderate/Large Pericardial Effusions

Despite the promising concept and good experimental efficiency, the initial clinical application was only partially successful in our experience. Similarly, in previously reported five patients with large to moderate pericardial effusions, the procedure was not successful despite good mediastinal access and capture of the pericardium [22]. Furthermore, in the study performed in patients who had undergone bypass surgery with a normal pericardium, the PerDUCER® procedure in patients with moderate/large pericardial effusions procedure was accomplished successfully in all of the eight patients studied in the open-chest setting [19].

However, in an additional four patients studied before sternotomy for aortocoronary bypass, pericardial access with the PerDUCER® procedure in patients with moderate/large pericardial effusions could be achieved only in two.

Potential Improvements of the Procedure

Apart from the appropriate selection of patients and the exclusion of those with a thickened pericardium, one of the major reasons for the limited success of the procedure thus far could be the inability to avoid fat tissue or adhesions in positioning the device under standard fluoroscopic control. Having had extensive personal experience with pericardioscopy [23–26], we applied the flexible percutaneous endoscope in the anterior mediastinal space for inspection and selection of the suitable pericardial surface. The addition of flexible endoscopy certainly complicates and increases the costs of the procedure, but we believe that its contribution was essential for the final success achieved in 2 patients.

The introduction of a large introducer-set into the mediastinal space is often painful despite local anesthesia and analgesia. It represents a further weak point of the technique. In the present design of the instrument, the size of the introducer set could be diminished from the current 19 F to 16.5 F, which would also fit the outer diameter of the device.

PeriAttacher® and AttachGuider®

The PeriAttacher for Accessing the Pericardial Space

The potential applications of a device using a controlled attachment of the pericardium with subsequent intrapericardial access are numerous. When pericardial effusion is present, such a device can be used for draining the pericardial fluid, taking biopsies and administering drugs. Contrary to the conventional puncture with a needle, no risk of injuring the epicardium and myocardium leading to cardiac tamponade is involved. In view of the recent progress in diagnostic procedures and treatment options involving intrapericardial instillation of various drugs, intrapericardial therapy would have already been extended to moderate effusions if a suitable, safe and reliable device were available. As an example for intrapericardial therapy in the absence of pericardial effusion, compounds releasing nitric oxide for treating restenosis could be instilled. Also various types of stem cells could be administered for myocardial regeneration (see Chapter 12). This section is therefore devoted to the description of the major features of the recent patent applications for the PeriAttacher and follow-up devices for pericardial access and intrapericardial navigation (DE 103 37 813.8, PCT/DE 2004/001806, EP 04762651.0-2318, US 10/568,430, DE 10 2005 057 479.3, PCT/DE 2006/002116 and DE 10 2006 058 447.3-35).

When the pericardial space is separated only by a few millimeters from the underlying epicardium which is characteristic of a healthy pericardium, the conventional needle approach is not applicable. Procedures are required which move the pericardium away from the epicardium before the pericardium can be punctured. Even in the case of pericardial effusion, an alternative to the needle approach would be very useful if it eliminates the risk of accidental puncture or laceration of the ventricular wall. While a number of new techniques have been disclosed in recent years, an alternative to the standard needle technique is not yet available. The reasons for this lack of progress include:

a) The procedure should be minimally invasive; in particular no open heart surgery involving deflation of a lung and general anesthesia should be required. Thus, procedures requiring an access perpendicular to the surface of the heart using minithoracotomy are not an alternative to the standard needle approach. Rather a procedure where the pericardium is accessed tangentially to the cardiac surface from the abdominal side, i.e. subxiphoidal approach, has to be used.

b) In a number of disease states such as infection, the pericardium becomes thickened thereby increasing also the stiffness of the tissue. As a consequence, the lifting of the pericardium away from the epicardium might work in healthy animals but not in patients with a pericardium which is thickened due to the underlying disease.

c) Excessive epicardial and pericardial fat represents a major obstacle for procedures involving lifting of the pericardium before the puncturing step. Any major progress in the development of a functioning device for puncturing the pericardium depends, therefore, on the approach used for moving the pericardium away from the epicardium.

In principal, moving or lifting of an organ or tissue can be achieved by mechanical devices such as clamps or forceps or by vacuum operated suction chambers as it is the case in PerDUCER device.

The device described here comprises a body with a distal and a proximal end. This body features a continuous bore. The distal end features several jaws which can be opened and closed. A needle for the tissue puncture is located in the jaws and is moveable within the continuous bore. Mechanical grasping devices have, however, the inherent risk of injuring the tissue. Thus grasping should be not stronger than required for tissue attachment to avoid unnecessary injury. Since in a minimally invasive approach for pericardial access, the space for tissue grasping is very limited, tissue injury represents a serious risk. Since the extent of tissue attachment by vacuum suction can be adjusted by the vacuum pressure used, suction heads were also developed for moving the pericardium. The PerDUCER device comprises a penetrating body which is located in a lumen of a guide tube. The guide tube features a deflection mechanism on its distal end for deflecting the distal end of the penetrating needle. Furthermore, the guide tube features a head on its distal end with a lateral opening for drawing in the tissue to be punctured. For this purpose, a vacuum source, which allows suction of the pericardium at the opening, however only when the head or the same opening is correctly positioned relative to the pericardium, is attached to the guide tube. When the attending physician is certain that the pericardium is attached to the side opening, the pericardium is punctured at an angle relative to the attached pericardial tissue.

A prerequisite of any suction device used for moving the pericardium is the maintenance of vacuum in the suction head by proper sealing of the vacuum from the environmental pressure. Since tissue in general has an uneven surface and deforms during attachment attempts were made for improving sealing during tissue attachment and during the process of tissue puncture which pushes the attached tissue away from the suction head. In this instrument, the "bleb" formed in the distal end of the guide tube is buttressed by a shoulder in a position that reduces the likelihood of the pericardium moving away from the distal tip of the guide tube and breaking the point of the vacuum seal when the bleb is contacted by the distally advancing piercing tip of the needle.

For a minimally invasive approach, a tangential approach is required whereby the suction head is placed in parallel and not perpendicular to the surface of the beating heart. The tangential alignment of the suction head on the pericardium is described in the PerDUCER device (see previous section) [19–22]. The suction results in movement of the pericardium into the suction head, i.e. it is lifted away from the epicardium. This is followed by puncture of the attached pericardium. If the pericardium is thin enough so that part of the pericardial space is also within the suction head, the needle reaches the underlying pericardial space. Although such a device has been used successfully in pigs, it failed in 4 out of 6 patients with myopericarditis and small (132 ± 49 ml) pericardial effusion [21]. The reasons for the failure can be manifold:

1. The suction is achieved manually by a syringe and any loss of vacuum during the puncturing step results in tissue detachment and thus failure of accessing the pericardial space. This problem is inherent also in the aforementioned devices where the attachment of bodily tissues or an organ to the

device is not reliably recognized and signaled, so that the user is always uncertain if attachment is reached successfully. We have tried in our patent application DE 103 37 813 A1 to enable exact control and display of the vacuum which is a considerable improvement of the technical state of the art of both aforementioned specifications. With this device (Marburg Attacher for tissue manipulation in general or PeriAttacher for pericardial access) it is possible to reliably recognize and signal satisfactory attachment of the tissue or organ for successful puncture or other type of manipulation. The device comprises a vacuum source, a suction head with a recess, a needle and an attachment detection device, as well as a display device (Fig. 5.5a). The attachment detection device can possess one or more means of detection, amongst others, acoustic, optical, as well as pressure dependent (Fig. 5.5b). By means of a display device signals, which are detected by the attachment detection device, are converted into display signals using e.g. a Schmitt trigger with hysteresis (Fig. 5.5c).

2. The PerDUCER device is expected to function when the pericardium is thin and the formed "bleb" in the suction head permits entry of the penetrating needle into the underlying pericardial space. This is expected to be case in inbred pigs kept under conditions which prevent infection affecting also the pericardium with subsequent pericardial thickening. Also fat deposition on the pericardium can block the suction head. Various other ill-defined pathologies can result in thickened pericardium. Even in patients without pericardial effusion, locally thickened pericardium can occur and a clinically useful device has, therefore, to cope with an unpredictably thickened pericardium. A modification of the above mentioned devices cannot overcome the problems of locally thickened pericardium. While the addition of a multitude of suction channels in the suction head as described in the PeriAttaccher patent specification US 5,071,412 could be expected to better fill the suction head. The vacuum channels within the capture mechanism are provided to hold a captured body duct and to open the duct interior to facilitate introduction of a fluid into the lumen of the duct. Also in this

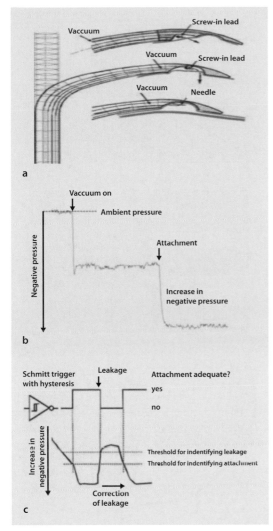

a

b

c

□ **Fig. 5.5a–c.** Various types of suction heads of a (flexible) Peri-Attacher device (**a**). Attachment of tissue results in an increased negative pressure (**b**). Any temporarily occurring leakage can be detected and corrected. The monitoring device for tissue attachment can consist of e.g. a Schmitt trigger with hysteresis (**c**)

device, a needle is disposed within an axial passage in the shaft and punctures the duct within the suction head. In the case of a thickened pericardium, the pericardium would be captured and held by the vacuum channels within the suction head. When the needle is advanced, it would, however, only travel into the thickened pericardium and not into the underlying pericardial sac.

There is thus a need for devices which are suitable for accessing the space between two tissues which closely overlay each other, whereby the thickness of the upper tissue is variable. The extent of thickening can vary locally and is not known when the procedure is started.

The AttachGuider for the Guidance of Instruments in Cavities, in Particular the Pericardial Space

A significant progress has been made by resynchronization therapy in patients with dilated cardiomyopathy and heart failure [27, 28]. The currently preferred procedure involves insertion of pacing leads into a tributary vein of the coronary sinus. A coronary sinus-lead implantation can, however, fail and require conversion to the implantation of an epicardial lead involving left-lateral thoracotomy. When taking into account the number of patients with unsuccessful implantations and patients whose leads become dysfunctional during follow-up, the clinical failure may approach 50% [29]. It has been shown by Mair et al. [30] that surgical epicardial lead placement revealed excellent long-term results and a lower complication rate compared to coronary sinus leads. Although, the approach via limited thoracotomy for biventricular pacing is associated with "more surgery", it is a safe and reliable technique and should be considered as an equal alternative. Therefore, the need for epicardial lead implantation is growing.

In view of the unresolved technical problems related to implantation of the left ventricular lead, we addressed a novel technique for intrapericardial navigation and left or right epicardial lead implantation after successful pericardial access. Contrary to minithoracotomy, the procedure does not require lung deflation and general anesthesia. Epicardial lead(s) could be implanted after mapping for functional improvement. While further development is required, the epicardial approach appears to be applicable at least to 15–20% of patients in whom resynchronization failed due to the suboptimal coronary sinus anatomy.

Another disadvantage of the known devices is that the feeding of the devices occurs mostly in an uncontrolled manner, e.g. in predominantly canal-shaped cavities except for the coincidental guidance through the walls of the cavities. An AttachGuider device as specified in the invention DE 10 2005 057 479.3 and PCT/DE 2006/002116 was, therefore, developed which allows fixation of the device within the cavity, e.g. the pericardial space, via means of attachment assigned to the device. The means of attachment provide for fixation of the device relative to at least one part of the wall of the cavity to be examined, in which the device must be at least partially inserted. The means of attachment are designed in such a way that they come into contact with at least one part of the cavity wall upon activation, e.g. frictional contact, and thus fix the device relative to this part of the wall. The device fixed in this way offers improved fixation for subsequent movement of the instrument, which is, e.g. guided within the device in order to conduct reliable manipulations or visual examinations etc. within the cavity or starting from its walls. Embodiment of the device offers much improved guidance compared to the current state of the art. For this, the device features at least two means of attachment separated from each other in the direction of the desired movement (e.g. forwards or backwards) which are affixed to the device and designed able to be activated one after another for the guidance of the forward movement.

Figure 5.6a–c schematically shows steps of the temporally and spatially staggered movement of the outer and the inner wall or the instrument, preferably in the pericardial space. In a), the device is inserted into the pericardial space. Both means of attachment (2) are not activated. In b), activation of the means of attachment (2a) on the outer wall is executed. In c), bending to the right occurs by continuous attachment (2a) with the help of a means of bending. In the embodiment of a flexible tube, the head section can e.g. feature a notch of different sizes, depending on the desired deflection angle. The head section is bent, e.g. a control wire lying in the device. In d) and e), the movement of the inner wall or the guided instrument in the direction of the bending occurs with continuous attachment (2a). In f), the inner wall or the guided instrument is also attached (2a). In g), the attachment (2) of the outer wall is detached. In h) and i), the outer wall is moved along the attached inner wall or the attached instrument. In j), attachment (2a) of the outer wall occurs, then, in k), the

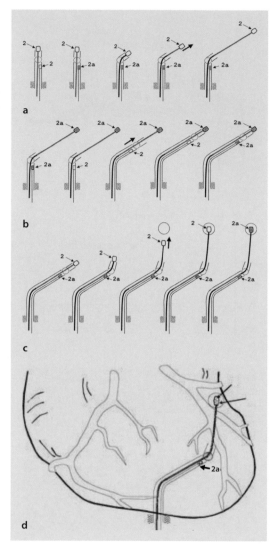

Fig. 5.6a–d. Schematic procedure of intrapericardial navigation using an AttachGuider® device for epicardial leads implantation or epicardial ablation

attachment (2) of the inner wall or the instrument is detached. In l), the head section of the outer wall is bent to the left, and in m) and n), the inner wall or the instrument is pushed in the direction of the bending. In o), the target destination is reached and the instrument can be attached.

These steps can be repeated as desired, whereby the direction of the bending is adjustable. Figure -5.6d shows the situation of the device depicted on the right in Fig. 5.6c O) projected onto the sur-

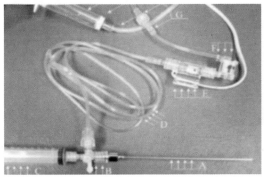 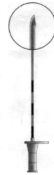

Fig. 5.7. *Left side:* Subxyphoid pericardial access system: a blunt-tip epidural (Tuohy-17) needle (*A*) (also shown enlarged in the right-sided image) is attached to a syringe (*C*) via a 3-way stopcock (*B*) hooked through high-pressure tubing (*D*) to a transducer (*F*) to monitor pericardial pressure. The system is attached to an intraflow valve (*F*) hooked to a pressurized saline bag (*G*). An electrode is also attached to needle for continuous electrocardiographic monitoring (ST- segment elevation). Reproduced with permission from Mannam et al. (2002) [32]. *Right side:* Tuohy needle (detail)

face of the heart. Right coronary artery, circumflex and left-anterior descending branch of the left coronary artery are illustrated. Tissue manipulation, e.g. an epicardial lead implantation which is indicated by the corkscrew-like arrangement of the instrument (5), occurs with the instrument pushed forward. The wall situated nearest to the instrument is attached (2a), in order to make the electrode head recognizable, the hatching of the activated means of attachment was removed during the implantation.

Pericardial Access Using a Blunt-Tip Needle

An elegant approach for pericardiocentesis of moderate/small pericardial effusions, actually intended for access of the normal pericardium was proposed by Mannam et al. [32]. His system consists of an epidural blunt-tip introducer needle (Tuohy-17) connected to a saline infusion via an intraflow system under continuous positive pressure of 20 to 30 mmHg (Fig. 5.7). Subxiphoid pericardial access using this technique, was applied in local anesthesia in 12 patients with pericardial effusion as a first step to evaluate feasibility of the procedure for further potential access of the normal pericardium (see Chapter 6). In the studied patients, the mean size of the effusion in echocardiography was 2.1 ± 0.8 cm).

During the procedures arterial pressure was continuously monitored through a femoral or radial arterial cannula. Right-sided cardiac catheterization was performed to measure right atrial, right ventricular, and pulmonary capillary wedge pressure, and cardiac output and index were measured using Fick's method.

The concept of this approach is to use positive pressure at the tip of the needle maintained by the running infusion to push the right ventricle away from the needle's pathway after the entry in the pericardial space.

Although electrocardiographic monitoring for ST-segment elevation from the pericardiocentesis needle is regarded as obsolete and unreliable, Mannam et al. have used it in this study in an attempt to increase the safety of the procedure. Upon successful entry in the pericardial space, access was confirmed by the injection of 1 ml of diluted contrast under fluoroscopy (Fig. 5.8). Pericardial pressure was then measured and compared with the right atrial pressure to evaluate the hemodynamic significance of the gradient. A soft floppy-tip 0.025-inch guidewire was then advanced to the pericardial space and the needle exchanged for a pericardial drainage catheter.

Pericardial access was achieved in all but 1/12 patients (8.3%), who had a loculated effusion, which required surgical drainage in the later stage of the management. No ST-segment elevation was noted on the lead attached to the pericardiocentesis needle during the procedure. There were no procedural complications. During the 6-month follow-up one patient (8%) had recurrent pericardial effusion (5 days after the initial procedure) and underwent the second pericardiocentesis. Three patients (25%) died within 1 month after index pericardiocentesis from their underlying malignancies.

The combination of a blunt-tip needle, pressurized saline flow, and fluoroscopic guidance could have the potential to decrease the procedural complication rate of pericardiocentesis and enable access to small effusions and normal pericardium. It is a

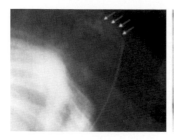
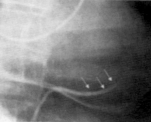

▫ **Fig. 5.8.** Subxyphoid access of the pericardial space in a patient with a pericardial effusion (*left-sided image*). The intrapericardial location of the blunt-tip needle is confirmed by the injection of angiographic contrast (*arrows*) under fluoroscopy. The needle is then exchanged for a drainage catheter (*arrows*) using a 0.025-in soft floppy-tip guidewire (*right-sided image*). Reproduced with permission from Mannam et al. (2002) [32]

simple, inexpensive technique, which uses equipment and material widely available in any catheterization laboratory.

Feasibility and Safety of the Procedure

Safety and efficacy of the subxyphoid access of the normal pericardium using a blunt-tip needle was first demonstrated in animal models used for angiogenic drug delivery studies [33, 34]. The feasibility of access to the normal pericardium with this system was previously shown in the experimental setting in 49 Yorkshire pigs [33] and in the numerous electrophysiological studies dealing with epicardial mapping and ablations (more than 300 procedures) [35–38].

Transbronchial Approach

Most of the loculated posterior pericardial effusions cannot be safely evacuated using the standard subxiphoid or apical, intercostal approach. In the presence of large, symptomatic effusions or if the pericardial drainage is regarded essential for diagnostic purposes, such patients are usually referred to surgery. Occasionally, in the presence of both left pleural and posterior pericardial effusion echocardiographically guided pleuro-pericardial drainage can be safely performed using the left axillary, intercostal route [39].

An exceptionally unusual, alternative approach for pericardiocentesis has been applied by Ceron et al. [40] in three patients with loculated posterior pericardial effusion. The authors used a transbronchial access through the left lower lobe bronchus. This access allowed both the diagnostic sampling and the evacuation of pericardial effusion. Patients, in whom the size of pericardial effusion has widened

the pleural fissure, are best suited for this technique, which brings the pericardium near or in contact with the left bronchial tree (usually left lower-lobe bronchus). Alternatively, for diagnostic purposes only, the pericardium can be also approached through the distal trachea.

By puncturing through the anterior tracheal wall at the level between the first and the third intercartilage space up from the carina even small posterior effusions can be reached. In computed tomography these small effusions are seen as a small homogenous, hypodense "half-moon" suspended from the ascending aorta (Fig. 5.9). The proper selection of the patients requires computed tomography to confirm that the pericardium is in contact with the large airway. Application of endobronchial ultrasound can facilitate the procedure but is not absolutely necessary.

The puncture of the tracheal or bronchial wall can be performed without fluoroscopic or ultrasonographic guidance by the "pushing technique" [41]. The

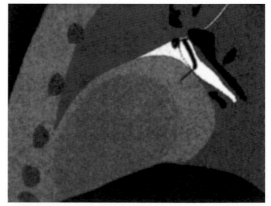

▫ **Fig. 5.9.** Transbronchial pericardiocentesis. Access of the posterior, loculated pericardial effusion is performed puncturing the anterior wall of the left lower bronchus. Adapted with permission from Ceron et al. (2003) [40]

needle tip is advanced so that the entire length of the needle protrudes out of the tip of the bronchoscope. The operator than pushes the bronchoscope and the catheter into the bronchial wall in the direction of the pericardial effusion, as one unit (holding at the same time the proximal end of the catheter to the bronchoscope with one or two fingers)). Suction and further drainage are performed with the same catheter providing 10, 220, and 700 ml of pericardial effusion in three patients.

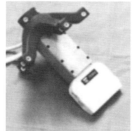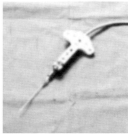

◨ **Fig. 5.10.** "Echostar", ultrasonic probe equipped with 24 infrared diodes (*left side*), the needle equipped with a "rigid body" (*right side*). Reproduced with permission from Chavanon et al. (2000) [43]

Safety of the Transbronchial Pericardiocentesis

The approach requires experience and skill in transbronchial needle aspiration as well as the accurate pre-procedural computerized tomography. In selected patients there is no risk of myocardial lesion, since only pericardium approaches the bronchial tree in the presence of the large effusion. Therefore, during the evacuation of the effusion, pericardium will move away from the bronchus until the needle cannot reach it any more. Therefore, it is useful to perform an echocardiographic control during the evacuation of the fluid, in order to obtain information about the quantity and distribution of the residual effusion.

Purulent pericarditis is theoretically the most important risk of the above described procedure since the puncturing needle is approaching the pericardium from a non-sterile environment (bronchial lumen). However, no such complication was noted in the follow-up of three patients described by Ceron et al. [40]. Similarly, experience from more than 700 patients who underwent the transbronchial needle aspiration of the mediastinal lymph nodes also resulted in no fever or bacteriaemia, even in the absence of the antimicrobial treatment or prophylaxis.

Computer-guided Pericardiocentesis

In order to improve the accuracy of access to smaller and/or loculated effusions Chavanon et al. [42–44] have applied and original concept and developed a new system for computer-guided pericardiocentesis. The pericardiocentesis is guided in this complex method-based on a model of the pericardial effusion,

constructed from the 3D reconstruction of echocardiography data, recorded preoperatively. In addition to the ultrasonic device and a needle the system also includes a 3-D localizer and a computer (Fig. 5.10). Current experience with this system includes studies on the experimental model, and in animals with an experimental pericardial effusion. The procedure comprises 3 steps: perception, decision, and action, all coordinated by the dedicated computer system.

Perception

The first step in the computer guided pericardiocentesis is to obtain and record a set of echocardiography data using a B-mode ultrasound probe connected to a 3-D localizer (Optotrak™ localizer, Northern Digital Inc, Ontario, Canada). At the time when this study was performed no 3D echocardiography machines were available yet.

Decision

The second step of the computer-guided pericardiocentesis is the calculation of the shortest and the safest route to enter the pericardial effusion. As a part of these calculations, the position, shape, and movements of the effusion are constructed as a computer model in this plane. The problem of systolic and diastolic movements of the heart is solved by defining a stable area in the effusion, independent of the cardiac cycle, the so-called "stable region".

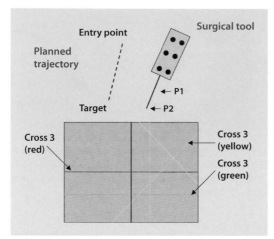

Fig. 5.11. Computer-guided pericardiocentesis. Principle of the passive guidance system. Reproduced with permission from Chavanon et al. (2000) [43]

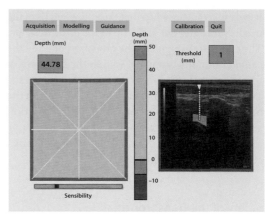

Fig. 5.12. Computer-guided pericardiocentesis. User-interface of the passive-guidance system: the 3 crosses (superimposed in this case), numerical data (concerning mainly the penetration depth) are displayed over the crosses. On the right, the reference echocardiographic plane with the outlined needle path. In the middle, the penetration depth scale. Reproduced with permission from Chavanon et al. (2000) [43]

Action

The third step of computer-guided pericardiocentesis is based on the real-time guidance of the pericardiocentesis needle in the direction of the previously defined "stable region" in the pericardial effusion. The operator is assisted by a passive guidance system based on superimposed crosses on the user interface (Fig. 5.11): on the screen, a green and a yellow cross correspond to two points located on the needle. The crosses move in real time according to the position of the needle. A third (red) cross is marking the planned trajectory. The operator has to guide the needle in order to superimpose the yellow and the green crosses. Further on, these two crosses must be superimposed over the red cross, positioning the tip of the needle at the entry point (Fig. 5.12). The operator must then push the needle in the established direction, precisely for the distance needed to reach the "stable region".

Protocol

The first tests of the above described system were performed on a 2-D model. After an echocardiographic examination, the physician selected a plane displaying a safe puncture site, and acquired a set of almost parallel planes in its surrounding. The ultra-

sound probe was tracked by the Optotrak™ during the acquisition. The "stable region", the target and the route were defined (Step 2 – Decision) and then the Step 3 – Action was performed in the referential plane.

Feasibility of the Computer-Guided Pericardiocentesis

After a feasibility study on a dynamic phantom which mimicked cardiac movement [42] the same protocol was successfully applied using a dog and a porcine model [45].

On the dynamic phantom it was possible to obtain 1-mm accuracy for pericardiocentesis [45]. The procedure was also successful in mongrel dogs with a 1 cm large serous pericardial effusion [46]. In the experimental study performed on 8 pigs (20–35 kg) 10 successful pericardiocentesis procedures were subsequently achieved [42]. The pericardial effusion ranged in these experiments from 5–12 mm (mean 7.5 mm, stable region: 5 mm) to 9–15 mm (average: 12.6 mm, stable region: 9 mm). The duration of the procedure was 10–15 minutes.

A new 3-D localizer system (Polaris™ Northern Digital Inc, Ontario, Canada) was applied by Cha-

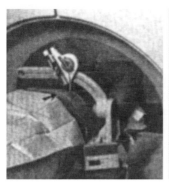

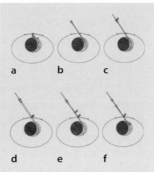

◘ **Fig. 5.13.** CT-guided pericardiocentesis. Reproduced with permission from Duvernoy and Magnuson (1996) [47]

vanon et al. in the second series of experiments on computer-guided pericardiocentesis [43] with the advantage of wireless infrared connections between the segments and the improved computer system allowing the surgeon to be in "enhanced reality" with direct visual access to both the operative field and the displayed data. The development of new, improved CASPER software enabled the first successful clinical application of computer-guided pericardiocentesis [44]. The system has achieved an accuracy for pericardiocentesis guidance of at least 2.5 mm.

Advantages and Drawbacks of the Procedure

The passive guiding system gives the operator feedback on his current action. It allows him to determine the optimal path for the needle used for pericardiocentesis, and to accurately reach previously defined "safety zone" at the center of effusion. Problems in development of the computer-guided pericardiocentesis system were mainly related to the physiological movements of the heart, lungs and the chest wall, unexpected motion of the patient, and deformability of soft tissues.

Pericardiocentesis Guided by Computed Tomography

After cardiac surgery pericardial effusions are often loculated, the residual pericardial space is interrupted with wide adhesions, and the effusion can be difficult to reach for diagnostic evaluation but even more

for the treatment. In such a condition, computed tomography (CT)-guided pericardiocentesis has been suggested as a potential alternative to fluoroscopy or echo-guided pericardial taps (Fig. 5.13) [47]. In contrast to echocardiography, CT imaging is not affected by postoperative mediastinal emphysema and pain, swelling, or scars from the surgical wounds. Therefore, Duvernoy and Magnuson [47] have developed a methodology for CT-guided pericardiocentesis and performed this procedure in ten patients using a stereotactic device and a 0.9-mm needle. The base of the stereotactic guidance device (CT-Guide, Bard (black-curved arrow in Fig. 5.13)) was placed underneath the patient at the level of the entry site. After disinfection of the skin, a sterile radiopaque grid (small black arrow in Fig. 5.13) was placed over the chest wall. Several levels were imaged in order to obtain a safe trajectory for the puncturing needle and avoid damage of the mammarian arteries, pleura, and the lung. When located and crosschecked, the entry point was marked on the skin.

Previously calculated depth and angle of the puncture were set at the stereotactic guidance device. The needle holder with the 0.9-mm needle was positioned over the marked entry point on the skin. The patient was asked to suspend respiration in the same phase as during previous scanning. Then the puncture was performed in one quick step (Fig. 5.13, right). When the needle tip reached the pre-determined puncture depth, the motion of the instrument was automatically stopped by the depth regulator. After verification of the position of the needle by CT-imaging a J-tip guidewire was introduced and the needle replaced with a 6F pigtail catheter with multiple side-holes.

Both the subxiphoid and parasternal approaches were suitable for this procedure, depending of the distribution of the loculated effusion. The procedure was successful in all patients, both regarding the effusion access and drainage, with no complications.

However, the technique is time-consuming and more expensive than the traditional methods utilizing fluoroscopy or echocardiography guidance. Although CT-guidance offers an alternative approach for pericardial drainage when conventional techniques fail in pericardiocentesis, the inability of real-time imaging remains the major disadvantage of the procedure.

CT-Fluoroscopy

CT-fluoroscopy has been successfully used for targeting of biopsies of the mediastinum, lung [48–50], and abdomen [51]. Bruning et al. recently applied CT-fluoroscopy for pericardiocentesis in eight patients with loculated pericardial effusions, that would be otherwise not reachable for echocardiography-guided pericardiocentesis. Out of these eight patients two had pericardial effusion of unknown origin, another two secondary acute myeloid leukemia, one patient had Wegener's granulomatosis, one Non-Hodgkin lymphoma, one had Dressler's syndrome, and one patient had lung cancer.

For all patients a Somatom Plus 4 CT scanner with a 6 frames/s CT-fluoroscopy system was used (C.A.R.E. Vision package, Siemens Medical Solutions, Forchheim, Germany). For the helical scans before the procedures, 120 KV and 240 mA were applied, 35 seconds following an injection of 120 ml of non-ionic contrast material. In fluoroscopy mode, tube voltage was 120 kV, tube current 90 mA, rotation time 0.75 s. The highest possible fluoroscopic current of 90 mA was chosen to optimally delineate the effusion from the pericardium and the myocardium. After reconstruction of a helical CT scan of the region (Fig. 5.14) the slice position that appeared most suitable for the interventional approach was determined and used further as a reference level for the intervention.

In seven procedures the drainage was performed using a medial (subxiphoidal) approach (Fig. 5.15 left), and in four procedures a lateral, intercostal approach (Fig. 5.15 right). The previously selected most suitable point of entry was marked on the chest wall and local anesthesia applied in this region. After a small incision of the skin the 18-gauge needle was inserted and verified by CT-fluoroscopy. As the needle was advanced CT-fluoroscopy was used to verify its position and the distance from the heart. When a sample of the pericardial effusion was drawn a 0.035" guidewire was introduced through the needle into the pericardial space and than exchanged for 4 to 6 F pigtail catheter for drainage of the pericardial effusion.

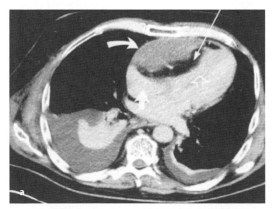 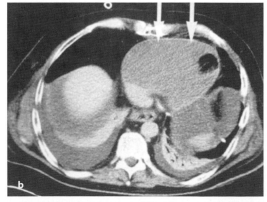

Fig. 5.14a,b. Helical CT-scan with contrast enhancement. **a** Section at the level of the ventricles revealing a localized effusion over the right ventricle (*curved arrow*). **b** Localized pericardial effusion observed at the caudal slices of the heart (*arrows*). Reproduced with permission from Bruning et al. (2002) [52]

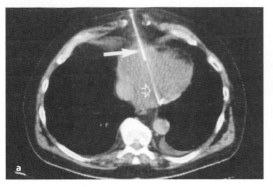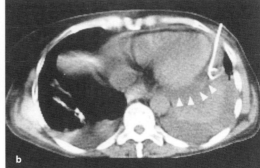

⬛ Fig. 5.15a,b. CT-fluoroscopy-guided pericardiocentesis. Medial (subxyphoidal) approach (**a**), and lateral approach (**b**). Reproduced with permission from Bruning et al. (2002) [52]

Feasibility and Safety

Pericardiocentesis guided by CT-fluoroscopy was technically successful in all of the 11 studied patients (11/11) and sufficient fluid could be aspirated in 10 out of 11 cases.

The catheters were left in place for an average of 2.7 days. As the investigators gained experience with the approach, the total procedure time decreased from initial 35 minutes to an average 10 to 13 minutes.

Ten of 11 procedures were performed without complications. In one procedure an epicardial laceration occurred. The patient underwent surgical treatment including pericardial fenestration.

The same approach was previously applied for the drainage of pleural effusions [48, 53, 54] with a complication rate between 2% and 42% [55, 56]. Most of the reported complications were pneumothoraces, which could be monitored by consecutive CT [57] and drained within the same session. However, this complication did not occur during CT-fluoroscopy-guided pericardial puncture and drainage.

One of the major obstacles for the wider application of this approach is radiation of both patient and the operator of approximately 70 cGy [58]. A second important problem may be the presence of highly viscous pericardial effusions that cannot be aspirated [53, 54, 59]. However, the density of the pericardial effusion can be measured by CT and intrapericardial hematomas and purulent effusions can be dissolved with the intrapericardial application of fibrinolytic therapy.

Pericardiocentesis Guided by a Pacing Capture

One of the alternative approaches attempting to increase the safety of pericardiocentesis was the one by Tweddell and coworkers [60] who developed a dog experimental model for pericardiocentesis guided by pacing. The pacing current was applied through the pericardiocentesis needle in comparison to the technique of electrocardiographic monitoring for the ST segment elevation from the needle tip electrogram, as initially introduced by Bishop et al. [61].

Pacing Needle Electrode

The pacing needle electrode consisted of an 18 or 20 gauge spinal needle, insulated along the length of the barrel with shrinkable Teflon tubing so that only 3 mm of the tip was exposed. The hub of the needle was soldered to a multistranded stainless steel insulated wire that could be connected alternatively to a current source or to the ECG set to record a precordial lead (Fig. 5.16).

Technique

The study was performed in four groups of anesthetized Mongrel dogs (25–35 kg). In group I open chest electrograms were recorded using the precordial lead connected to the puncturing needle. ST segment elevation was measured at 3 mm from the epicardium,

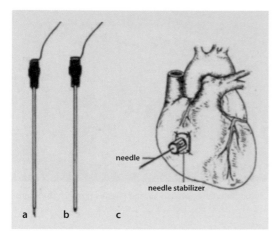

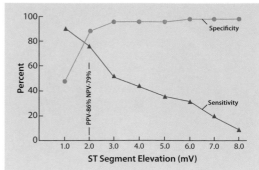

□ **Fig. 5.17.** Sensitivity and specificity of the various level of ST-segment elevation to distinguish between the needle contact with the epicardium and the absence of contact during pericardiocentesis. PPV positive predictive value; NPV negative predictive value. Reproduced with permission from Tweddel et al. (1989) [60]

□ **Fig. 5.16a–c.** The pacing needle electrode for closed-chest studies (**a**) consisted of an 18 or 20 gauge spinal needle insulated along the length of the barrel with shrinkable Teflon tubing so that only 3 mm of the tip was exposed. The hub of the needle was soldered to a multistranded stainless steel insulated wire. For open chest studies (**b**) a blunt-tip pacing needle electrode was used. The needle stabilizer (**c**) consisted of a rectangular base 1.5´2 cm with a 1 cm diameter hole, connected to two struts, 2 cm tall, which supported a rubber diaphragm. The pacing needle electrode was introduced through the rubber diaphragm, which supported the pacing electrode and held it at any chosen distance from the heart. Reproduced with permission from Tweddel et al. (1989) [60]

after epicardial contact, after epicardial penetration and again at 3 mm from the epicardium after epicardial penetration. Six, open-chest dogs were studied at 26 different sites (14 over the right ventricle, 12 over the left ventricle). The pericardium was arranged in a sling and filled with lactated Ringer's solution which imitated pericardial effusion. The needle stabilizer was attached to the epicardial surface.

With a needle electrode in light contact with the epicardial surface, a spinal needle stiletto was advanced through the barrel of the electrode and the epicardial surface was intentionally penetrated to a depth of 2 mm. The stiletto was then removed and the ECG recorded. At the distance of 3 mm from the epicardial surface an average ST-segment elevation of 1.2 ± 1.1 mV was noted. After light contact with the blunt-tipped electrode, an average ST elevation of 3.6 ± 4.0 mV was recorded.

After intentional epicardial penetration an average ST elevation of 4.8 ± 4.6 mV was recorded. When the needle was withdrawn to 3 mm after epicardial

puncture, an average ST elevation of 2.2 ± 1.1 mV was recorded. The highest combined positive and negative predictive values were obtained with 2.0 mV of ST segment elevation (Fig. 5.17).

In group II the pacing study was performed in the open-chest and open-pericardium setting in five dogs. To determine the optimal stimulus strength, pacing studies were performed using 2, 4, 6, 8 and 10 mA electrical current, with a pacing rate 50–100 ms. The pacing studies were performed both with and without a hemodynamically significant pericardial effusion to determine if increased pericardial pressure altered the pacing threshold. Cathodal unipolar stimulation was tested at six sites (three over the left and three over the right ventricle) and anodal unipolar stimulation at seven sites (four in the left and three in the right ventricle). With anodal unipolar pacing capture was achieved at all seven sites at all stimulus strengths only with direct contact of the pacing needle electrode with the epicardial surface. With cathodal unipolar pacing the results were more variable. A 2 mA and 4 mA unipolar cathodal stimulus captured the ventricle only with direct contact of the epicardium, but stimulus strengths of 6 mA and higher resulted occasionally in capture of the ventricle from the distance of 4-6 mm from the epicardial surface.

In group III, open-chest, closed-pericardium pacing study was performed to verify that increased pericardial pressure did not alter the pacing thresholds determined in group II dogs. A Ringer solution was infused into the pericardium until hemodynamic decompensation occurred. The pulse generator, stimulus strengths, and pacing rates were the same as in group II. Nine sites were tested using anodal unipolar stimulation and eight sites were tested with use of cathodal unipolar stimulation. At current strengths of 2, 4, and 6 mA anodal unipolar pacing achieved capture only with direct contacts, but at currents of 8 and 10 mA captures were recorded at distances of 1–2 mm at one of the nine pacing sites. Cathodal unipolar pacing at strengths of 2 and 4 mA captured only with direct contact. As the pacing stimulus strength increased capture was likely to occur at a distance from the epicardial surface.

Group IV underwent closed-chest studies (10 dogs) in simulated cardiac tamponade using the same methodology for pacing and ST segment elevation recording as in the open-chest studies. In five dogs a cathodal unipolar stimulus was used (4 mA, 2 ms duration); in the other five, an anodal unipolar stimulus of equal magnitude and duration was applied. In all 10 dogs, the effusion was punctured and the epicardium was contacted as indicated by capture. No myocardial perforation or coronary artery or venous injuries were produced. However, ST segment monitoring was not reliable enough in the determination of the needle-epicardial contact since it could only differentiate between the absence of epicardial contact and epicardial penetration. Importantly, ST segment can be altered by medications, pericardial inflammation, ventricular hypertrophy, ischemia and infarction, which would further limit the usefulness of ECG monitoring as a safeguard. Based on this reasons the direct ECG monitoring from the pericardiocentesis needle was not recommended in the European Society of Cardiology Guidelines.

Future Perspectives and Recommendations

Pericardiocentesis in patients with small pericardial effusions by use of a blunt tip Touhy needle and applying the halo phenomenon could provide an easy access to the pericardium and potential application of intrapericardial therapy in patients with autoreactive and neoplastic pericardial disease. The epicardial halo sign is sensitive enough to be used for fluoroscopic guidance of pericardiocentesis as a demarkation line for the puncturing needle. Seeking for the changes of the sign could also facilitate the recognition of complications during invasive or interventional procedures. Sudden occurrence or intensification of the epicardial halo after endomyocardial biopsy or pacemaker lead implantation might indicate cardiac perforation and imminent cardiac tamponade.

Pericardioscopy performed from the anterior mediastinum significantly contributed to the success of the PerDUCER® procedure, enabling visualization of the portions of the pericardium suitable for puncture with the device. Human pericardium is obviously significantly different in comparison to the evaluated animal models regarding the important features of the PerDUCER® procedure. However, the principle of action of the device is promising as seen with the Marburg Attacher system.

The blunt-tip Touhy needle is nowadays the standard instrument for pericardiocentesis. Mannam et al. have shown that pressurized saline flow gives additional safety in effusions of 300 ml and more. This method shows promise for use in smaller effusions and even in permitting access in patients with no effusion at all.

The transbronchial approach to the pericardium is possible, but needed in very rare cases only. It should be reserved for extremely experienced centers and operators trained both in bronchoscopy and pericardial access.

After recent modifications (CASPER system) computer-assisted pericardiocentesis has the potential to improve the current pericardiocentesis technique, to make it safer in small pericardial effusions, and to extend the range of indications: draining pericardial effusion for early diagnosis or therapy, for smaller or poorly accessible, typically loculated postoperative pericardial effusions. Simplification of the procedure is still necessary in order to make its routine clinical application feasible.

CT-fluoroscopy allows safe access to loculated pericardial effusions. However, radiation exposure is significant, both for the patient and for the physician. The clinical setting in which this approach would have the advantage over a much less expensive echocardiography- or standard fluoroscopy-guided pericardiocentesis is very rare.

The use of a pulse generator to guide pericar-diocentesis has an advantage of reliably localizing the needle tip to the epicardium, except in loculated posterior effusions and in tamponade secondary to the hemopericardium with clotted blood. There were no significant difference in the pacing threshold between experiments performed with and without hemodynamically significant pericardial effusions. Due to its lower potential to cause arrhythmias only cathodal stimulation should be used in further potential human studies. This method, however, did not reach any wider clinical application.

Reference

1. Botsch H. Pericardial effusion: its demonstration through the epicardial fat. Fortschr Geb Rontgenstr Nuklearmed 1977; 127(2): 170–174

2. Carsky EW, Mauceri RA, Azimi F. The epicardial fat pad sign: analysis of frontal and lateral chest radiographs in patients with pericardial effusion. Radiology 1980; 137(2): 303–308

3. Heinsimer JA, Collins GJ, Burkman MH, et al. Supine cross-table lateral chest roentgenogram for the detection of pericardial effusion. JAMA 1987; 257(23): 3266–3268

4. Ristić AD. Pericardiocentesis and intrapericardial treatment: Advances of the technique, diagnostic, and therapeutic value. Doctoral Thesis. Faculty of Medicine, Philipps Universty Marburg, Germany, 2002

5. Eisenberg MJ, Dunn MM, Kanth N, et al. Diagnostic value of chest radiography for pericardial effusion. J Am Coll Cardiol 1993; 22: 588–593

6. Torrance DJ. Demonstration of subepicardial fat as an aid in the diagnosis of pericardial effusion or thickening. Am J Roentgenol 1955; 74: 850–855

7. Goebel N. Pericardial shadows caused by fatty tissue – the chest image and computer tomography. Prax Klin Pneumol 1985; 39(9): 309–314

8. Tehranzadeh J, Kelley MJ. The differential density sign of pericardial effusion. Radiology 1979; 133(1): 23–30

9. Taguchi R, Takasu J, Itani Y, et al. Pericardial fat accumulation in men as a risk factor for coronary artery disease. Atherosclerosis 2001; 157(1): 203–209

10. Kremens V. Demonstration of the pericardial shadow on the routine chest roentgenogram: a new roentgen finding. Radiology 1955; 64: 72–80

11. Maisch B, Ristić AD. Practical aspects of the management of pericardial disease. Heart 2003; 89(9): 1096–1103

12. Kanth N, Eisenberg M, Gamsu G. Effect of varying kVp on visibility of epicardial fat stripe in pericardial effusions [letter]. Am J Roentgenol 1995; 164(2): 510

13. Lane EJ Jr, Carsky EW. Epicardial fat: Lateral plain film analysis in normals and in pericardial effusion. Radiology 1968; 91(1): 1–5

14. Jorgens J, Kundel R, Lieber A. The cinefluorography approach to the diagnosis of pericardial effusion. Am J Roentgenol 1962; 87: 911–916

15. Duvernoy O, Borowiec J, Helmius G, et al. Complications of percutaneous pericardiocentesis under fluoroscopic guidance. Acta Radiol 1992; 33(4): 309–313

16. Krikorian JG, Hancock EW. Pericardiocentesis. Am J Med 1978; 65: 808–812

17. Rodeheffer RJ. Pericardiocentesis. In: Holmes DR, Vlietstra RE, eds. Interventional Cardiology. F.A. Davis Company, Philadelphia, 1989, pp 210–217

18. Tsang TS, Enriquez-Sarano M, Freeman WK, et al. Consecutive 1127 therapeutic echocardiographically guided pericardiocenteses: clinical profile, practice patterns, and outcomes spanning 21 years. Mayo Clin Proc 2002; 77(5): 429–436

19. Macris PM, Igo SR. Minimally invasive access of the normal pericardium: Initial clinical experience with a novel device. Clin Cardiol 1999; 22 (Suppl 1): I-36–39

20. Rieger PJ, Beaurline CM, Grabek JR. Intrapericardial therapeutics and diagnostics. In: Seferovic PM, Spodick DH, Maisch B, Maksimovic R, Ristic AD (eds) Pericardiology: Contemporary Answers to Continuing Challenges. Science, Belgrade, 2000, pp 393–406

21. Maisch B, Ristić AD, Rupp H, Spodick DH. Pericardial access using the PerDUCER® and flexible percutaneous pericardioscopy. Am J Cardiol 2001; 88(11): 1323–1326

22. Seferovic PM, Ristic AD, Maksimovic R, et al. Initial clinical experience with PerDUCER®: promising new tool in the diagnosis and treatment of pericardial disease. Clin Cardiol 1999; 22(suppl I): I-30–35

23. Maisch B, Drude L. Pericardioscopy – a new diagnostic tool in inflammatory diseases of the pericardium. Eur Heart J 1991; 12 (Suppl D): 2–6

24. Maisch B, Bethge C, Drude L, Hufnagel G, Herzum M, Schoenian U. Pericardioscopy and epicardial biopsy-new diagnostic tools in pericardial and perimyocardial disease. Eur Heart J 1994; 15 (Suppl C): 68–73

25. Maisch B, Pankuweit S, Brilla C, et al. Intrapericardial treatment of inflammatory and neoplastic pericarditis guided by pericardioscopy and epicardial biopsy – results from a pilot study. Clin Cardiol 1999; 22 (Suppl I): I-17–22

26. Seferovic PM, Ristic AD, Maksimovic R, Ostojic M, Simeunovic D, Petrovic P, Maisch B. Flexible percutaneous pericardioscopy: inherent drawbacks and, recent advances. Herz 2000; 25: 741–747

27. Grimm W, Sharkova J, Funck R, Maisch B. How many patients with dilated cardiomyopathy may potentially benefit from cardiac resynchronization therapy? Pacing Clin Electrophysiol 2003; 26 (1 Pt 2): 155–157

28. Funck RC, Blanc JJ, Mueller HH, Schade-Brittinger C, Bailleul C, Maisch B; BioPace Study Group. Biventricular stimulation to prevent cardiac desynchronization: rationale, design, and endpoints of the 'Biventricular Pacing for Atrioventricular Block to Prevent Cardiac Desynchronization (BioPace)' study. Europace 2006; 8(8): 629–635

29. Steinberg JS, Derose JJ. The rationale for nontransvenous leads and cardiac resynchronization devices. Pacing Clin Electrophysiol 2003; 26: 2211–2212

30. Mair H, Sachweh J, Meuris B, et al. Surgical epicardial left ventricular lead versus coronary sinus lead placement in biventricular pacing. Eur J Cardiothorac Surg 2005; 27: 235–242

31. Ota T, Patronik N, Riviere C, Zenati MA. Percutaneous subxiphoid access to the epicardium using a miniature crawling robotic device. Innovations 2006; 1(5): 227–231

32. Mannam AP, Ho KK, Cultip DE, et al. Safety of subxyphoid pericardial access using a blunt-tip needle. Am J Cardiol 2002; 89(7): 891–893

33. Laham R, Rezaee M, Post M, et al. Intrapericardial delivery of fibroblast growth factor-2 induces neovascularization in a porcine model of chronic myocardial ischemia. J Pharmacol Exp Ther 2000; 292: 795–802

34. Laham R, Hung D, Simons M. Subxyphoid access of the normal pericardium: a novel drug delivery technique. Catheter Cardiovasc Diagn 1999; 47: 109–111

35. Sosa E, Scanavacca M, d'Avila A, Pilleggi F. A new technique to perform epicardial mapping in the electrophysiology laboratory. J Cardiovasc Electrophysiol 1996; 7(6): 531–536

36. Kiser AC, Nifong LW, Raman J, Kasirajan V, Campbell N, Chitwood WR Jr. Evaluation of a novel epicardial atrial fibrillation treatment system. Ann Thorac Surg 2008; 85(1): 300–303

37. Shivkumar K. Percutaneous epicardial ablation of atrial fibrillation. Heart Rhythm 2008; 5(1): 152–154

38. Brugada J, Berruezo A, Cuesta A, et al. Nonsurgical trans-thoracic epicardial radiofrequency ablation: an alternative in incessant ventricular tachycardia. J Am Coll Cardiol 2003; 41(11): 2036–2043

39. De Divitlis M, Dialleto G, Covino FE, et al. An unusual pro-cedure for the treatment of simultaneous pericardial and pleural effusions. G Ital Cardiol 1999; 29: 796–798

40. Ceron L, Manzato M, Mazzaro F, Bellavere F. A new diagnostic and therapeutic approach to pericardial effusion: trans-bronchial needle aspiration. Chest 2003; 123(5): 1753–1758

41. Wang KP. How I do it: transbronchial needle aspiration. J Bronchol 1994; 1: 63–68

42. Chavanon O, Barbe C, Troccaz J, et al. Accurate guidance for percutaneous access to a specific target in soft tissues: preclinical study of computer-assisted pericardiocentesis. Laparoscop Adv Surg Tech 1999; 9: 259–266

43. Chavanon O, Carrat L, Pasqualini C, Dubois E, Blin D, Troc-caz J. Computer guided pericardiocentesis: experimental results and clinical perspectives. Herz 2000; 25(8): 761–768

44. Marmignon C, Chavanon O, Troccaz J. CASPER, a Computer ASsisted PERicardial puncture system: first clinical results. Comput Aided Surg 2005; 10(1): 15–21

45. Barbe C, Carrat L, Chavanon O, et al. Computer-assisted pericardiac surgery. In: Computer assisted radiology. Else-vier, Amsterdam, 1996, pp 781–786

46. Chavanon O, Barbe C, Troccaz J, et al. Computer-assisted pericardial puncture: work in progress. Comput Aided Surg 1997; 2: 356–364

47. Duvernoy O, Magnusson A. CT-guided pericardiocentesis. Acta Radiol 1996; 37(5): 775–778

48. Meyer CA, White CS, Wu J, et al. Real-time CT. fluoroscopy: usefulness in thoracic drainage. AJR 1998; 171: 1097–1101

49. White CS, Meyer CA, Templeton PA. CT fluoroscopy for thoracic interventional procedures. Radiol Clin North Am 2000; 38: 303–322

50. White CS, Templeton PA, Hasday JD. CT-assisted transbron-chial needle aspiration: usefulness of CT fluoroscopy. AJR 1997; 169: 393–394

51. Kirchner J, Kickuth R, Walz MV, et al. CTF-guided puncture of an unenhanced isodense liver lesion during continuous intravenous injection of contrast medium. Cardiovasc Intervent Radiol 1999; 22: 528–530

52. Bruning R, Muehlstaedt M, Becker C, et al. Computed tomography-fluoroscopy guided drainage of pericardial effusions: Experience in 11 cases. Invest Radiol 2002; 37: 328–332

53. Daly B, Krebs TL, Wong-You-Cheong JJ, et al. Percutaneous abdominal and pelvic interventional procedures using CT fluoroscopy guidance. AJR 1999; 173: 637–644

54. Katada K, Kato R, Anno H, et al. Guidance with real-time CT fluoroscopy: early clinical experience. Radiology 1996; 200: 851–856

55. Cox JE, Chiles C, McManus CM, et al. Transthoracic needle aspiration biopsy: variables that affect risk of pneumotho-rax. Radiology 1999; 212: 165–168

56. Laurent F, Latrabe V, Vergier B, et al. CT-guided transtho-racic needle biopsy of pulmonary nodules smaller than 20 mm. Results with an automated 20-gauge coaxial cut-ting needle. Clin Radiol 2000; 55: 281–287

57. Bungay HK, Berger J, Traill ZC, et al. Pneumothorax post CT-guided lung biopsy: a comparison between detection on chest radiographs and CT. Br J Radiol 1999; 72: 1160–1163

58. Silverman SG, Tuncali K, Adams DF, et al. CT Fluoros-copy-guided abdominal interventions: techniques, results, and radiation exposure. Radiology 1999; 212: 673–681

59. Cooper JP, Oliver RM, Currie P, et al. How do the clinical findings in patients with pericardial effusions influence the success of aspiration? Br Heart J 1995; 73: 351–354

60. Tweddell JS, Zimmerman AN, Stone CM, Rokkas CK, Schuessler RB, Boineau JP, Cox JL. Pericardiocentesis guided by a pulse generator. J Am Coll Cardiol 1989; 14(4): 1074–1083

Pericardiocentesis in the Absence of Effusion

Introduction

The idea of nonsurgically entering the normal pericardial sac for diagnostic or therapeutic purposes was unrealistic until recently. This was largely due to the perception that access to the pericardial space by a pericardial puncture was only safely possible in the presence of a sizable pericardial effusion.

Novel techniques have been developed to access the pericardial space even with small or no effusion. These techniques might enable us to make use of this space to treat cardiovascular disease in the near future [1]. Two techniques have been applied to achieve percutaneous access into the normal pericardial sac in humans and additional two were investigated in animal studies. These techniques will be reviewed in the following sections [1–8].

Subxiphoid Pericardiocentesis Using a Tuohy Needle and Fluoroscopy

Pericardial access in the absence of effusion was first reported by Sosa et al. [9] in 1996 in three patients undergoing epicardial mapping for ventricular tachycardia. He used a Tuohy needle and fluoroscopy control for subxiphoid pericardiocentesis. The same methodology was subsequently used by other authors [10–12] to access the normal pericardium. Mannam et al. [13] used this technique to evacuate small pericardial effusions. The Marburg center has followed this approach also in selected patients with very small or no effusion for intrapericardial treatment.

Technique and Potential Complications

The needle is introduced at the 45° angle in the direction of the left scapula. As the needle approaches the heart under fluoroscopic guidance, small amounts of contrast media are injected to document the penetration of the needle tip into the pericardial space. The angle of the needle can be further adjusted in order to perform the pericardiocentesis at the area of the medial third of the right ventricle and avoid major coronary vessels. The proper positioning of the needle is associated with layering of the contrast in the pericardial space. Catheters placed at the right ventricular apex and in the coronary sinus are useful markers to guide the needle tip.

The needle can occasionally perforate the right ventricle, which is noticed by the lack of layering of the contrast in the pericardial space and its prompt disappearance in the outflow tract of the right or rarely left ventricle. In case that happens, the needle is slightly retrieved and contrast medium is injected until the pericardial space is reached. Once the needle tip is in the pericardial space, a soft floppy-tip guidewire is introduced in the pericardial space. The guidewire position is also monitored by fluoroscopy. Standard electrocardiography can provide another important clue about the position of the guidewire since an intrapericardially placed guidewire will not cause any arrhythmias in contrast to the guidewire placed intracardially. No lateral manipulations of the distal end of the needle should be performed in order to avoid laceration of the right ventricle or coronary veins.

Finally, the guidewire is exchanged for an introducer sheath and catheter and the pericardial fluid is aspirated to check for potential hemorrhage. Only a trivial amount of translucent pericardial fluid is expected. Subsequently an ablation catheter is passed into the pericardial space [14] or a pigtail catheter for application of intrapericardial treatment.

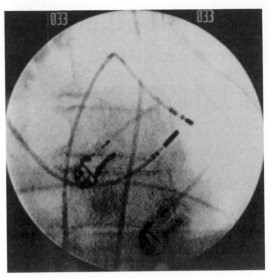

Fig. 6.1. Radioscopic anteroposterior view showing a quadripolar diagnostic catheter in the right ventricle and an 8-mm tip ablation catheter in the pericardial space. Angiographic contrast accumulation is confirming intrapericardial access. Reproduced with permission from Brugada et al. (2003) [12]

Feasibility and Safety

In the early phase of this study Sosa et al. [9, 15, 16] used electrocardiographic monitoring for ST-segment elevation from the precordial lead attached to the puncturing needle. Along with the accumulation of the experience (~250 patients with ventricular tachycardia and atrial fibrillation), this step became unnecessary. Actually, a good fluoroscopy and feeling of the heart beat touching the blunt needle tip became the most crucial step for the safety of this approach. It should be further evaluated if the use of continuous infusion of saline to create positive pressure to push the right ventricle away from the needle tip has significant impact on the safety or feasibility of the procedure.

In the initial report by Sosa et al. [9] the subxiphoid pericardial access was feasible and safe in all three patients. In the subsequent experience published in 1998 Sosa et al. [15] described in 1/10 patients hemopericardium requiring drainage, and retrosternal discomfort and pericardial friction rub in another 3/10 patients [15]. Reporting on the safety of the procedure in 2000 Sosa et al. [17] have mentioned accidental right ventricular perforation in 4/53 patients (7.5%) and in 3 of them a small hemopericardium of up to 50 ml which could be drained with a pigtail

catheter at the electrophysiology laboratory. Three out of 53 patients complained of precordial discomfort and two of these had a pericardial rub. These patients were successfully treated with non-steroid anti-inflammatory drugs.

When the results of the same pericardial access technique were analyzed in a consecutive series of 173 patients, there was an 8% rate of self-limiting hemopericardium that resolved with aspiration of the pericardial space and one instance of hemoperitoneum that required surgical ligation (0.6%) [18]. All patients underwent echocardiography after pericardiocentesis and on discharge from the hospital. No other complications were noted.

The same procedure was used by Schweikert et al. [19] in 48 patients with previously failed endocardial ablation. Pericardial access was possible in all patients without any major complications that would require intervention or treatment during or after the procedure.

Josep Brugada et al. [12] reported in 2003 on the successful access to the normal pericardium in 10/10 patients indicated for an epicardial ablation procedure. There were no significant complications (Fig. 6.1). Two patients had chest pain for three days after the procedure, which resolved with acetaminophen. The control echocardiogram did not show a relevant pericardial effusion, and cardiac enzymes were not increased. In an experimental setting, the subxiphoid pericardial access using the same methodology as above was achieved in 10 normal goats and 7 pigs with healed myocardial infarctions [11].

Limitations of the Approach

Patients with previous cardiac surgery are not suitable for this approach due to the presence of adhesions that could limit the access to the pericardial space. In addition, this approach should not be attempted in anticoagulated patients. If during the epicardial mapping an additional endocardial electrode became necessary its placement should be performed only after pericardiocentesis is performed without any complications. With this restriction the administration of 5000 IU + 1000 IU/h of heparin can be taken into account, since it is needed for the endocardial mapping. Although the subxiphoid needle approach is feasible in the absence of pericardial effusion, as demonstrated by several independent investigators, the risks of myocardial or coronary laceration cannot be ignored and may be increased as compared with standard subxiphoid pericardiocentesis, where the pericardial space has been expanded by the presence of fluid.

Pericardial Access in the Absence of Effusion Using the PerDUCER® Technique

The PerDUCER® instrument for pericardiocentesis (Comedicus Inc., Columbia Heights, Minnesota) was developed to enable percutaneous pericardial access in the absence of pericardial effusion [20, 21]. Pericardial access with the PerDUCER® was successfully performed in a cadaver study, in several animal studies, and in patients with normal pericardium undergoing cardiac surgery for other reasons.

Experimental Experience

Animal experiments with the PerDUCER® device included
1. feasibility and safety studies,
2. studies of intrapericardial therapy of restenosis,
3. epicardial electrophysiology,
4. studies of intrapericardial application of angiogenic growth factors,
5. hypothermic pericardial perfusion studies, and
6. studies on intrapericardial anti-arrhythmic therapy.

Our own experimental experience comprises 30 procedures performed in 5 F1 white pigs [mean weight 30 ± 2 kg) under fluoroscopic control and in general anesthesia [3]. Respiration and electrocardiogram were monitored during the experiments. After the procedures, animals were killed and the heart and the pericardium were examined for eventual damage or lesions. Access to the mediastinal space, pericardial capture, and puncture were possible in all animal experiments (Table 6.1).

Insertion of the guidewire was feasible in 28 of 30 procedures, and it was possible to advance the pericardial catheter over the wire in 26 of 30 procedures. There were no complications during the experiments, apart from minor cardiac rhythm disturbances. Examination of the pericardium and pig hearts after the experiments revealed no significant damage to

Table 6.1. Feasibility of mediastinal access, pericardial capture and puncture, guidewire and pericardial catheter insertion in pig experiments (total of 30 procedures in 5 pigs). Reproduced with permission from Maisch et al. (2001) [3]

	Access to the mediastinal space	Pericardial capture and puncture	Insertion of the guidewire	Insertion of the pericardial catheter
Feasibility	100%	100%	93%	87%
Complications	0	0	VPCs in 77%	no

VPCs ventricular premature contractions.

any of the structures. The pericardium was thin and translucent in 4 of 5 pigs, and in 1 there were minor adhesions and fibrotic changes.

Our animal experiments with the PerDUCER® were focussed on the procedural technique, the extent of myocardial and pericardial trauma, and the possible therapeutic applications of the method. Because of the excellent fluoroscopic control and the thin pericardium in the pigs, the procedure was highly successful. Only 2 of 30 experimental attempts of pericardial guidewire insertion and 4 of 30 intrapericardial catheter insertions were unsuccessful in a pig that had some pericardial adhesions and a slightly thickened pericardium [3].

Using the same methodology Tio et al. [5] successfully applied the PerDUCER® for access of the normal pericardium in 10 pigs. Four pigs were injected with a mixture of 10 ml Evans blue and 10 ml saline. Four other pigs were injected with a mixture of 10 ml Indian ink and 10 ml saline. Before and after injection the position of the introducer was checked with a small contrast injection under fluoroscopic guidance. After injection the introducer was removed and the skin incision closed. Pigs were monitored for 3 h and then either sacrificed (2 from each group) or taken back to their cages and sacrificed after 3 days (remaining two from each group). In two additional pigs, the PerDUCER® procedure was performed under endoscopic guidance (Ethicon, Amersfoort, The Netherlands) connected to an online computer system (Contec Medical, Waalwijk, The Netherlands). In all pigs pericardial access could be obtained (in six through the left thoracic cavity and in four animals via the right thoracic cavity. During the procedure no adverse reactions with respect to hemodynamic parameters or serious arrhythmias were noted. In all pigs sacrificed after 3 h traces of Indian ink (n = 2) or Evans blue (n = 2) could be seen in the thoracic cavity at the side of the access route to the pericardium. In the pigs sacrificed after 3 days (n = 2) neither Indian ink nor Evans blue were present. The microscopical examination of tissue sections of epimyocardial, lung and mediastinal lymph nodes and of liver-tissue sections did not show any local impregnation or distal dissemination of Indian ink. In particular, no Indian ink was seen in macrophages in the lung, the lymph node and liver tissue. Endoscopic observation of the procedure was performed in two pigs in order to in-

vestigate its contribution to the selection of the proper position of the device. Access to the pericardium may be prevented by pericardial fat since no reliable vacuum suction can be obtained in such a region. If the PerDUCER® is moved too far laterally due to the curve of the heart, good contact of the hemispherical well at the distal tip of the instrument with the pericardium will be lost. The same problem is faced when the PerDUCER® is advanced too far or retracted too far. The combination of thoracoscopic monitoring with the PerDUCER® technique can resolve the potential obstacles caused by epicardial fat or pericardial adhesions.

The largest experimental experience with the PerDUCER® device applied in 53 pigs was reported by Hou and March [4]. In contrast to Tio et al. who used the lateral approach, in this study, as well as in ours [3, 21, 22], the subxiphoid approach was implemented. Capture, puncture of the pericardium, and intrapericardial insertion of the guidewire was possible in all animals. The procedure was well tolerated and caused no major complications or adverse hemodynamic effects. The mean arterial pressure and heart rate were maintained during the entire pericardial access. As in our study, most of the animals had occasional ventricular premature contractions. Twelve animals were sacrificed immediately after the experiment, while 41 animals were sacrificed 28 days after the procedure. Histological examination showed no occurrence of epicardial vessel or myocardial damage. In addition, no late complications related to the pericardial access were found [4].

Access of the Human Pericardium in the Absence of Effusion Using PerDUCER®

Five trials on closed-chest human cadavers were conducted to demonstrate and verify the performance of the PerDUCER® device in human anatomy and to develop an optimal closed-chest procedure for use in clinical trials. All studies were successful and supported the plan to proceed in clinical trials. The ease of mediastinal access and the sequential procedural steps (capture, puncture, guidewire insertion) of the PerDUCER® were confirmed [23].

Clinical experience in accessing normal pericardium with the PerDUCER® comprises semi-closed chest attempts (direct vision) performed in eight patients prior to an elective surgical intervention requiring a sternotomy [20]. Additional four patients underwent a closed-chest, fluoroscopy-assisted procedure. In all patients, the PerDUCER® was inserted into the chest, via the 19F sheath, and positioned over the pericardium. The pericardium was captured by suction and a bleb was formed within a side-hole on the distal tip of the PerDUCER® device. A sheathed needle was advanced, puncturing the isolated bleb of the pericardium. A guidewire was placed through the needle into the pericardial space and the PerDUCER® was removed. Guidewire insertion was successful in 10/12 patients (7 on first attempt, 3 on second) without adverse hemodynamic effects or arrhythmia.

Pericardial Access Via Transatrial Approach

Transatrial pericardiocentesis is an alternative approach for the access of the normal pericardium. The catheter system applied for this purpose is inserted using a percutaneous approach from the femoral vein to pierce the right atrial appendage [6, 7, 24]. A small perforation is made in the right atrial appendage using a 21-gauge, hollow radiopaque needle mounted at the tip of a 4 F catheter (Fig. 6.2) or, as recently reported, a new streamlined catheter system (Fig. 6.3) [7].

Catheter System with a Pre-Mounted Needle

In the initial version of the procedure [6, 24], after perforation of the right atrial appendage with a needle mounted at the tip of a 4-F catheter, a soft, 0.014 guidewire with a second radiopaque marker was advanced through the needle catheter into the pericardial space. The guidewire is used not only to secure the point of entry, but also to give support and enable easier manipulation with the application catheter and confirm its position in the pericardial space (Fig. 6.2c). The needle catheter is then withdrawn over the wire and exchanged for a 4-F catheter with multiple side holes at its distal end, which is positioned and left in the pericardial space (Fig. 6.2d) for delivery of drugs. Radiopaque markers at the tip of catheter improve visualization during fluoroscopy.

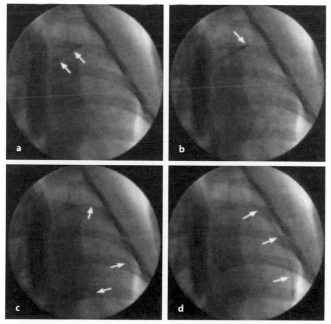

□ **Fig. 6.2a–d.** Transatrial access to the normal pericardial space. Fluoroscopic images were obtained with Diasonics OEC 902 clinical unit. **a** The 8-F guide catheter (*arrows*) rests against the wall of the right atrial appendage. **b** The needle catheter (*arrow*) is protruding through the wall of the right atrial appendage into the pericardial space. **c** The guide wire (*arrows*) has been advanced through the needle catheter into the pericardial space. **d** The 4-F delivery catheter (*arrows*) has been advanced over the wire through the appendage wall and positioned in the pericardial space. Reproduced with permission from Waxman et al. (1999) [24]

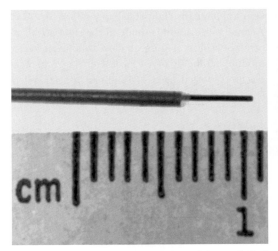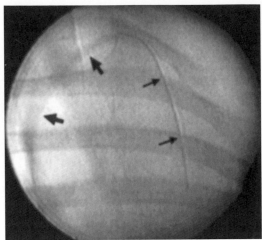

◻ **Fig. 6.3.** Wire system to access the pericardial space (*left*). The inner (0.014″) guidewire is pre-mounted inside a 0.038″ infusion guidewire protruding 2 mm from the tip. The penetration through the atrial appendage is carried out with the smaller wire tip and then both wires are advanced simultaneously. Fluoroscopy in the right anterior oblique projection demonstrates the 8-F guiding catheter (*large arrows*) positioned in the right atrium and the infusion guidewire (*small arrows*) positioned inside the pericardial space (*right-side image*). Reproduced with permission from Waxman et al. (2000) [7]

The procedure was performed in six dogs of either sex weighing 15 to 25 kg and 13 Yorkshire pigs of either sex weighing 25 to 35 kg were used. The animals were pre-anesthetized with ketamine 5 mg/kg i.v., xylazine 2.2 mg/kg i.v., and atropine 0.04 mg/kg i.v. and anesthetized with isoflurane or alpha-chloralose 100 mg/kg i.v. Arterial blood pressure was recorded through a femoral or carotid arterial sheath. Precordial ECGs and arterial blood pressure were monitored with a Gould recorder [6].

After placement of the 6-F or 8-F guide catheter, accessing the normal pericardial space in experimental animals required 3 to 5 minutes and was confirmed fluoroscopically. Multiple repetitions of the access procedure were successfully performed in each of 19 large experimental animals (6 dogs and 13 pigs). No hemodynamic or electrocardiographic changes resulted from transatrial pericardial access. In acute studies in 17 of the animals, direct inspection of the pericardial space after thoracotomy revealed no hemopericardium, laceration, or bleeding on catheter withdrawal. In 24-hour survival studies performed in 2 of the dogs, the animals exhibited no behavioral signs of discomfort or untoward consequences on recovery from anesthesia. Histology revealed only a small (~1 mm) fibrinous plug at the site of puncture. There were no complications from pericardial access and no notable bleeding.

Waxman et al. [24] confirmed the same results in additional 5 pigs. Transatrial pericardial access required 1 to 3 min in all animals with no complications.

Streamlined Catheter System

Waxman et al. [7] investigated the safety of a modified percutaneous method for the transatrial approach to the normal pericardium. In contrast to the previous studies, a new streamlined catheter system was used instead of the needle catheter to access to the normal pericardial space via the right atrial appendage. The study was performed on 20 anesthetized Yorkshire pigs of either sex weighing 25 to 35 kg. Instead by a needle-catheter, penetration through the atrial appendage is carried out with the wire system (Fig. 6.3). The wire system consisted of a 0.014″ guidewire (300 cm length) pre-mounted inside of a 0.038″ infusion guidewire (Bard, Billerica, MA).

The stiff end of the smaller guidewire was allowed to protrude 2 mm from the distal tip of the larger infusion wire. Under fluoroscopic guidance, both wires were advanced until the wall of the right atrial appendage was pierced with the 0.0140 wire. The guidewire's position in the pericardial space is confirmed by conforming to the contour of the heart. It secures the point of entry and allows over-the-wire exchanges of other catheters. Both wires are then advanced into the pericardial space as a single unit. The inner 0.0140 wire is removed, and pericardial fluid aspirated and analyzed immediately for the hematocrit level. Confirmation of the presence of the wire inside the pericardial space is obtained by fluoroscopy, and by aspiration of pericardial fluid, avoiding the need to inject contrast material. The infusion wire was left in the pericardial space for 5 minutes and then removed. The guide was kept in position inside the right atrial appendage for 2 additional minutes and then removed. The femoral vein sheath was immediately removed and manual compression was applied to achieve hemostasis. The animals were returned to their cages and allowed to recover.

Access was successfully accomplished in all animals within 3 minutes of guide catheter positioning and was documented by fluoroscopic imaging and pericardial fluid sampling. The animals were sacrificed at 24 h (n = 10) and 2 weeks (n = 10) for histopathologic analysis. At 24 h, there was local inflammatory reaction in the atrial wall in 5/10 animals and a small thrombus at the site of puncture in all animals. At two weeks, no significant inflammatory changes or pericarditis were evident. The technique was well tolerated with no apparent adverse complications.

Safety of the Transatrial Approach

The safety of the transatrial technique reported in the literature [6, 7, 24] can be related to a number of factors that are unique to this experimental approach. First, in the modified approach when only the 0.014" guidewire is used for puncture, it remains tangential to the heart as it crosses the right atrial appendage. This minimizes the risk of coronary laceration and myocardial perforation. Second, the dimensions and flexibility of the wire allow it to curve naturally over the surface of the heart. When the wire is removed, three possible mechanisms account for sealing the exit site and prevent bleeding. First is the rapid action of clotting factors and platelet aggregation at the

site of injury. A small thrombus is observed within 24 h after puncture. Second, the pressure within the right atrium is relatively low, and third, the tone and contractility of the atrial appendage act to close the puncture site immediately. It is possible that the latter factor may be the most important, as the rapid closure of the puncture site was noted under direct vision. Moreover, no increased bleeding was observed following aspirin pretreatment and in the setting of experimental pulmonary hypertension, suggesting that neither clotting nor atrial pressure appears to be the main factor in rapid sealing of the puncture site [7].

The lack of a relevant amount of blood in the pericardium after 24 h and of any evidence of pericarditis for up to 2 weeks supports the safety of this technique. As expected from a stab wound, a localized inflammatory response in the right atrial appendage at the puncture site was found on histopathologic analysis. It is unlikely that such an injury will be of any clinical relevance, since recovery of the animals following the procedure was uneventful.

Limitations of the transatrial approach

Experimental data obtained by the transatrial pericardiocentesis systems appear promising for feasible and safe local drug delivery or diagnostic sampling of pericardial fluid. However, to avoid possible complications, only small-size catheters (4F) were used so far. If larger catheters are required, such as those used in electrophysiologic studies, another route for access to the pericardial space may be required, unless such equipment can be miniaturized. Despite the favorable preliminary experience in animals taking aspirin and those with pulmonary hypertension, the safety of this method and the setting of anticoagulation or severely elevated right heart pressures need further testing. Finally, it remains to be determined whether the human right atrial appendage will respond in a manner similar as the porcine heart.

Clinical Implications

Verrier et al. [6] and Waxman et al. [7, 24] have demonstrated the feasibility of nonsurgical, percutaneous access to the normal pericardial space through the right atrial appendage. The transatrial technique could be used for relief of pericardial effusion, diagnostic fluid sampling, and local cardiac drug delivery in the absence of pericardial effusion. Repeated access and topical applications of agents is also feasible and safe. The modified transatrial method using the streamlined catheter system provided a less invasive approach for access of the normal pericardium, with the same feasibility and safety as the system with premounted needle.

Since the pericardial fluid reflects myocardial interstitial fluid its sampling and analyses could aid in the early identification of myocardial and pericardial disease markers. The most intriguing application of transatrial access to the pericardial space is local cardiac drug delivery, for which it may afford efficient, sustained delivery to perivascular and myocardial tissue while minimizing the loss of an agent into the circulation.

Right Ventricular Approach

In a study of pericardial gene transfer March et al. [2] implemented the transventricular percutaneous pericardial approach in seven Mongrel dogs using a hollow, helical-tipped catheter designed for con-

trolled penetration into or through the right ventricular myocardium during fluoroscopic visualization (Fig. 6.4).

All procedures were performed in general anesthesia with thiopental-sodium (25 mg/kg). Following induction, animals were intubated and ventilated with oxygen containing 2% isoflurane for maintenance of anesthesia.

After a 7-F sheath was placed into the right jugular vein, a catheter was inserted through the sheath and advanced under fluoroscopic guidance into the right ventricle to the cardiac apex, with the catheter tip directed inferiorly. An infusion of normal saline through the delivery lumen was maintained at 0.5–1 ml/min throughout the procedure in order to avoid clotting of the helical penetration tip with blood elements. Upon firm contact with the ventricular wall, the catheter tip was advanced through the myocardium using a gentle turning motion. After advancement over several millimeters, hand infusion of a 2:1 meglumine/normal saline mixture was initiated and contrast location was monitored fluoroscopically.

Successful intrapericardial tip placement was identified by the accumulation of contrast in the pericardium, at which point the catheter was fixed in position and flushed with 2 ml of saline prior to the delivery of a suspended vector for gene transfer.

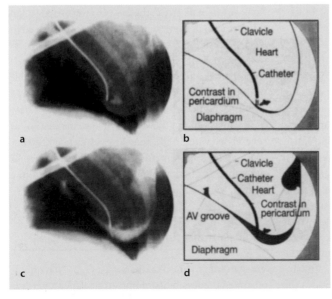

◨ Fig. 6.4a–d. Transventricular approach for pericardial access. Right anterior oblique projection. a Cardiac silhouette with the helix catheter in place transmurally in the right ventricular wall. The instillation of contrast had just begun at the time of angiography; a thin layer of contrast is seen outlining the cardiac edge, confirming pericardial loculation. b Line drawing of a. c The same projection after the infusion of approximately 15 ml of a mixture of radiographic contrast and vector suspension. d Line drawing of c. Reproduced with permission from March et al. (1999) [2]

Following delivery the final catheter position was confirmed by fluoroscopic visualization of a bolus of air instilled into the pericardial space, after which the catheter was removed.

Future Perspectives and Recommendations

Transthoracic pericardiocentesis of the normal pericardium is clearly feasible with a Tuohy needle under fluoroscopic guidance and has been successfully performed in humans not only in the group of Sosa et al. but also in other groups for the last ten years, thus allowing drug delivery to the pericardial space and epicardial access for left ventricular mapping [1, 9-19].

Despite promising experimental data, clinical experience in application of the PerDUCER® instrument for pericardial access in the absence of effusion remained very limited. A large multicenter-trial was planned but was never conducted. However, if the further experimental studies would give support for clinical trials of intrapericardial therapy for nonpericardial disease, the PerDUCER® approach might be attractive for its implementation. At present a technical modification of the device (Periattacher, see Chapter 5) is being tested in the Marburg experimental cardiology laboratory.

It remains to be demonstrated if the transatrial approach can be implemented in human subjects. If the results of the experimental studies would be confirmed in humans, this approach may provide a new opportunity for identification of diagnostic markers in the pericardial fluid and administration of angiogenic, myogenic, and antiarrhythmic intrapericardial therapy.

The right ventricular approach was successful and well tolerated in all animals. There were no electrocardiographic changes and no clinical sequels of the myocardial puncture. However, the study by March et al. [2] is the only one applying the transventricular approach for access to the normal pericardium. Having the experience with perforations after right-ventricular endomyocardial biopsy and pericardial hemorrhage it is our opinion that this approach should not be used in humans.

References

1. Sosa E, Scanavacca M, d'Avila A. Different ways of approaching the normal pericardial space. Circulation 1999; 100(24): e115–116

2. March KL, Woody M, Mehdi K, Zipes DP, Brantly M, Trapnell BC. Efficient in vivo catheter-based pericardial gene transfer mediated by adenoviral vectors. Clin Cardiol 1999; 22 (Suppl I): I-23–29

3. Maisch B, Ristić AD, Rupp H, Spodick DH. Pericardial access using the PerDUCER® and flexible percutaneous pericardioscopy. Am J Cardiol 2001; 88(11): 1323–1326

4. Hou D, March KL. A novel percutaneous technique for accessing the normal pericardium: a single-center successful experience of 53 porcine procedures. J Invasive Cardiol. 2003; 15(1): 13–17

5. Tio RA, Grandjean JG, Suurmeijer AJ, van Gilst WH, van Veldhuisen DJ, van Boven AJ. Thoracoscopic monitoring for pericardial application of local drug or gene therapy. Int J Cardiol 2002; 82(2): 117–121

6. Verrier RL, Waxman S, Lovett EG, Moreno R. Transatrial access to the normal pericardial space: a novel approach for diagnostic sampling, pericardiocentesis, and therapeutic interventions. Circulation 1998; 98(21): 2331–2333

7. Waxman S, Pulerwitz TC, Rowe KA, Quist WC, Verrier RL. Preclinical safety testing of percutaneous transatrial access to the normal pericardial space for local cardiac drug delivery and diagnostic sampling. Cathet Cardiovasc Intervent 2000; 49: 472–477

8. Laham RJ, Simons M, Hung D. Subxyphoid access of the normal pericardium: a novel drug delivery technique. Cathet Cardiovasc Intervent 1999; 47: 109–111

9. Sosa E, Scanavacca M, d'Avila A, Pilleggi F. A new technique to perform epicardial mapping in the electrophysiology laboratory. J Cardiovasc Electrophysiol 1996; 7: 531–536

10. Socjima K, Stevenson WG, Sapp JL, Selwyn AP, Couper G, Epstein LM. Endocardial and epicardial radiofrequency ablation of ventricular tachycardia associated with dilated cardiomyopathy: the importance of low-voltage scars. J Am Coll Cardiol 2004; 43(10): 1834–1842

11. d'Avila A, Houghtaling C, Gutierrez P, et al. Catheter ablation of ventricular epicardial tissue: a comparison of standard and cooled-tip radiofrequency energy. Circulation 2004; 109(19): 2363–2369

12. Brugada J, Berruezo A, Cuesta A, et al. Nonsurgical transthoracic epicardial radiofrequency ablation: an alternative in incessant ventricular tachycardia. J Am Coll Cardiol 2003; 41(11): 2036–2043

13. Mannam AP, Ho KKK, Cutlip DE, et al. Safety of subxyphoid pericardial access using a blunt-tip needle. Am J Cardiol 2002; 89: 891–893

14. Sosa E, Scanavacca M, d'Avila A. Gaining access to the pericardial space. Am J Cardiol 2002; 90(2): 203–204

15. Sosa E, Scanavacca M, d'Avila A, et al. Endocardial and epicardial ablation guided by nonsurgical transthoracic epicardial mapping to treat recurrent ventricular tachycardia. J Cardiovasc Electrophysiol 1998; 9: 229–239

16. Sosa E, Scanavacca M, d'Avila A, Bellotti G, Pilleggi F. Radiofrequency catheter ablation of ventricular tachycardia guided by non-surgical epicardial mapping in chronic Chagasic heart disease. Pacing Clin Electrophysiol 1999; 22: 128–130

17. Sosa E, Scanavacca M, d'Avila A, Oliveira F, Ramires JAF. Nonsurgical transthoracic epicardial catheter ablation to treat recurrent ventricular tachycardia occurring late after myocardial infarction. J Am Coll Cardiol 2000; 35: 1442–1449

18. D'Avila A, Scanavacca M, Sosa E, Ruskin JN, Reddy VY. Pericardial anatomy for the interventional electrophysiologist. J Cardiovasc Electrophysiol 2003; 14(4): 422–430

19. Schweikert RA, Saliba WI, Tomassoni G, et al. Percutaneous pericardial instrumentation for endo-epicardial mapping of previously failed ablations. Circulation 2003; 108: 1329–1335

20. Macris PM, Igo SR. Minimally invasive access of the normal pericardium: Initial clinical experience with a novel device. Clin Cardiol 1999; 22(Suppl 1): I-36–39

21. Seferovic PM, Ristic AD, Maksimovic R, Spodick DH. New percutaneous pericardial access device: early clinical data. Seferovic PM, Spodick DH, Maisch B, Maksimovic R, Ristic AD (eds) Pericardiology: contemporary answers to continuing challenges. Science, Belgrade, 2000, pp 407–416

22. Seferovic PM, Ristic AD, Maksimovic R, et al. Initial clinical experience with PerDUCER®: promising new tool in the diagnosis and treatment of pericardial disease. Clin Cardiol 1999; 22 (Suppl I): I-30–35

23. Rieger PJ, Beaurline CM, Grabek JR. Intrapericardial therapeutics and diagnostics. In: Seferovic PM, Spodick DH, Maisch B, Maksimovic R, Ristic AD (eds) Pericardiology: Contemporary Answers to Continuing Challenge. Science, Belgrade, 2000, pp 393-406

24. Waxman S, Moreno R, Rowe K, Verrier RL. Persistent primary coronary dilation induced by transatrial delivery of nitroglycerin into the pericardial space: a novel approach for local cardiac drug delivery. J Am Coll Cardiol 1999; 33: 2073–2077

Diagnostic Value of Pericardial Fluid Analyses

Introduction

Pericardial effusion is the result of an increased production and/or decreased clearance of pericardial fluid. Samples of the fluid can be obtained for analyses by either needle pericardiocentesis, catheter drainage or surgical pericardiectomy. While laboratory analyses of pleural effusion are well established, the diagnostic approach to pericardial fluid is less clearly defined. An etiologically correct diagnosis of pericardial diseases can often be based on a positive fluid analysis alone but the sensitivity may vary between 24–93%, depending on the patient cohort and the diagnostic methods [1].

In routine clinical practice the fluid analyses of pericardial effusion should be oriented according to the clinical presentation and the suspected etiology as well as pre-test probabilities for some rare diseases in the specific population. Laboratory results are supplementary but often important findings to the clinical diagnosis. A targeted and sometimes stepwise analyses of pericardial fluid can still establish the specific diagnosis of viral, bacterial, tuberculous, fungal, cholesterol, and malignant pericarditis, and the cost-benefit ratio for the analyses can be still kept in the favorable range [2].

Volume and Appearance of Pericardial Effusion

In the absence of the disease, only a minute amount of pericardial fluid is present in the pericardial space. It is a clear, pale, sometimes yellow fluid. If fluid is detectable by echocardiography pericardial disease is suggestive. If the pericardial fluid is turbid, infection or malignancy must be considered. Serosanginous, cloudy fluid is frequently associated with tumors and tuberculosis. If blood is drawn during pericardiocentesis cardiac rupture or the puncture of a ventricle is likely. In uremic pericarditis a clear or straw-colored fluid can be found most frequently. Chylopericardium is characterized by a milky effusion [3].

However, the macroscopic appearance of pericardial fluid is not diagnostic by itself. It even does not allow to differentiate between exudates and transudates in some cases. In the study of Meyers et al. [1] 72.6% of a broad spectrum of effusions including postpericardiotomy, rheumatologic, and traumatic effusions were found to be serosanguinous or hemorrhagic. But sanguineous effusions can also occur because of artificial lesions of blood vessels during pericardiocentesis and bleeding into an initially non-hemorrhagic effusion.

The determination of fluid volumes is routinely performed but is not useful to discriminate among specific etiologies of pericardial effusion.

Pericardial Fluid Cytology

Pericardial fluid cytology is one of the most important methods used for the laboratory assessment of pericardial effusion [1, 4–7]. It is performed by direct smears and/or cytocentrifuge spinning and sedimentation on cover slips with staining according to the established methods [4–7]. Smears are best made immediately after the pericardial fluid is obtained, since poor cell preservation reduces the accuracy of any interpretation. Samples of a pericardial effusion sent for cytology more than 24 h after pericardiocentesis are useless or misleading.

Despite the widespread use of pericardial fluid cytology in the clinical assessment of pericardial effusions, its diagnostic value is still controversial [8]. The diagnostic yield of cytology findings varies considerably ranging from very low 24% [9] and 26% [10] to considerably high 87% [1]. However, the diagnostic accuracy is generally high [7] and was found to be 94% [1] and 100% [9] for neoplastic pericardial effusions. After radiotherapy of a malignant disorder such as breast cancer or bronchus carcinoma the differential diagnosis between a malignant effusion or postradiation syndrome determines both the patient's prognosis and the intrapericardial treatment regimen.

The cytological analysis of large pericardial effusions gives better diagnostic results when compared to smaller effusions. In a study of 59 patients with massive pericardial effusion, the etiology of pericarditis could be determined in 93% [10]. In 7% no definite diagnosis was possible. Major diagnoses in this study were: malignancy in 23%, viral pericarditis in 14%, whereas various pericardial disorders were detected in the rest of the patients. This study published in 1993 could not make use of molecular methods such as PCR.

In the study of Maisch et al. [11] with 60 patients bacterial pericarditis was diagnosed in 13.9% of patients, and pericarditis associated with infective endocarditis and abscess formation in 5.5%. In an additional 5.5% of patients, acid-fast bacilli were recovered from the pericardial fluid. Lymphocytic effusions were found in 44.4%. Autoreactive effusions of the humoral type were seen in 16.7%, in whom the lymphocyte and leukocyte counts were minimal, anticardiac antibody titers were high, and cytolysis of isolated heart cells could be observed with or without addition of complement.

Number of Specimens Needed for Pericardial Fluid Cytology

The number of pericardial fluid specimens required for the determination of a specific diagnosis is controversial. In a four-year period, Garcia et al. [8] examined a total of 570 specimens from 215 patients. In the majority of these, two or more specimens were obtained from the same anatomic site, and from each individual specimen two direct smears and two cytospin preparations were made and examined. The cytological diagnosis of malignancy was established in at least one specimen in 26% of the cases. The first diagnosis of malignant cells was revealed already with the initial specimen in 89% of cases. This confirms that, in most cases, malignancy can be detected by the cytological examination of two specimens.

Detection of Malignancy by Pericardial Fluid Cytology

The most important issue in pericardial fluid cytology is the detection of neoplastic cells (Fig. 7.1). Cellular changes associated with neoplasia are a marked variation in cell size and shape, a striking variation in nuclear size and shape, nuclear atypia, coarse chromatin, abnormal mitoses, independent growth, and nuclear molding.

Pericardial fluid cytology positive for malignancy is highly specific, but the sensitivity of fluid examples in patients with or after treatment of a malignant growth may vary [4, 12]. Some authors believe that there is a high false negative rate in cytological examinations, so a negative report does not eliminate malignant pericardial effusion from the differential diagnosis [13, 14]. Other authors oppose this viewpoint and urge that 42–62% of patients with symp-

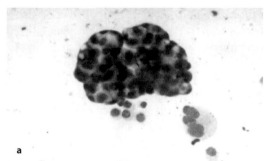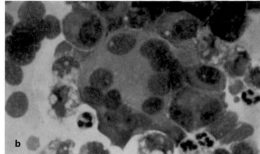

a   b

Fig. 7.1a,b. Pericardial effusion cytology in neoplastic pericardial effusion. Pericardial metastases of oat cell cancer (**a**) and Hodgkin's disease (**b**). Reproduced with permission from Maisch and Ristic (2003) [18].

tomatic pericardial disease and underlying cancer may have nonmalignant pericardial disease [9, 15]. This is to be considered in patients with a postradiation syndrome, which may occur even years after radiotherapy of breast cancer and bronchus carcinoma. Altogether the true incidence of a false-negative pericardial cytology is hard to determine because it is virtually impossible to identify the true reference or gold standard. The most appropriate standard used in the literature so far were the combination of pericardial biopsy findings (obtained with pericardioscopy guidance) and the clinical outcome of the patient during the long-term follow-up. Nevertheless, it is reasonable to assume that the false negative rate is similar to the one in pleural fluids, which was estimated to be 30–67% [16].

The differential diagnosis of pericardial effusions with a negative malignant cytology opens a broad spectrum from the false negative to various other causes of an effusion. In the meta-analysis from four studies Meyers and Boyska [6] found that among 93 patients, 51% were diagnosed as various types of primary and secondary malignancies, while in the remaining 49% other pericardial disorders were demonstrated, including 15% of "idiopathic" pericarditis. According to these data, the cytological examination of pericardial effusion had a sensitivity of 87% and a specificity of 100%. The positive predictive value was 100%, while the negative predictive value reached 83%. The cytological analysis confirmed either the presence or absence of malignancy in 94%.

In a later metaanalysis Meyers et al. [1] investigated the cytology of pericardial fluid in 165 patients with various underlying diseases. They found a sen-

sitivity for malignancies to be 92% and a specificity to be 100%. However, in a study that included 123 patients, Krikorian et al. [9] uncovered the etiology of pericardial disease in only 24%, whereas etiological entities were malignancy, bacterial infection, chylous effusion or hemopericardium. In their report etiological entities such as viral or autoreactive effusions were missing, thus leaving the term "idiopathic" effusion for to many unknown etiologies. Remarkably the diagnostic accuracy correlated with the values of venous pressure: pericardial fluid analyses were diagnostic in 27% of patients with an elevated, but only in 14% with a normal venous pressure. Malignant pericarditis was properly recognized by cytological examination in each instance, but false negative cytology occurred in patients with lymphoma and mesothelioma. Since many patients in their study underwent radiotherapy, the differential diagnosis of neoplastic versus radiation-induced pericardial disease remained unresolved in several "negative" cases.

Malamou-Mitsi et al. [7] analysed a total of 53 pericardial fluid specimens from 44 patients over a 7-year period in a similar setting. Their overall sensitivity was 100%, the overall specificity was 93.3%, and the overall cytological accuracy was 95.4%. The predictive value of the correct histological type of cancer by cytology was 77.7%.

The opposite example is the study of Corey et al. [10] in which pericardial fluid cytology was diagnostic in only 26% of patients, 21% all patients with a large effusion of had a malignant etiology.

Bardales et al. [17] analyzed pericardial fluids and pericardial biopsies. In 61 cases paired cytology and histology specimens were available. 45 showed a malignant and 16 benign cytology. In 7 cases cytology and histology gave discrepant results with respect to the underlying tumor. In 6 of those cases cytology demonstrated the original tumor after careful review. DNA diploidy obtained by flow cytometry in a subgroup of 34 cases correlated with benign cytology, whereas aneuploidy was associated with malignant cytology in a total of 32/34 cases.

Wilkes et al. [19] analyzed retrospectively the diagnostic and therapeutic aspects of malignancy-related pericardial effusions in 127 patients with proven malignancies. Pericardial fluid cytology was found malignant 55% of cases, pericardial biopsy carried out in parallel gave a lower yield with only 56%. In 45% of patients, the malignant nature of the effusion could not be confirmed.

Reactive Mesothelial Versus Adenocarcinoma Cells

In occasional cases, it could be difficult to recognize the exact nature of the cells in the pericardial fluid. The differential diagnosis of pericardial effusion or cardiac tamponade developing in a cancer patient includes in addition to malignant pericardial effusion, radiation pericarditis, drug-induced pericarditis, infection, hypothyroidism, and local autoreactive or systemic autoimmune disorders [15]. Cytological findings have to distinguish between cells reactive to an inflammatory process and those of a malignancy. This is especially true when reactive mesothelial and adenocarcinoma cells are to be differentiated.

Chen et al. [20, 21] investigated the value of immunocytochemical staining in malignant effusions obtained from three large body cavities in 99 patients. Five commercially available antibodies to the epithelial membrane antigen, the carcinoembryonal antigen, cytokeratin, vimentin and Leu-M1 were tested. No single marker was unconditionally reliable in differentiating between reactive mesothelial and malignant cells. However, a combination of epithelial membrane antigen, carcinoembryonal antigen, and vimentin proved to be helpful in identifying the real nature of a particular cell. Another useful method for the cytological identification of malignancy in pericardial effusions is DNA analysis [17, 22, 23]. In the study of Fischler et al. [22] all 12 patients with proven malignancy had cells with a DNA content of more than 5c (= hyperploid). In the eight patients with reactive cells only, a single diploid DNA peak and no cells more than 5c were demonstrated.

Pericardial effusion in patients with AIDS show a moderate cellularity with the presence of inflammatory cells. Zakowski et al. [24] investigated 15 cytology specimens obtained from 14 patients with AIDS and observed atypical or reactive mesothelial cells in 80% of cases, while in 13% of the patients cells suspicious for a malignant lymphoma were noticed. An accurate cytological diagnosis of inflammatory effusion in AIDS is essential to avoid the confusion with atypical cells seen in malignant effusions.

Prognostic and Therapeutic Implications

The relationship of the cytological findings in the pericardial fluid and the natural history as well as the survival of patients with malignancy has been the subject of several studies [25, 26, 27].

Edoute et al. [25] investigated cytological findings in 21 breast cancer patients with symptomatic pericardial effusion. Malignant cells were detected in pericardial effusion in 62%, suspected malignancy was revealed by cytology in 9%, whereas in 24% of patients no evidence of malignancy was observed. The average survival of patients with negative cytology was 12 months, while patients with suspicious cytology survived an average of 9 months. Patients with proven malignant effusion and treated by pericardiectomy had a mean survival of 22.3 months, while patients with malignant pericardial effusion, in whom surgery was deferred, survived only 4.7 months. Their data demonstrate, that symptomatic pericardial effusion in patients with breast cancer is not necessarily malignant, and underline the importance of fluid cytology in establishing a definite diagnosis. Cytology is crucial, not only as prognostic predictor, but even more importantly, as an indicator for the change or intensification of oncological treatment.

The natural history of patients with lung cancer and symptomatic pericardial effusion is even more rapid. In a study including 20 patients with lung cancer and pericardial effusion Edoute et al. confirmed malignant cells in 13 and suspected malignancy in 2 additional patients[26]. Seventeen patients died within less than 3 months and all patients were dead within 9 months after the appearance of pericardial effusion. Therefore, in lung cancer patients, the presence of pericardial effusion and the demonstration of neoplastic cells in the pericardial fluid are highly suggestive of a rapid disease progression and poor survival.

The impact of treatment after pericardiocentesis on the prognosis was emphasized by Wang et al. [28] in a retrospective post mortem analysis of 82 patients with non-small cell lung cancer (NSCLC). At the time of pericardiocentesis 60 patients had a malignant, 22 patients had a negative cytology. The prognosis was similarly poor in both groups of patients independent of a positive or negative pericardial cytology with a median survival time of 74,5 days for all patients. The survival was longest, however, in patients who went on to receive systemic chemotherapy in addition to pericardiocentesis; it was shortest, when only supportive treatment was carried out, and in between, when local sclerosing and/or radiotherapy and/or a pericardial window operation was carried out. Pericardial involvement as the direct or contributory cause of death was noted in 46% of these patients [28]. This is much less than in the autopsy series by Thurber et al. [29] in 1962, who reported pericardial involvement as the primary or contributory cause of death in 85% of patients. The lack of effective local treatment resulted in a higher mortality. With the improvements in the local management of pericardial effusion, the systemic treatment of the cancer became more important for the overall prognosis. This might also explain why chemotherapy prolonged the survival in the systemically treated patients [28].

Paramalignant Pericardial Effusion

If the tumor does not directly invade the pericardium ("true negative" cytology) malignancy still cannot be completely excluded. Pericardial effusions can result from inflammation or blockage of lymphatic or blood vessels [30-32]. These, paramalignant effusions are associated with and caused by the malignancy but do not result from direct tumor invasion [31].

Blood Cells in Pericardial Effusion

The proportion of normal blood cells in the pericardial effusion is not directly diagnostic for any etiology of the disease. Red blood cells (RBC) counts were even similar between exudate and transudate and were also not significantly different among the various etiologies in the study of Meyers et al. [1]. White blood cell (WBC) counts were highest in inflammatory diseases, particularly of bacterial and rheumatologic origin. High monocyte counts, and low neutrophil and WBC counts have been demonstrated in myxedema. Monocyte count was highest in malignant and hypothyroid effusions ($79 \pm 27\%$ and $74 \pm 26\%$), while rheumatoid and bacterial effusions had the highest proportions of neutrophils ($78 \pm 20\%$ and $69 \pm 23\%$) [1].

High lymphocyte counts can also be found in effusions secondary to connective tissue disorders and malignancies, particularly those secondary to hematological malignancies [1].

In addition, identification of RA and LE cells may help to correctly classify pericardial effusion associated with rheumatoid arthritis or systemic lupus erythematosus.

Polymorphs were the predominant population in all patients with bacterial effusions in the study of Maisch et al. [11]. The number of granulocytes in the effusion was substantially reduced ($<5000/mm^3$) in all viral and autoreactive effusions and in 13 out of 16 lymphocytic effusions. Lymphocytes were the predominant cell population ($>1000/mm^3$) in the lymphocytic effusions but counts of $>1000/mm^3$ were also found in both tuberculous and in two out of five bacterial effusions. Furthermore, polymorphs were also frequently observed in this kind of pericardial effusion. It should be noted, however, that in neoplastic effusions high counts of lymphocytes and granulocytes were frequently found, as well.

Staining for Bacteria in Pericardial Effusion

In pericarditis caused by bacterial infection, the cytology of the pericardial fluid is of considerable diagnostic value. The demonstration of a purulent infection often indicates the need for a more radical therapeutic approach e.g. the intrapericardial application of fibrinolytic agents, pericardiotomy and extensive drainage or even pericardiectomy.

For the microscopical evaluation of bacteria in the pericardial fluid gram, acid-fast, and silver staining are performed as baseline staining. The presence of acid-fast bacilli is virtually diagnostic for tuberculous pericarditis but they can be found in only 40–60% smears of patients with tuberculous pericardial effusions [33]. Compared with the positive growth on bacterial cultures of pericardial fluids as the reference standard, stained bacteria were noted in 3 of 8 culture-positive fluid samples and in 1 of 83 culture-negative samples in the study of Myers et al. [1]. The absence of stained bacteria had a specificity of 99%, but a sensitivity of only 38%.

Biochemical Analyses

Differentiation of Transudates and Exudates

The normal pericardial fluid originates from the visceral pericardium and is essentially an ultrafiltrate of plasma. In contrast to transudative fluids which result from the obstruction of fluid drainage, exudative fluids are caused by infectious or autoimmune inflammation or malignant processes within the pericardium [34].

It is clinically important to classify pericardial fluids into exudates and transudates because this is indicative of the underlying pathophysiological process [35]. Such a distinction allows appropriate investigations to be initiated, enabling a better patient management. There is no biochemical marker that alone allows a complete differentiation between transudates and exudates [1, 9, 10, 35–41]. Specific gravity >1016 is generally attributed to an exudates with a sensitivity of 90% [1]. Light et al. [37] used a fluid to serum total protein ratio >0.5, a fluid lactate dehydrogenase (LDH) value > 200 U/l, or a fluid to serum LDH ratio >0.6 to diagnose exudates (Table 7.1). This has been reported as the best method for discriminating between exudates and transudates [1], although other authors [9] have modified the cut off points used by Light et al. [37]. Based on the degree of inflammation alone, malignant and non-malignant pericardial effusions cannot be separated.

The differentiation between exudates and transudates may be confounded by treatment. In patients with pericardial effusion due to congestive heart failure, more rapid reabsorption of water than protein and LDH can convert the hydropericardium to a pseudoexudate [36]. This phenomenon has been described in patients with congestive heart failure and pleural effusions receiving diuretic therapy by Pillay [42] and Chakko et al. [43, 44]. It is probable that a similar mechanism exists in pericardial effusions as well.

◻ Table 7.1. Comparison of biochemical parameters used to differentiate between pericardial exudates and transudates

Methods	Efficiency [%]***	Sensitivity [%]	Specificity [%]	Positive predictive value [%]	Negative predictive value [%]
Light's criteria *[37]	94	98	72	95	87
SEAG (> 12 g/L)*	90	90	89	98	64
Cholesterol (> 1.55 mmol/l)*	73	71	83	95	38
Cholesterol (< 1.15 mmol/l)**	83	88	56	90	50
P/S cholesterol ratio (< 0.3)*	88	91	83	95	64
P/S bilirubin ratio (< 0,3)*	86	90	65	93	58

*characteristic for a transudate, **characteristic for an exudates, *** definition of efficiency (= diagnostic accuracy):
a = (nTP+nTN) : (nTP+nFP+nFN+nTN), whereby a = accuracy, n = number, T = True, P = Positives, N = Negatives, F = False
Light's criteria for an exudate: Fluid/Serum protein ratio >0,5; fluid LDH >200/U/L, F/S LDH ratio >0,6), if one is positive
Light's criteria are fulfilled.
P/S – pericardial / serum cholesterol < 0,3 are characteristic for a transudate; P/S bilirubin ratio < 0,3 characteristic for a transudate, SEAG – serum/effusion albumin gradient (if >12 g/l characteristic for a transudate, if < 12 g/L for an exudates); modified from Burges et al. (2002) [34].

Protein Concentration

Based on the data generally accepted for pleural effusions, a fluid protein level of > 3.0g/dl and a fluid to serum protein ratio of >0.5 had a sensitivity of 97% and 96% to correctly identify exudates, respectively. In tuberculous pericarditis effusion demonstrates high specific gravity, high protein levels, and high white-cell count (from $0.7–54 \times 10^9/l$) [1]. The measurement of the fluid to serum protein ratio substantially improves the sensitivity and specificity, especially in cases of malignancy, infection, and renal failure.

LDH

The measurement of fluid LDH was found to be especially helpful in those cases of congestive heart failure, when fluid total protein values are borderline. Determination of LDH was the most sensitive marker of an exudate in the study of Meyers et al. [1]. Levels of > 200 mg/dl had a sensitivity of 98% for an exudate. The serum to fluid LDH ratio of > 0.6 had a sensitivity of 94%, however with a low specificity of 30% and 40%, respectively.

Fluid LDH measurements were also better at classifying infective causes of an exudate compared with fluid total protein measurements alone. When both protein level and LDH concentration were increased beyond 3 g/dl and 200 mg/dl respectively the fluid was classified as exudates.

The criteria of Paramothayan et al. [35] are less strict: both a pericardial fluid LDH > 130 U/l or a fluid to serum total protein ratio > 0.4 indicated the presence of an exudate.

Glucose

Glucose concentration is significantly lower in exudates than in transudates (77.9 ± 41.9 vs. 96.1 ± 50.7 mg/dl respectively) [1]. In addition, purulent effusions with positive cultures have significantly lower fluid glucose levels (47.3 ± 25.3 vs. 102.5 ± 35.6 mg/dl) and fluid to serum ratios (0.28 ± 0.14 vs. 0.84 ± 0.23 mg/dl), than non-infectious effusions [1].

However, no differences in the pericardial fluid to serum ratio of glucose were found between exudates and transudates. Compared with parainfective pericardial fluids, infective effusions with positive cultures had significantly lower fluid glucose levels and fluid to serum ratios (47.3 ± 25.3 vs. 102.5 ± 35.6 mg/dl and 0.28 ± 0.14 vs. 0.84 ± 0.23, respectively).

Cholesterol

Both bacterial and malignant pericardial fluids have significantly higher cholesterol levels in comparison with controls (49 ± 18 vs. 121 ± 20 and 117 ± 33 mg/dl) [1]. Patients with uremic pericarditis may have an increased cholesterol value in the pericardial effusion as well.

Determination of pH in Pericardial Fluid

Lowest pH levels are noted in infective pericardial fluids. However, a variation of pH between the various etiological groups of patients with pericardial diseases is so large, that no discrimination based on pH values is possible.

Specific Gravity

Exudates are correctly detected by a specific gravity of >1015 in >90%. Moreover, there was a significant positive correlation between pericardial effusion total protein and pericardial effusion specific gravity ($r = 0.56$) [1]. No discrimination of the underlying etiology could be made by the determination of specific gravity, however.

Pericardial Cytokines

Cytokines are soluble proteins critical for the function of the immune system. Their expression may be altered in various disease states. They play an important role in the regulation of the growth, development, and activation of immune system and the mediation of the inflammatory response. Immunoregulatory cytokines are involved in the activation, growth, and differentiation of lymphocytes and monocytes (e.g., interleukin (IL)-2, IL-4, and transforming growth factor beta (TGF-beta). Pro-inflammatory cytokines are produced predominantly by mononuclear phagocytes in response to infectious agents (e.g., IL-1, tumor necrosis factor (TNF) alpha, and IL-6). The chemokine family of inflammatory cytokines includes IL-8, monocyte chemotactic protein (MCP)-1, MCP-2, MCP-3, macrophage inflammatory protein (MIP)-1-alpha, MIP-1-beta, and regulation-upon-activation, normal T expressed and secreted (RANTES). Major cytokines that regulate immature leukocyte growth and differentiation are IL-3, IL-7, and granulocyte-macrophage colony-stimulating factor (GM-CSF). In general, cytokines exert their effects by influencing gene activation, cellular activation, growth, differentiation, functional cell surface molecule expression, and cellular effector function. In this regard, cytokines can have dramatic effects on the regulation of immune responses and the pathogenesis of a variety of diseases.

In the pathophysiology of inflammatory and neoplastic processes of the pericardium local cytokine production or diffusion from systemic circulation plays a yet underestimated role [45]. So changes in the cytokine regulation could contribute to the induction of fibrosis during the organization and development of pericardial constriction. In the interferon (IFN)-gamma knock-out mice model the development of constrictive pericarditis could be demonstrated[46].

IL-6 and TNF-alpha in pericardial effusions were significantly increased when compared to sera of the same patients. In our own patients Pankuweit et al. demonstrated in 93 pericardial effusions dramatically and significantly increased levels of IL-6 and IL-8 independent of the respective etiology when fluid and serum levels were compared. In contrast IFN-gamma concentration was low in viral and malignant pericardial effusions in comparison to serum values. Effusion and serum values of IFN were comparable, however, in autoreactive pericarditis, and only slightly increased values were obtained in lymphocytic pericardial effusions [45]. Thus the local pericardial production of proinflammatory cytokines is, not unexpectedly, a hallmark of inflammatory or neoplastic pericardial disease.

In a subsequent analysis the following additional cytokine patterns were identified in patients with various forms of pericardial disease in the pericardial fluid:

a) A high TNF-alpha/low TGF-beta1 ratio was obtained in patients with viral pericarditis in addition to an increased IL-6.
b) An elevated IL-6 levels was characteristic for all forms of pericarditis, except for the autoreactive pericardial effusions [47]. Except in autoreactive pericarditis IL-6 was also significantly increased in all other forms of pericardial effusion when the fluid was compared to the "normal" pericardial fluid of bypass surgery patients at the time of surgery. The immunoregulatory cytokine, TGF-beta1 was found in strikingly lower concentrations in all pericardial effusions than in the serum of all pericarditis patients. However, the TGF-beta1 levels in pericardial effusion were still significantly higher in all pericarditis patients than in the pericardial fluid of aorto-coronary bypass surgery controls. The IFN-gamma concentrations did neither significantly differ between effusion and serum nor in comparison to the pericardial fluid of bypass surgery controls. GM-CSF was present only in a small proportion of patients with neoplastic and autoreactive pericardial effusions.

Concentrations of IL-6, TNF-alpha, and TGF-beta1 obtained in the pericardial fluid of bypass surgery controls in our study [47] were comparable to the findings of Riemann et al. [48] in 127 patients. At the time of surgery these authors analyzed the pericardial fluid in 23 patients who underwent heart valve replacement (group 1), 14 patients with congenital heart disease undergoing surgery(group 2) , and 32 patients with chronic ischemic heart disease undergoing bypass surgery.

These authors also observed a wide range of cytokine concentrations. Interestingly but of course not unexpectedly IL-6 levels were low (ranging from undetectable to 4500 U/ml), acid activated TGF-beta levels ranged from <3 ng/ml up to 80 ng/ml, and TNF-alpha levels from <3 pg/ml to 233 pg/ml in all 3 groups of surgical patients. There were no statistically significant differences in the level of either of the cytokines between the three groups of patients. When compared to the data in infective, malignant, lymphocytic or autoreactive pericardial effusions, their levels can be considered "baseline concentrations".

In collagen diseases few data are available. The pericardial effusion obtained from a 38 years old male patient with systemic lupus erythematosus and cardiac tamponade showed similar ratios and elevated concentrations [49] as the infective and autoreactive patients of our own studies [45, 47]; IL-6, TNF-alpha, and IFN-gamma concentrations were significantly increased when compared the sera [49]. In a patients with rheumatoid arthritis and pericardial effusion, the concentration of IL-6 in the pericardial fluid was notably increased when compared to the serum values [50]. In patients with aggressive multiple myeloma high IL-6 levels were noted in the pericardial effusion as well[51, 52]. In conclusion, increased IL-6 is a sensitive marker for exudative, neoplastic, autoreactive, infective and rheumatic pericardial effusions, but does not really distinguish between the respective etiological entities.

Significantly elevated levels of IFN-gamma were demonstrated in patients with tuberculous pericarditis when compared to those with both infective and malignant pericardial effusions [53], with a similar or slight decrease compared to serum values as in our study. So an elevated IFN-gamma concentration points to tuberculous pericarditis. Since in patients with tuberculous pleural and peritoneal effusions an increased IFN-gamma has also been reported in a number of studies [37, 38] as well, this has lead to the proposal that an IFN-gamma concentration in whatever fluid can used as a diagnostic tool for a tuberculous exudates. Using a cut-off level of 200 pg/l for the diagnosis of tuberculous pericarditis both 100% sensitivity and 100% specificity could be achieved.

Mistchenko et al. [54] reported on the fatal case of adenoviral pericarditis in a 10-months old under-nourished boy. Pericardial fluid IL-6 and IFN-alpha concentrations were three times higher than serum levels. In one of our patients with viral pericarditis IFN-gamma was detectable neither in the pericardial effusion nor in the serum. This points to a lack of immunoreactivity in these individuals with a poor prognostic outcome.

These findings are also in concordance with experimental data by Nakayama et al. [55] who found elevated levels of IL-1beta and IL-6 in the pericardial effusion in a rat model of Coxsackie virus B3 myo-pericarditis, when compared to the serum cytokines at the peak of inflammation. IFN-gamma in the pericardial effusion and the serum was not elevated.

In contrast to the limited experience on pericardial cytokines in pericardial effusion, there are numerous studies concerning cytokines in pleural effusion. Some of these findings may be extrapolated for pericardial effusion. Dore et al. [56] evaluated IL-6 levels in sera and pleural effusions from 42 patients with metastatic carcinoma, non-Hodgkin's lymphoma, tuberculosis, cardiac failure and miscellaneous diseases. Pleural IL-6 levels measured by ELISA were very high in all patient groups without permitting a differentiation of the diseases. Serum IL-6 levels were low and did not correlate with pleural fluid levels. In lung cancer patients, concentrations of IL-6 and IL-8 were significantly higher in the pleural effusion in comparison to serum levels [57]. Remarkably, in pleural effusion caused by pleural mesothelioma the concentration of IL-6 was strikingly higher than in lung adenocarcinoma. This quantitative aspect is underlined by the fact that the IL-6 concentrations in the pleural effusion were 60-1400 times higher than in serum [58]. But also serum levels can be found elevated, when the tumor mass increases by the number of metastases: In a population of 46 Japanese patients with metastatic breast cancer Zhang and Adachi [59] detected significantly higher IL-6 serum levels in patients with more than one metastatic site and with dominant metastatic visceral disease than in those with one metastatic site or with dominant metastatic bone or soft tissue disease. The patients with liver metastasis and pleural effusion showed significantly higher serum IL-6 levels than those without liver metastases or pleural effusion. In addition, patients unresponsive to chemoendocrine therapy showed significantly higher serum IL-6 levels than those who responded to chemoendocrine therapy. Moreover, the patients with high IL-6 serum levels had a significantly shorter survival time than patients with low IL-6 levels. Multivariate analysis revealed that IL-6, as well as a disease-free interval, is an independent prognostic factor of metastatic breast cancer. When IL-6 in malignant pleural effusions was compared to tuberculous pleural effusions both were elevated but IL-6 in tuberculous pleural effusion was significantly higher when compared to metastatic pleural fluid

[60]. In pleural effusion of infectious etiology levels of IL-6 were increased both in serum and pleural effusion but with no significant difference in septic vs. non-septic patients [61].

Weissflog et al. [62] found lower concentrations of TNF-alpha, GM-CSF, and IL-10 in malignant pleural effusion in comparison to the pleural effusions of other etiologies. Another important finding that could be further investigated and extrapolated to pericardial pathology was made by De Pablo et al. [63]: patients with tuberculous pleuritis that develop extensive pleural thickening have high concentrations of TNF-alpha in their pleural effusion. Correspondingly in a recent study Hua et al. [64] found the levels of TNF-alpha in 33 tuberculous patients significantly higher than in the malignant pleural effusions of 30 patients. Residual pleural thickening was found in nine of 33 patients (27.3%) with tuberculous pleurisy. Pleural TNF-alpha was significantly higher in tuberculous pleurisy patients with residual pleural thickening. If this is also valid for pericardial effusion, TNF-alpha could be a valuable prognostic marker of constrictive pericarditis.

Maeda et al. [65] described three to six-times higher TGF-beta concentrations in pleural effusions caused by malignant mesothelioma in comparison to the effusions caused by primary lung cancer. Ikubo et al. described in 10 effusion samples from patients with various types of carcinoma cells considerably elevated TGF-beta levels [66]. Concentrations ranged from 0.90 to 8.75 ng/ml, which is comparable to our findings in pericardial effusion [47].

Adenosine Deaminase Activity in Pericardial Effusion

Adenosine deaminase (ADA) is a polymorphic enzyme that is involved in purine metabolism. It catalyzes the deamination of adenosine to inosine and ammonium [67]. ADA levels are believed to reflect T-cell activity. Although it is found in most tissues, ADA activity is greatest in the lymphoid tissues, its activity being 10 to 20 times more active in T lymphocytes than in B lymphocytes [68]. The presence of ADA in pleural fluid and other fluids reflects the cellular immune response in the fluid compartment, especially the activation of T lymphocytes [69].

Burgess et al. [53] found pericardial ADA levels to be highest among patients with tuberculous pericardial effusion. Although other infective conditions may also be associated with high ADA levels, a relative cell count can be used to distinguish between tuberculous and other forms of effusion[70]. Tuberculous effusions are also characterized by a relative lymphocytosis, and non-tuberculous infective effusions are characterized by a neutrophil predominance [1].

Table 7.2 summarizes the results of studies conducted to evaluate the use of ADA for the diagnosis of tuberculous pericarditis [53, 71–76]. Based on relative operating characteristic curves (ROC) [71] the best results are yielded at a cutoff level of 30 U/l, which corresponds to a sensitivity, specificity, positive predictive value, negative predictive value, and diagnostic accuracy of 94, 68, 80, 89, and 83%, respectively.

Table 7.2. Studies reporting the diagnostic utility of determination of adenosine deaminase activity in patients with tuberculous pericarditis

Author	No. of TBC pts	ADA [U/l]	Sensitivity [%]	Specificity [%]	Positive predictive value [%]	Negative predictive value [%]	Diagnostic accuracy [%]
Komsougly 1995 (n = 108) [72]	20	70	100	91	71	100	93
Telenti 1991 (n = 35) [73]	8	60	100	80	62	100	86
Koh 1994 (n = 26) [71]	14	40	93	97	93	97	96
Martinez-Vazquez 1986 (n = 56) [74]	3	*	100	100	100	100	100
Burgess 2002 (n = 110) [53]	64	35	89	74	83	83	83

*No ADA cutoff level was suggested, however, all patients with non-tuberculous effusions had ADA levels <20 U/l, while the mean ADA level for the three patients with pericardial tuberculosis was 92.4 ± 29.4 U/l. Reproduced with permission from Burges et al. (2002) [53].

Table 7.3. Comparison of the different methods used to diagnose tuberculous pericarditis

Methods	Sensitivity [%]	Specificity [%]	Positive predictive value [%]	Negative predictive value [%]	Diagnostic accuracy [%]
Positive pericardial fluid culture and/or biopsy	52	100	100	60	72
Positive sputum ZN stain and/or culture	23	98	94	48	55
Empirical anti-tuberculous therapy	39	91	86	52	61
Pericardial ADA>30 U/l	94	68	80	89	83
Pericardial ADA > 35 U/l	89	74	83	88	83
IFN-gamma > 200 pg/l	100	100	100	100	100

ADA adenosine deaminase; *IFN* interferon; *ZN* Ziel-Nielsen – acid-fast bacilli staining. Reproduced with permission from Burgess et al. (2002) [53]

Using a cut-off value of ADA activity of 40 U/l, the sensitivity and specificity of ADA testing in one series of nine patients with proven and of five patients with suspected tuberculous pericarditis were 93 and 97 percent, respectively [71]. In addition, very high ADA (>100 IU/l) levels are prognostic for pericardial constriction [72].

Tuberculous pericarditis is traditionally diagnosed by the identification of Mycobacterium tuberculosis in the pericardial fluid or in the biopsy specimens. In an comparative analysis of available diagnostic methods tuberculous pericarditis was diagnosed in only 33 of 64 patients (52%) in this manner by Burgess [53]. Further 15 patients (23%) were characterized by a positive result of sputum Ziel-Nielsen acid-fast bacilli staining in the presence of clinical and radiological evidence of TBC. 9 of these patients also had a pericardial fluid or biopsy specimen positive for M. tuberculosis. The diagnosis of tuberculosis in the remaining 25 patients (39%) was based on clinical and radiological evidence associated with a response to empirical antituberculous therapy. These findings are summarized in Table 7.3 and compared with pericardial ADA levels and IFN-gamma concentration > 200 pg/l.

The use of pericardial ADA levels and pericardial IFN-gamma concentrations thus provides a rapid and accurate means of detecting tuberculous pericarditis, especially in high-prevalence areas, thereby expediting the initial decision making process. IFN-gamma should be used to aid in the rapid diagnosis

of tuberculous pericarditis. When IFN-gamma is not routinely available as a diagnostic test, ADA can be used as a screening test and IFN-gamma as a confirmatory test, if diagnostic uncertainty for tuberculous pericarditis still remains particularly in cases of concomitant HIV infection in Africa.

The European Society of Cardiology Guidelines gave a class I recommendation to the use of pericardial ADA testing for the diagnosis of tuberculous pericarditis [77]. However, as with the interpretation of pericardial fluid polymerase chain reaction (PCR) testing for mycobacterial DNA, interpretation of pericardial ADA levels must take into consideration the pretest probability of a diagnosis of tuberculous pericarditis [78]. In areas where the prevalence of tuberculosis is low, the utility of the pericardial ADA test is correspondingly low. In addition, ADA testing is not widely available and is, at present, limited to specialized centers.

Virology of Pericardial Fluid

Viral pericarditis is the most common infection of the pericardium. Inflammation may due to direct damage caused both by the virus (entero-, echo-, adeno-, cytomegalo-, Ebstein Barr, herpes simplex, herpes humanus 6, influenza, parvo B19, hepatitis C, human immunodeficiency virus, etc.; Table 7.4) and the antiviral and anticardiac immune response [11]. Cytomegalovirus pericarditis has an increased incidence

▢ Table 7.4. Etiology and incidence of infectious pericarditis

Etiology	Incidence [%]	Pathogenesis
Viral (Coxsackie A9, B1-4, Echo 8, Mumps, EBV, CMV, Varicella, Rubella, HIV, Parvo B19, Herpes humanus 6, Herpes simplex)	30a	Multiplication and spread of the causative agent and release of toxic substances in pericardial tissue cause serous, serofibrinous or hemorrhagic (bacterial, viral, tuberculous, fungal) or purulent inflammation
Bacterial (Staphylococcus aureus, Klebsiella pneumoniae, Pneumo-, Meningo-, Gonococcosis, Hemophilus, Pseudomonas, Legionella, Myco-plasma, Peptostreptococcus, Prevotella, Propionibacterium, Bacteroides fragilis, Clostridium spp., Fusobacterium spp., Bifidobacterium spp., Salmonella, Campylobacter, Listeria, Treponema pallidum, Borreliosis, Chlamydia, Tuberculosis...)	5a	
Fungal (Candida, Histoplasma ...)	Rare	
Parasitary (Entameba histolytica, Echinococcus, Toxoplasma ...)	Rare	

aPercentage related to the population of 260 subsequent patients undergoing pericardiocentesis, pericardioscopy, and epicardial biopsy (Marburg pericarditis registry)[11]. *EBV* Epstein-Barr virus, *CMV* cytomegalovirus, *HIV* human immuno-deficiency virus

in immunocompromised hosts [79]. The diagnosis of viral pericarditis is not possible without the evaluation of pericardial effusion and/or pericardial or epimyocardial tissue, preferably by PCR or in-situ hybridization. In small effusions inaccessible to pericardiocentesis, endomyocardial biopsy with PCR for (peri)cardiotropic viruses can be attempted to establish viral etiology of the inflammatory cardiac process [77]. Viral cultures from a site other than the pericardial fluid, such as the stool or throat, can be used to diagnose the likely cause of concomitant pericarditis. A four-fold rise in serum antiviral antibody levels is suggestive but not diagnostic [77]. Viral serology for antimicrobial antibodies is helpful in particular for the diagnosis of rickettsiae, borrelia burgdorferi, HIV and mycoplasma, or for other (peri) cardiotropic agents where PCR of cardiac tissue and pericardial fluid is not available. IgM-titers signal an acute infection, that should be followed a later assessement for the conversion to an IgG antibody.

Polymerase Chain Reaction (PCR)

PCR is the most important diagnostic tool for the detection of viral infection both from the pericardial fluid and/or myocardial or pericardial tissue in the contemporary medical practice. Therefore the detailed methodology applied for PCR at the Laboratory for cardioimmunology of the Philipps University in Marburg will be reviewed in this section.

Viral DNA/RNA Extraction

Obtained pericardial fluid specimens or peri- or myocardial tissue are snap-frozen and conserved in liquid nitrogen until the final PCR analysis. Lymphocytes are prepared from the peripheral blood by the use of ficoll gradient centrifugation. PCR for the following cardiotropic viruses (influenza A/B, cytomegalovirus, enterovirus, adenovirus, herpes simplex virus, herpes humanus 6, Epstein Barr virus, Parvo B19), as well as for the bacteria Borrelia burgdorferi, Chlamydia pneumoniae, and Mycobacterium tuberculosis are routinely performed. Total DNA or RNA is obtained by the use of QIAamp Kit (Quiagen). The samples are incubated in 180 µl buffer ATL and 20 µl Proteinase K (stock solution) for 4 hours at 55 °C. 200 µl buffer AL is added to each sample, they are mixed thoroughly by vortexing and incubated for 10 min at 70 °C. 210 µl ice cooled ethanol is added and the complete mixture including the DNA/RNA precipitate is placed on a spin column and centrifuged at 6000 g for 2 min. The DNA/RNA now placed on the filter is washed three times with 500 µl buffer AW by centrifugation with full speed for 3 min. For elution of the DNA/RNA 70 µl preheated (70 °C) distilled water is added, incubated for 5 min and then centrifuged for 1 min at 6000 g. For long term storage buffer AE instead of distilled water is used for elution. For positive control viral genome is extracted from viral stock solutions obtaining between 100-300 ng total RNA or DNA.

Polymerase Chain Reaction and Southern Blot Hybridization

All primers for PCR are synthesized by TipBiomol Co. using published viral sequences:

1) region "5'NTR" for Entero virus   198 bp
2) region "US10/11" for Cytomegalo virus   360 bp
3) region "Hexon" for Adeno viruses   308 bp
4) region matrix protein for Influenza viruses   625 bp
5) region DNA polymerase for Herpes simplex viruses   229 bp
6) region VP1of parvo virus B 19   699 bp
7) region "EBNA-1" for Epstein-Barr virus   80 bp
8) region "chromosomal-Ly-1" and "anonymous gene" for Borrelia   224/357 bp

For DNA-Virus-PCR 5µl of total extracted DNA is combined with 50 pmol of the appropriate primer, 10 µl 10 × PCR buffer (1.5 mmol MgCl2), 10 mmol dNTP's and 2.5 U Taq polymerase Gold each in a 50 µl reaction volume. After an initial incubation at 94 °C for 3 to 5 min forty rounds of amplification are performed on following conditions: 94 °C (denaturation) for 1 min, 60 °C (annealing temperature for adenovirus-primer pairs), 57 °C (annealing temperature for cytomegalovirus, EBV-and Parvo B 19 primer pairs), 65 °C (annealing temperature for herpes virus and Borrelia primer pairs) for 1 min, 72 °C (extension) for 2 min. A final cycle for 5 min and 72 °C for complete polymerization is added. For Enterovirus-and Influenza virus-PCR the Titan One Tube PCR-System is used with two Mastermix combined: Mastermix 1: 6.5 µl distilled water, 50 pmol of the appropriate primer, 10 mmol dNTP's and 2.5 µl DTT and 5 µl of the extract, Mastermix 2: 14 µl distilled water, 10 µl 5 × RT-PCR-buffer with Mg^{2+} and 1 µl enzyme mix). After 60 °C for 30 min for reverse transcription and an initial incubation at 94 °C for 2 min, ten cycles with following conditions: 94 °C (denaturation) for 2 min, 58 °C (annealing temperature for enterovirus primer pairs), 60 °C (annealing temperature for influenza virus primer pairs) for 2 min, 72 °C (extension) for 2 min and 40 cycles with following conditions: 94 °C for two minutes, 50 °C for 2 min are performed. A final cycle for 5 min and 72°C for complete polymerization is added. Ten microliters of each reaction are analyzed on a 1.5% agarose gel containing 0.5 µg/ml ethidium bromide. All samples run with a simultaneous positive and negative control for the virus analyzed. Southern blotting and hybridization with specific probes are used to confirm positive results. For each primer pair a digoxigenin labeled hybridization probe has to be available.

Bacteriology of Pericardial Effusion

A wide variety of bacterial organisms have been reported as causative agents of pericarditis. The infection can be endogenous or exogenous. The endogenous infection often occurs in hosts predisposed by age (neonates or the elderly), alcoholism, injection drug abuse, diabetes mellitus, immunosuppressive therapy with corticosteroids or cytotoxic drugs, or underlying malignancy [80–82]. The causative bacterial agents can be isolated best by fluid cultures from the pericardium, or as described in special cases also by PCR from fluid or cardiac tissue (see previous paragraph).

Although some reports suggested an increased incidence of Gram-negative organisms, the recent series reported that the most commonly isolated organisms were Gram-positive cocci [83–86]. The bacteria include Staphylococcus aureus, Neisseria meningitidis, Streptococcus pyogenes, Streptococcus pneumoniae, Haemophilus influenzae, Escherichia coli, Klebsiella spp., Salmonella spp., Pseudomonas aeruginosa, Staphylococcus epidermidis, and anaerobic bacteria. Other organisms include: Mycobacterium tuberculosis, Mycoplasma pneumoniae, Coxiella burnetti, and protozoa (Amoebas, and Toxoplasma gondii).

However, the role of anaerobic bacteria was not well studied in many previous investigations, as methods for the recovery of the bacteria were inadequate [87–91] or not used consistently [83]. Out of 15 cases of bacterial pericarditis reported by Brook and Frazier [92] aerobic or facultative bacteria alone were present in 7 specimens (47%), anaerobic bacteria alone in 6 specimens (40%), and mixed aerobic-anaerobic flora in 2 specimens (13%). In total, there were 21 isolates: 10 aerobic or facultative bacteria and

11 anaerobic bacteria, an average of 1.4 per specimen. Anaerobic bacteria predominated in patients with pericarditis who also had mediastinitis that followed esophageal perforation and in patients whose pericarditis was associated with orofacial and dental infections. The predominant aerobic bacteria were S. aureus (3 isolates) and Klebsiella pneumoniae (2 isolates), and the predominant anaerobic bacteria were Prevotella spp. (4 isolates), Peptostreptococcus spp. (3 isolates), and Propionibacterium acnes (2 isolates). Skiest et al. [93] presented 1 case and reviewed 29 cases of anaerobic pericarditis previously reported in the English language literature. In 17 cases, only anaerobic bacteria were isolated, while in 13 cases anaerobes were isolated with a mixture of facultative and/or aerobic bacteria. The predominant anaerobes were: Bacteroides spp. (mostly of the B. fragilis group), anaerobic streptococci, Clostridium spp., Fusobacterium spp., and Bifidobacterium spp. Five of the patients were children, 2 of whom had pneumonia. The pathogenesis of inflammation following infection of the pericardial sac is based on a sequence of events: fibrin exudation is accompanied by an influx of mononuclear cells and/or polymorphonuclear leukocytes, which are followed by a fluid exudates into the pericardial space. Proliferation of fibrous tissue, neovascularization, and scarring also occur. This induces a loss of elasticity, a consecutive restriction of cardiac filling, and finally constrictive pericarditis [94], if not interrupted by treatment or spontaneous improvement. Infectious pericarditis often results from contiguous extension of pneumonia, empyema, myocarditis, suppurative mediastinal lymphadenitis, myocardial abscess, and infective endocarditis. Pericarditis can also result from spread during bactereimia, especially in pericarditis due to S. aureus and H. influenzae in children.

Anaerobic infection of the pericardium can result from (1) a spread from a contiguous focus of infection, either de novo or after surgery or trauma (pleuropulmonary, esophageal fistula or perforation, and odontogenic); (2) a spread from a focus of infection within the heart, most commonly from endocarditis; (3) a hematogenous infection, and (4) a direct inoculation as a result of a penetrating injury or cardiothoracic surgery [95, 96].

The microbiological evaluation of pericardial fluid retrieved by pericardiocentesis should include gram, acid-fast, and silver stains as well as cultures for aerobic and anaerobic bacteria, isolation of or PCR for pericardiotropic viruses, mycobacteria, and fungi. Latex agglutination tests for bacterial antigens can facilitate diagnosis. Blood cultures should also be performed, as they can be positive in 40–70% of the instances [96].

Complete identification and testing for antimicrobial susceptibility and lactamase production are essential for the management of bacterial infections of the pericardium.

Bacteriology of Pericardial Effusion in Tuberculous Pericarditis

The diagnosis of tuberculous pericarditis is made by the identification of Mycobacterium tuberculosis in the pericardial fluid or tissue, and/or the presence of caseous granulomas in the pericardium [33, 97]. Staining for acid-fast bacilli, a positive mycobacterium culture, preferably with radiometric growth detection (e.g., BACTEC-460), increased levels of adenosine deaminase (ADA >40 IU/l), interferon-gamma (> 200 pg/l), and pericardial lysozyme (> 6.5 microg/dl), as well as positive PCR findings are also highly accurate [36, 53, 69–76, 78].

However, it should be noted that PCR is as sensitive (75% vs. 83%), but more specific (100% vs. 78%) than ADA estimation for tuberculous pericarditis [98, 99]. Importantly, PCR can identify DNA of Mycobacterium tuberculosis rapidly from only 1 ml of pericardial fluid [100]. Despite these promising findings, the interpretation of PCR findings and pericardial ADA levels must take into consideration the pretest probability of a diagnosis of tuberculous pericarditis as already pointed out above. In areas where the prevalence of tuberculosis is low, the cost/benefit ratio for these tests is rather low.

Standard mycobacterial cultures (Loewenstein-Jensen medium), have a high diagnostic yield, but 4–6 weeks may be needed for definitive results. Positive cultures for M. tuberculosis from the pericardial fluid have varied from 30–100% [97–101]. The use of liquid media and radiometric methods (e.g., BACTEC) permits the detection and identification of M. tuberculosis in 10–14 days. Drug sensitivity testing can be simultaneously performed on the same specimen; thus, an accurate microbiological diagnosis is available in most patients in 14–18 days. Roberts et al. [102] showed that the BACTEC method shortened the detection of M. tuberculosis and subsequent drug sensitivity testing from an average of 38.5 days with conventional solid media testing to only 18 days.

Strang et al. [103] were able to culture M. tuberculosis from all patients using a double strength Kirchner culture medium after bedside inoculation and also conventional culture in Stonebrink medium. M. tuberculosis was cultured in all 10 patients, in Kirchner medium in nine and in conventional medium only in one.

Since culture of the organism is a prerequisite for susceptibility testing which is essential for proper clinical management of tuberculosis, bacteriologic confirmation and susceptibility testing should be attempted in all cases with suspected tuberculous pericarditis. In addition, HIV test should be performed within two months of the diagnosis of tuberculous pericarditis [104], since in many areas of the world, predominantly in Africa, the association of HIV with TBC is very high.

Cegielski et al. [36] compared PCR, culture, and histopathology in the diagnosis of tuberculous pericarditis. PCR was performed with both pericardial fluid and tissue with IS6110 based primers specific for the M. tuberculosis complex. The overall accuracy of PCR approached the results of conventional methods, although PCR was faster. However, the sensitivity for pericardial fluid was poor and false positive results with PCR remained a concern [98].

In 2004, European Society of Cardiology Guidelines on the diagnosis and management of pericardial disease gave a class I recommendation to the use of PCR for diagnosis of tuberculous pericarditis [77]. However, this recommendation should be interpreted with the following limitations in mind [105]:

Most studies on the validity of PCR in the diagnosis of extrapulmonary tuberculosis have been performed in highly endemic areas and have involved small numbers of patients. The utility of such methods for extrapulmonary tuberculosis in nonendemic areas has not been extensively studied.

The positive predictive value of PCR testing in extrapulmonary tuberculosis is determined not only by the sensitivity and specificity of the test, but also by the pretest likelihood that tuberculosis is present.

In situations in which the pretest probability of tuberculosis is low, PCR testing should be interpreted with caution.

PCR testing for tuberculosis should be undertaken only by laboratories with high standards in performance and quality assurance [99].

Bacteriology of Pericardial Effusion in Patients with AIDS

The aquired immune deficiency syndrome (AIDS) predisposes patients to infection by multiple organisms. Many of them are opportunistic. AIDS has become a leading cause of infectious pericardial disease worldwide [106], but was rarely found in a large cohort of the German Competence Net in Heart Failure (personal communication Dr. Neumann). In AIDS pericarditis, the incidence of bacterial infection is much higher than in the general population, where it is below 23%. A high proportion of Mycobacterium avium-intracellulare infection was described with 35% of all patients with bacterial pericarditis [107, 108]. Immune deficiency during AIDS also imposes an increased risk for infection with S. aureus, K. pneumoniae, M. tuberculosis, and some rare bacterial species [109–111]. In progressive disease the incidence of echocardiographically detected pericardial effusion is up to 40% [112, 113], but cardiac tamponade is rare [114]. The rate of HIV and tuberculosis co-infection varies widely among different geographic areas and may be up to 58% in patients with tuberculosis [115]. Patients with HIV infection and tuberculosis can usually be treated with standard antituberculous regimens, with good results, although prolonged therapy may be warranted in some cases [116] and multidrug-resistant tuberculosis could cause serious additional problems [117]. Patients with tuberculosis and HIV may also have a more rapid resolution of their tuberculosis if the HIV infection is treated concurrently. Since treatment of HIV may require protease inhibitors or non-nucleoside reverse transcriptase inhibitors, the use of rifampicin may be precluded [52]. The use of corticosteroid therapy as an adjunct to tuberculostatic treatment is recommended but their safety in HIV-infected patients has not been established conclusively [77, 118, 119].

Tumor Markers

Our current knowledge on the diagnostic utility of the determination of tumor markers in pericardial effusion is limited by the small series of patients in studies available so far. Furthermore, tumor markers are highly suggestive of malignant effusions when antigen levels are very high in the effusion, but are of limited value, if they are only modestly increased [120–122].

In addition, the number of tumor markers tested in pericardial effusion is relatively small (carcinoembryonic antigen (CEA), neuron-specific enolase (NSE), and carbohydrate antigen 125 (CA125), cytokeratin-19 fragments (CYFRA 21-1)), as well are the studied populations of patients. According to the experience from analyses of other body fluids (pleural effusion, ascites) several other tumor markers are of potential interest. Elevated ascitic hyaluronic acid levels have been associated with mesothelioma [123]. Squamous cell carcinoma antigen [120, 124], CA 19-9 [125, 126], tissue polypeptide antigen (TPA) [120, 125, 126], alpha-fetoprotein [120], and cytokeratin fragments 21-1 (CYFRA 21-1) [127, 128] were studied as potential diagnostic parameters for neoplastic pleural effusion.

Carcinoembrionic Antigen (CEA)

Carcinoembrionic antigen (CEA) is used in the assessment and follow-up of tumors of the colon, liver, pancreas and lung, when measured in the serum of patients. Serum CEA can be elevated, however, also in inflammatory processes of these organs as well as in smokers. It is therefore of limited value in the early detection of cancer in these organs. But it has been used to identify malignant pericardial effusions [71, 129–131]. Koh et al. [71] have shown that the pericardial CEA level in benign fluids is significantly lower than in malignant pericarditis. With a cut-off level of 5 ng/ml, the sensitivity was 75% and the specificity 100% in the diagnosis of malignant pericarditis. Differentiation of tuberculous from neoplastic effusion is virtually absolute with low levels of ADA and high levels of CEA [71].

In the study of Szturmowicz et al. [131] the median CEA value in malignant effusions was 80 ng/ml (range 0–305 ng/ml) and in non-malignant ones 1.26 ng/ml (range 0.2–18.4 ng/ml), resulting in a p-value < 0.01. The sensitivity of a CEA elevation above 5 ng/ml for the recognition of malignant pericarditis was 73% and the specificity was 90%. Pericardial fluid cytology was positive in 22 of 26 patients with malignant pericarditis (85%). CEA exceeding 5 ng/ml or a positive cytology were seen in 96% of the patients with malignant pericarditis.

Neuron-Specific Enolase (NSE)

NSE (neuron-specific enolase) is found predominantly in nerve cells, in neuroendocrine cells of the gastrointestinal tract. It is an accepted marker for children with neuroblastoma. It is also found increased in the blood of patients with oat cell carcinoma of the lung, metastatic seminoma, but also „nonspecifically" elevated in various infectious lung diseases. Szturmowicz et al. [131] have shown that neuron-specific enolase (NSE) is associated with malignant pericardial effusions. The median value of NSE in malignant pericardial effusions was 41.8 µg/l (range 2–172 µg/l) and in non-malignant ones 5.85 µg/l (range 1–83.9 µg/l), p <0.3 due to a large overlap of values. Due to methodological problems, the measurement of NSE in hemorrhagic pericardial fluid is of limited value, since the fragmentation of erythrocytes also causes increased NSE levels.

Carbohydrate Antigen 125 (CA125)

Carbohydrate antigen 125 (CA125) is a tumor marker associated with ovarian cancer and to a lesser extend with pancreas and choledochus carcinoma. Its serum value can be non-specifically increased in liver cirrhosis, acute pancreatitis and cholecystitis and benign processes in gynecology.

Seo et al [132] examined the relationship between serum levels of CA125 and the presence or severity of pericardial effusion. Fifty-seven patients (25 with heart failure, 22 with pericardial metastasis, 4 with hypothyroidism, 4 with renal failure, and 2 with other diseases) in whom pericardial effusion was confirmed by echocardiography or autopsy, were included in the study. Thirty-seven of these patients (65%) tested positive for CA125 in the serum. Of these, no significant differences in serum levels of CA125 were found between patients with benign and those with malignant underlying diseases or between those with, or without, pericarditis. However, CA125 values were higher in the patients with larger pericardial effusions and the serum level decreased when the pericardial effusion was reduced. In some cases, the serum level normalized before the effusion had resolved. Pericardial drainage was performed on 6 patients with cardiac tamponade. Four of these 6 patients had high serum CA125 levels and recurrent pericardial effusion. The other 2 patients had normal serum CA125 levels and no recurrence of effusion.

An immunohistological study showed that a positive stain of pericardial tissues reacting to CA125 antibodies correlated to higher serum and pericardial fluid levels of CA125 than the levels of groups staining negative to the antibody.

These results suggest that CA125 can be useful in assessing the status and clinical course of this disease. However, false positive neoplastic findings in biopsy samples and high levels of CA125 were noted in systemic lupus erythematosus [133].

Alpha-Fetoprotein

Elevated alpha-fetoprotein (AFP) in serum and pericardial fluid was noted in several cases of intrapericardial teratoma [134–136]. Its serum levels can be also elevated in hepatocellular cancer, seminoma, and ovarian cancer. Pericardial metastases of these tumors are, however, extremely rare.

Other Tumor Markers

Studies on other tumor markers with respect to pericardial effusion such as PSA (prostate-specific antigen), CA 15-3 characteristic for breast and ovarian cancer, CA 19-9 characteristic for tumor of the colon, the stomach, the pancreas and liver, or SCC (squamous cell carcinoma antigen) or HCG (human chorionic gonadotropin) are at present not available.

Immunology of the Pericardial Fluid

In autoreactive and viral pericardial effusion lymphocytes represent the predominant cell population. Lymphocytes are also found in tuberculous and some bacterial effusions in counts up to 1000/mm^3 [10]. When higher lymphocyte counts are found in the pericardial fluid, a malignant hematological disease must also be considered.

Latex agglutination of rheumatoid antigen, immunoglobulin complexes, and diminished fluid complement concentration and presence of RA cells in pericardial fluid have been demonstrated. In case reports, increased levels of IL-6 have been reported and associated with disease progression [137–141].

Mixed type cryoglobulins consisting of IgG, IgM, and C1q have been demonstrated in pericardial effusion of patients with systemic lupus erythematosus. Selective concentrations of antinuclear antibodies in the pericardial fluid and cryoglobulin have been demonstrated in case reports. Moreover, anti-DNA antibodies were found in the serum and in the pericardial fluid . Pericardial fluid from the same patient contained immune complexes. Although a negative antinuclear antibody test makes a diagnosis of lupus serositis unlikely, even high antinuclear antibodies titers in pericardial fluid are not diagnostic of lupus serositis. An unexplained high antinuclear antibodies titer in pericardial effusion also warrants the search for malignancy [142].

In autoreactive (virus negative) pericardial effusions antibodies directed against the sarcolemma (ASA), the myolemma (AMLA), fibrils (AFA), and extracellular matrix antigens (ECA) can be found both in the circulating blood and in the exudative effusion and demonstrated by the indirect immunofluorescence test [11, 77]. ASAs, ECAs and AMLAs of the IgG-type are a regular finding in up to 90% of serum and fluid samples (titers > 1:20), AFAs are found in up to 45%, AIDA in less than 3%. AIDA can be found in >50% in the serum of patients with constrictive pericarditis (pers. communication A. Caforio 2010). They may be also complement fixing and thus upholding the activity of an underlying immunological process. In the pericardial effusion in comparable or lower titers when compared to the serum levels antiviral antibodies can be detected. They are a reflection of a serum filtrate into the pericardial sac.

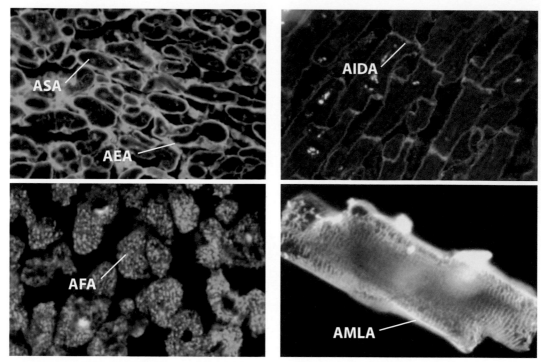

Fig. 7.2. Demonstration of anticardiac serum autoantibodies in autoreactive pericardial effusion, which can also be detected in the pericardial fluid. *ASA* Antisarcolemmal antibodies, *AEA* antiendothelial antibodies, *AFA* antifibrillary antibodies, *AIDA* antiintercalated disk antibodies, *AMLA* antimyolemmal antibodies

Lymphocyte subpopulations in the pericardial effusion can be differentiated most efficiently by means of flow cytofluorometry on fluorescence-activated cell sorters (FACS). Flow cytofluorimetry provides a precise and objective means of quantifying both the number of cells expressing a given surface marker (cluster of differentiation (CD) antigens, adhesion molecules and other activation markers) and the extent of the expression [1]. Certain combinations of surface CD antigens are specific not only for various lymphocyte subsets and various life stages, but also for the inflammatory activation of cells and the specific forms of lymphomas and leukemia [7].

Cytofluorometric analysis of pericardial fluid lymphocytes was performed by Riemann et al. [48] in 127 patients undergoing open cardiac surgery (45 with heart valve disease, 27 with congenital heart defects, and 55 with chronic ischemic heart disease). In the entire study population B cells ranged from 0–40% (mean 5%), natural killer (NK) cells from 4–67% (mean 18%) and T cells from 29–95% (mean 76%).

Among the T cells, the ratio between CD4 (helper) and CD8 (effector) cells varied between 0.2 and 7.0 (mean 1.0). Between 1 and 42% of cells showed the $CD4^+CD8^+$ phenotype (mean 11%) and only 2–6% of T cells were $CD4^--CD8^-$. Similar to T cells of body fluids other than in the peripheral blood, a high percentage of pericardial fluid T cells expressed CD45R0 and activation-associated molecules such as HLA-DR, -DQ, CD69, CD54, and CD26. In addition, it was previously shown that $CD45R0^+$ cells migrate preferentially from the peripheral blood to the sites of inflammation. These cells are considered to be memory cells and have increased expression of adhesion/activation molecules that facilitate cell-matrix and cell-to-cell interactions, as well as antigen recognition. This finding is also characteristic for inflammatory cardiomyopathy, when in endomyocardial biopsy the specific subset of T-cells is determined.

Among the three studied groups of patients, T lymphocytes of patients with congenital heart disease showed the highest proportion of CD69+ and CD11b+ and the lowest number of CD25+ cells. CD11b has been suggested as possible marker of CD8+ cytotoxic T cell activation and memory in virus infection. The highest percentage of aminopeptidase N/CD13+ T cells could be observed in patients with valvular disease. The observed differences could be explained by the type and extent of T-cell activation in a specific local environment. The difference among the groups was not significant for other investigated CD markers.

The studies comparing the immunophenotype of pericardial fluid lymphocytes in different forms of pericarditis with patients undergoing cardiac surgery for valvular or ischemic heart disease are currently under way. In addition to their undoubted value in recognizing hematological malignancies [7], FACS analyses are expected to reveal the role of diverse lymphocyte subsets in pathophysiology of the various forms of pericardial inflammation.

Serodiagnosis of Tuberculous Pericarditis

Ng et al. [143] tested a solid phase antibody competition sandwich ELISA (SACT-CE) for the serodiagnosis of tuberculous pericarditis. A monoclonal antibody (CDC/WHO reference number IT39), raised against a specific epitope on the M. tuberculosis 30 kDa antigen was used. All but one of the patients had a negative sputum microscopy for acid-fast bacilli. A sensitivity of 61% with a 96% specificity was reported. More recently a broad clonal heterogeneity of antigen specific CD4+ T-cells localizing at the site of tuberculous disease were observed [143].

A radioimmunoassay for detecting tuberculous antigens and antibodies have been standardized for cerebrospinal, pleural and ascitic fluids, but their sensitivity and specificity for the diagnosis of pericardial tuberculosis has not yet been established because of the lack of a "gold standard" [105].

Future Perspectives and Recommendations

The analyses of a pericardial effusion in conjunction with the clinical presentation may be very helpful in uncovering the etiology of the disease. They can directly establish the diagnosis of viral, bacterial, tuberculous, fungal, cholesterol, and malignant pericarditis.

The future development of the pericardial fluid analyses will have to include a more precise diagnosis of neoplastic disease based on immunocytochemical evaluations. In non-malignant pericarditis their analysis shows that cascades of the immune system are involved and that the term "idiopathic" pericardial effusion is just the label for ignorance. Further research on pericardial cytokines in various etiological forms of the disease is promising and might elucidate the pathophysiology and pathogenesis further. Similar to the sets of surface immunocytochemical markers currently available to identify inflammatory or neoplastic cells, it will be possible in the future to determine specific cytokine patterns characteristic for the pathogenesis and the etiology of the underlying disease. This will enable the selection of an appropriate causative treatment for the individual patient.

References

1. Meyers DG, Meyers RE, Prendergast TW. The usefulness of diagnostic tests on pericardial fluid. Chest 1997; 111: 1213–1221
2. Spodick DH. Diagnostic interpretation of pericardial fluids. Chest 1997; 111: 1156–1157
3. Kjeldsberg CR, Knight JA (eds) Body fluids. 3rd edition. American Society of Clinical Pathologists Press, Chicago, 1993, pp. 159–254
4. Wiener HG, Kristensen IB, Haubek A, Kristensen B, Baandrup U. The diagnostic value of pericardial cytology. An analysis of 95 cases. Acta Citol 1991; 35(2): 149–153
5. King DT, Nieberg RK. The use of cytology to evaluate pericardial effusions. Ann Clin Lab Sci 1979; 9: 8–23
6. Meyers DG, Boyska DJ. Diagnostic usefulness of pericardial fluid cytology. Chest 1989; 95: 1142–1143
7. Malamou-Mitsi VD, Zioga AP, Agnantis NJ. Diagnostic accuracy of pericardial fluid cytology: an analysis of 53 specimens from 44 consecutive patients. Diagn Cytopathol 1996; 15(3): 197–204
8. Garcia LW, Ducatman BS, Wang HH. The value of multiple fluid specimens in the cytological diagnosis of malignancy. Mod Pathol 1994; 7(6): 665–668
9. Krikorian JG, Hancock EW. Pericardiocentesis. Am J Med 1978; 65: 808–814
10. Corey GR, Campbell PT, Van Trigt P, et al. Etiology of large pericardial effusions. Am J Med 1993; 95: 209–213

11. Maisch B, Bethge C, Drude L, Hufnagel G, Herzum M, Schönian U. Pericardioscopy and epicardial biopsy – new diagnostic tools in pericardial and perimyocardial disease. Eur Heart J 1994; 15(Suppl C): 68–73

12. Reyes CV, Strinden C, Banerji M. The role of cytology in neoplastic tamponade. Acta Cytol 1981; 26: 299–302

13. Theologides A. Neoplastic cardiac tamponade. Semin Oncol 1978; 5: 181–192

14. Johnson WD. The cytological diagnosis of cancer in serous effusions. Acta Cytol 1966; 10: 161–172

15. Posner WR, Cohen GI, Skarin AT. Pericardial disease in patients with cancer: the differential diagnosis of malignant from idiopathic and radiation-induced pericarditis. Am J Med 1981; 71: 407–413

16. Decker DA, Dines DE, Payne WS, et al. The significance of a cytologically negative pleural effusion in bronchogenic carcinoma. Chest 1978; 74: 640–642

17. Bardales RH, Stanley MW, Schaefer RF, Liblit RL, Owens RB, Surhland MJ. Secondary pericardial malignancies: a critical appraisal of the role of cytology, pericardial biopsy, and DNA ploidy analysis. Am J Clin Pathol 1996;106(1): 29-34.

18. Maisch B, Ristić AD. Practical aspects of the management of pericardial disease. Heart 2003; 89: 1096–1103

19. Wilkes JD, Fidias P, Vaickus L, Perez RP. Malignancy-related pericardial effusion. 127 cases from the Roswell Park Cancer Institute. Cancer 1995; 76(8): 1377–1387

20. Chen CJ, Chang SC, Tseng HH. Assessment of immunocytochemical and histochemical stainings in the distinction between reactive mesothelial cells and adenocarcinoma cells in body effusions. Chung Hua Hsueh Tsa Chih Taipei 1994; 54(3): 49–55

21. Chen LM, Chao TY, Chiang JH, et al. Examination of pericardial effusions by cytology and immunocytochemistry. Chung Hua Hsueh Tsa Chih Taipei 1996; 58(4): 248–253

22. Fischler DF, Wongbunnate S, Johnston DA, Katz RL. DNA content by image analysis. An accurate discriminator of malignancy in pericardial effusions. Anal Quant Cytol Histol 1994; 16(3): 167–173

23. Rijken A, Dekker A, Taylor S, Hoffman P, Blank M, Krause JR. Diagnostic value of DNA analysis in effusions by flow cytometry and image analysis. A prospective study on 102 patients as compared with cytologic examination. Am J Clin Pathol 1991; 95(1): 6–12

24. Zakowski MF, Lanuale S, Shanerman A. Cytology of pericardial effusions in AIDS patients. Diagn Cytopathol 1993; 9(3): 266–269

25. Edoute Y, Kuten A, Ben Haim SA, Moscovitz M, Malberger E. Symptomatic pericardial effusion in breast cancer patients: the role of fluid cytology. J Surg Oncol 1990; 45(4): 265–269

26. Edoute Y, Malberger E, Kuten A, Moscovitcz M, Ben Haim SA. Symptomatic pericardial effusion in lung cancer patients: the role of fluid cytology. J Surg Oncol 1990; 45(2): 121–123

27. Edoute Y, Malberger E, Kuten A, Ben Haim SA, Moscovitz M. Cytologic analysis of pericardial effusion complicating extracardiac malignancy. Am J Cardiol 1992; 69(5): 568–571

28. Wang PC, Yang KY, Chao JY, Liu JM, Perng RP, Yen SH. Prognostic role of pericardial fluid cytology in cardiac tamponade associated with non-small cell lung cancer. Chest 2000; 118: 744–749

29. Thurber DL, Edwards JE, Achor RWP. Secondary malignant tumors of the pericardium. Circulation 1962; 26: 228–241

30. Johnson WD. The cytological diagnosis of cancer in serous effusions. Acta Cytol 1966; 10: 161–172

31. Sahn SA. Malignant pleural effusion. Semin Respir Med 1987; 9: 43–53

32. Chernow B, Sahn SA. Carcinomatous involvement of the pleura: an analysis of 96 patients. Am J Med 1977; 63: 695–702

33. Fowler NO. Tuberculous pericarditis. JAMA 1991; 266: 99–103

34. Burgess LJ, Reuter H, Taljaard JJ, Doubell AF. Role of biochemical tests in the diagnosis of large pericardial effusions. Chest 2002; 121(2): 495–499

35. Paramothayan NS, Barron J. New criteria for the differentiation between transudates and exudates. J Clin Pathol 2002; 55: 69–71

36. Cegielski JP, Devlin BH, Morris AJ, et al. Comparison of PCR, culture and histopathology for the diagnosis of tuberculous pericarditis. J Clin Microbiol 1997; 35: 3254–3257

37. Light RW, MacGregor MI, Luchsinger PC, et al. Pleural effusions: the diagnostic separation of transudates and exudates. Ann Intern Med 1972; 77: 507–513

38. Light RW. Diagnostic principles in pleural disease. Eur Respir J 1997; 10: 476–481

39. Jay SJ. Diagnostic procedures for pleural diseases: symposium on pleural diseases. Clin Chest Med 1985; 6: 33–48

40. Roth BJ, O'Meara TF, Cragun WH. The serum-effusion albumin gradient in the evaluation of pleural effusions. Chest 1990; 98: 546–549

41. Hamm H, Brohan U, Bohmer R, et al. Cholesterol in pleural effusions: a diagnostic aid. Chest 1987; 92: 296–302

42. Pillay VKG. Total proteins in serous fluids in cardiac failure. S Afr Med J 1965; 39: 142–143

43. Chakko SC, Caldwell SH, Sforza PP. Treatment of congestive heart failure: its effect on pleural fluid chemistry. Chest 1989; 95: 978–982

44. Chakko S. Pleural effusion in congestive heart failure. Chest 1990; 95: 521–522

45. Pankuweit S, Wadlich A, Meyer E, Portig I, Hufnagel G, Maisch B. Cytokine activation in pericardial fluids in different forms of pericarditis. Herz 2000; 25(8): 748–754

46. Afanasyeva M, Georgakopoulos D, Fairweather D, Caturegli P, Kass DA, Rose NR. Novel model of constrictive pericarditis associated with autoimmune heart disease in interferon gamma-knockout mice. Circulation 2004; 110: 2910–2917

47. Ristić AD, Pankuweit S, Meyer E, et al. Proinflammatory and immunoregulatory cytokines in neoplastic, autoreactive, and viral pericarditis. Eur Heart J 2004; 25(Suppl.): P673

48. Riemann D, Wollert HG, Menschikowski J, Mittenzwei S, Langner J. Immunophenotype of lymphocytes in pericardial fluid from patients with different forms of heart disease. Int Arch Allergy Immunol 1994; 104(1): 48–56

49. Vila LM, Rivera del Rio JR, Rios Z, Rivera E. Lymphocyte populations and cytokine concentrations in pericardial fluid from a systemic lupus erythematosus patient with cardiac tamponade. Ann Rheum Dis 1999; 58(11): 720–721

50. Shikama N, Terano T, Hirai A. A case of rheumatoid pericarditis with high concentrations of interleukin-6 in pericardial fluid. Heart 2000; 83(6): 711–712

51. Abe Y, Muta K, Kato S, et al. A high serum level of interleukin-6 in a patient with aggressive multiple myeloma. Rinsho Ketsueki 1991; 32(11): 1458–1462

52. Takahashi R, Ashihara E, Hirata T, et al. Aggressive myeloma with subcutaneous tumor and pericardial involvement. Rinsho Ketsueki 1994; 35(3): 291–295

53. Burgess LJ, Reuter H, Carstens ME, Taljaard JJF, Doubell AF. The use of adenosine deaminase and interferon-gamma as diagnostic tools for tuberculous pericarditis. Chest 2002; 122: 900–905

54. Mistchenko AS, Maffey AF, Casal G, Kajon AE. Adenoviral pericarditis: high levels of interleukin 6 in pericardial fluid. Pediatr Infect Dis J 1995; 14(11): 1007–1009

55. Nakayama R, Yoneyama T, Takatani O, Kimura K. A study of metastatic tumors to the heart, pericardium and great vessels. Jpn Heart J 1966; 7: 227–234

56. Dore P, Lelievre E, Morel F, et al. IL-6 and soluble IL-6 receptors (sIL-6R and sgp130) in human pleural effusions: massive IL-6 production independently of underlying diseases. Clin Exp Immunol 1997; 107(1): 182–188

57. Hoheisel G, Izbicki G, Roth M, et al. Proinflammatory cytokine levels in patients with lung cancer and carcinomatous pleurisy. Respiration 1998; 65(3): 183–186

58. Nakano T, Chahinian AP, Shinjo M, et al. Interleukin 6 and its relationship to clinical parameters in patients with malignant pleural mesothelioma. Br J Cancer 1998; 77(6): 907–912

59. Zhang GJ, Adachi I. Serum interleukin-6 levels correlate to tumor progression and prognosis in metastatic breast carcinoma. Anticancer Res 1999; 19(2B): 1427–1423

60. Yokoyama A, Maruyama M, Ito M, Kohno N, Hiwada K, Yano S. Interleukin 6 activity in pleural effusion. Its diagnostic value and thrombopoietic activity. Chest 1992; 102(4): 1055–1059

61. Marie C, Losser MR, Fitting C, Kermarrec N, Payen D, Cavaillon JM. Cytokines and soluble cytokine receptors in pleural effusions from septic and nonseptic patients. Am J Respir Crit Care Med 1997; 156(5): 1515–1522

62. Weissflog D, Kroegel C, Luttmann W, Grahmann PR, Hasse J. Leukocyte infiltration and secretion of cytokines in pleural drainage fluid after thoracic surgery: impaired cytokine response in malignancy and postoperative complications. Chest 1999; 115(6): 1604–1610

63. De Pablo A, Villena V, Echave-Sustaeta J, Encuentra AL. Are pleural fluid parameters related to the development of residual pleural thickening in tuberculosis? Chest 1997; 112(5): 1293–1297

64. Hua CC, Chang LC, Chen YC, Chang SC. Proinflammatory cytokines and fibrinolytic enzymes in tuberculous and malignant pleural effusions. Chest 1999; 116(5): 1292–1296

65. Maeda J, Ueki N, Ohkawa T, et al. Transforming growth factor-beta 1 (TGF-beta 1)- and beta 2-like activities in malignant pleural effusions caused by malignant mesothelioma or primary lung cancer. Clin Exp Immunol 1994; 98(2): 319–322

66. Ikubo A, Morisaki T, Katano M, et al. A possible role of TGF-beta in the formation of malignant effusions. Clin Immunol Immunopathol 1995; 77(1): 27–32

67. Van der Weyden MB, Kelley WN. Human adenosine deaminase distribution and properties. J Biol Chem 1976; 251: 5448–5456

68. Bovornkitti S, Pushpakom R, Maranetra N, et al. Adenosine deaminase and lymphocytic populations. Chest 1991; 99: 789–790

69. Ocaña I, Martinez-Vazquez JM, Segura RM, et al. Adenosine deaminase in pleural fluids: test for diagnosis of tuberculous pleural effusion. Chest 1983; 84: 51–53

70. Burgess LJ, Maritz FJ, Le Roux I, et al. Use of adenosine deaminase as a diagnostic tool for tuberculous pleurisy. Thorax 1995; 50: 672–674

71. Koh KK, Kim EJ, Cho CH, et al. Adenosine deaminase and carcinoembryonic antigen in pericardial effusion diagnosis, especially in suspected tuberculous pericarditis. Circulation 1994; 89: 2728–2735

72. Komsuoglu B, Goldeli O, Kulan K, Komsuoglu SS. The diagnostic and prognostic value of adenosine deaminase in tuberculous pericarditis. Eur Heart J 1995; 16(8): 1126–1130

73. Telenti M, Fdez J, Susano R, et al. Tuberculous pericarditis: diagnostic value of adenosine deaminase. Presse Med 1991; 20: 637–640

74. Martinez-Vazquez JM, Ribera E, Ocaña I, et al. Adenosine deaminase activity in tuberculous pericarditis. Thorax 1986; 41: 888–889

75. Aggeli C, Pitsavos C, Brili S, et al. Relevance of adenosine deaminase and lysozyme measurements in the diagnosis of tuberculous pericarditis. Cardiology 2000; 94: 81–85

76. Dogan R, Demircin M, Sarigul A, et al. Diagnostic value of adenosine deaminase activity in pericardial fluids. J Cardiovasc Surg 1999; 40: 501–504

77. Maisch B, Seferovic PM, Ristic AD, et al. The Task force on the diagnosis and management of pericardial diseases of the European society of cardiology. Guidelines on the diagnosis and management of pericardial diseases (executive summary). Eur Heart J 2004; 25: 587–610

78. Arroyo M, Soberman JE. Adenosine deaminase in the diagnosis of tuberculous pericardial effusion. Am J Med Sci 2008; 335(3): 227–229

79. Campbell PT, Li JS, Wall TC, O'Connor CM, et al. Cytomegalovirus pericarditis: a case series and review of the literature. Am J Med Sci 1995; 309(4): 229–234

80. Rolston KV. Group G streptococcal infections. Arch Intern Med 1986; 146: 857–858

81. Lam K, Bayer AS. Serious infections due to group G streptococci. Am J Med 1983; 75: 561–570

82. Fujita NK, Lam K, Bayer AS. Septic arthritis due to group G streptococcus. JAMA 1982; 247: 812–813

83. Rubin RH, Moellering RC Jr. Clinical, microbiologic and therapeutic aspects of purulent pericarditis. Am J Med 1975; 59: 68–78

84. Klacsmann PG, Bulkley BH, Hutchins GM. The changed spectrum of purulent pericarditis: an 86 year autopsy experience in 200 patients. Am J Med 1977; 63: 666–673

85. Sagrista-Sauleda J, Barrabes JA, Permanyer-Miralda G, Soler-Soler J. Purulent pericarditis: review of a 20-year experience in a general hospital. J Am Coll Cardiol 1993; 22: 1661–1665

86. Ricardo Z, Manuel A, Francisco T, et al. Incidence of specific etiology and role of methods for specific etiologic diagnosis of primary acute pericarditis. Am J Cardiol 1995; 75: 378–382

87. Gould K, Barnett JA, Sanford JP. Purulent pericarditis in the antibiotic era. Arch Intern Med 1974; 134: 923–927

88. Klacsmann PG, Bulkley BH, Hutchins GM. The changed spectrum of purulent pericarditis. Am J Med 1975; 59: 68–78

89. Ilan Y, Oren R, Ben-Chetrit E. Acute pericarditis: Etiology, treatment and prognosis. Jpn Heart J 1991; 32: 315–321

90. Soler-Soler J, Permanyer-Miralda G, Sagrista-Sauleda J. A systematic diagnostic approach to primary acute pericardial disease: The Barcelona experience. Cardiol Clin 1990; 8: 609–620

91. Connolly DC, Burchell HB. Pericarditis: A 10-year survey. Am J Cardiol 1961; 7: 7–14

92. Brook I, Frazier EH. Microbiology of acute purulent pericarditis. A 12-year experience in a military hospital. Arch Intern Med 1996; 156: 1857–1860

93. Skiest DJ, Steiner D, Werner M, Gamer JG. Anaerobic pericarditis: Case report and review. Clin Infect Dis 1994; 19: 435–440

94. Aikat S, Ghaffari S. A review of pericardial diseases: Clinical, ECG and hemodynamic features and management. Cleve Clin J Med 2000; 67: 903–914

95. Kim NH, Park JP, Jeon SH, et al. Purulent pericarditis caused by group G streptococcus as an initial presentation of colon cancer. J Korean Med Sci 2002; 17(4): 571–573

96. Kennedy C, McEvoy S. Purulent pericarditis. Ir J Med Sci 2009; 178: 97–99

97. Mayosi BM, Wiysonge CS, Ntsekhe M, et al. Mortality in patients treated for tuberculous pericarditis in sub-Saharan Africa. S Afr Med J 2008; 98(1): 36–40

98. Lee JH, Lee CW, Lee SG, et al. Comparison of polymerase chain reaction with adenosine deaminase activity in pericardial fluid for the diagnosis of tuberculous pericarditis. Am J Med 2002; 113: 519–521

99. Piersimoni C, Scarparo C. Relevance of commercial amplification methods for direct detection of Mycobacterium tuberculosis complex in clinical samples. J Clin Microbiol 2003; 41: 5355–5365

100. Seino Y, Ikeda U, Kawaguchi K, et al. Tuberculous pericarditis presumably diagnosed by polymerase chain reaction analysis. Am Heart J 1993; 126: 249–251

101. Sagrista-Sauleda J, Permanyer-Miralda G, Soler-Soler J. Tuberculous pericarditis: ten-year experience with a prospective protocol for diagnosis and treatment. J Am Coll Cardiol 1988; 11: 724–728

102. Roberts GD, Goodman NL, Heifets L, et al. Evaluation of the BACTEC radiometric method for recovery of mycobacterium tuberculosis from acid-fast smear-positive specimens. J Clin Microbiol 1983; 18(3): 689–696

103. Strang JI. Rapid resolution of tuberculous pericardial effusions with high dose prednisone and anti-tuberculous drugs. J Infect 1994; 28(3): 251–254

104. Horsburgh CR Jr, Feldman S, Ridzon R. Infectious Diseases Society of America. Practice guidelines for the treatment of tuberculosis. Clin Infect Dis 2000; 31(3): 633–639

105. Mayosi BM, Burgess LJ, Doubell AF. Tuberculous pericarditis. Circulation 2005; 112(23): 3608–3616

106. Harmon WG, Dadlani GH, Fisher SD, Lipshultz SE. Myocardial and pericardial disease in HIV. Curr Treat Options Cardiovasc Med 2002; 4(6): 497–509

107. Goodman LJ. Purulent pericarditis. Curr Treat Options Cardiovasc Med 2000; 2(4): 343–350

108. Estok L, Wallach F. Cardiac tamponade in a patient with AIDS: a review of pericardial disease in patients with HIV infection. Mt Sinai J Med 1998; 65(1): 33–39

109. DeCastro S, Migliau G, Silvestri A, et al. Heart involvement in AIDS: a prospective study during various stages of the disease. Eur Heart J 1992; 13: 1452–1459

110. Nathan PE, Arsura EL, Zappi M. Pericarditis with tamponade due to cytomegalovirus and the acquired immunodeficiency syndrome. Chest 1991; 99: 765–766

111. Toma E, Poisson M, Claessens MR, et al. Herpes simplex type 2 pericarditis and bilateral facial palsy in patients with AIDS. J Infect Dis 1989; 160: 553–554

112. Chen Y, Brennessel D, Walters J, et al. Human immunodeficiency virus-associated pericardial effusion: report of 40 cases and review of literature. Am Heart J 1999; 137: 516–521

113. Fink L, Reicheck N, Sutton MG. Cardiac abnormalities in acquired immune deficiency syndrome. Am J Cardiol 1984; 54: 1161–1163

114. Silva-Cardoso J, Moura B, Martins L, et al. Pericardial involvement in human immunodeficiency virus infection. Chest 1999; 115: 418–422

115. Onorato IM, McCray E. Prevalence of human immunodeficiency virus infection among patients attending tuberculosis clinics in the United States. J Infect Dis 1992; 165(1): 87–92

116. Centers for Disease Control and Prevention. Prevention and treatment of tuberculosis among patients infected with human immunodeficiency virus: principles of therapy and revised recommendations. MMWR Morb Mortal Wkly Rep 1998; 47(RR-20): 1–51

117. Wells CD, Cegielski JP, Nelson LJ, et al. HIV infection and multidrug-resistant tuberculosis: the perfect storm. J Infect Dis 2007; 196 (Suppl 1): S86–107

118. Evans DJ. The use of adjunctive corticosteroids in the treatment of pericardial, pleural and meningeal tuberculosis: do they improve outcome? Respir Med 2008; 102(6): 793–800

119. Syed FF, Mayosi BM. A modern approach to tuberculous pericarditis. Prog Cardiovasc Dis 2007; 50(3): 218–236

120. San José NE, Alvarez D, Valdés L, et al. Utility of tumour markers in the diagnosis of neoplastic pleural effusion. Clin Chim Acta 1997; 265: 193–205

121. Hanley KZ, Facik MS, Bourne PA, et al. Utility of anti-L523S antibody in the diagnosis of benign and malignant serous effusions. Cancer 2008; 114(1): 49–56

122. Szturmowicz M, Tomkowski W, Fijalkowska A, et al. Diagnostic utility of CYFRA 21-1 and CEA assays in pericardial fluid for the recognition of neoplastic pericarditis. Int J Biol Markers 2005; 20(1): 43–49

123. Kjeldsberg CR, Knight JA, editors. Body fluids. 3rd edition. American Society of Clinical Pathologists Press, Chicago, 1993, pp 159–254

124. Conejo JR, Benedito JE, Jiminez A, et al. Diagnostic value of three tumor markers determined in pleural effusions. Eur J Clin Chem Biochem 1996; 34: 139–142

125. Niwa Y, Kishimoto H, Shimokata K. Carcinomatous and tuberculous pleural effusions; comparison of tumour markers. Chest 1985; 87: 351–355

126. Mezger J, Permanetter W, Gerbes AL, et al. Tumour-associated antigens in diagnosis of serous effusions. J Clin Pathol 1988; 41: 633–643

127. Salama G, Miedouge M, Rouzard P, et al. Evaluation of pleural CYFRA 21-1 and carcinoembryonic antigen in the diagnosis of malignant pleural effusions. Br J Cancer 1998; 77. 472–476

128. Lee YC, Knox BS, Garrett JE. Use of cytokeratin fragments 19.1 and 19.21 (Cyfra 21-1) in the differentiation of malignant and benign pleural effusions. Aust N Z J Med 1999; 29: 765–769

129. Koh KK, In HH, Lee KH, et al. New scoring system using tumour markers in diagnosing patients with moderate pericardial effusions. Int J Cardiol 1997; 61: 5–13

130. Tatsuta M, Yamamura H, Yamamoto R, et al. Carcinoembryonic antigens in the pericardial fluid of patients with malignant pericarditis. Oncology 1984; 41: 328–330

131. Szturmowicz M, Tomkowski W, Fijalkowska A, et al. The role of carcinoembryonic antigen (CEA) and neuron-specific enolase (NSE) evaluation in pericardial fluid for the recognition of malignant pericarditis. Int J Biol Markers 1997; 12: 96–101

132. Seo T, Ikeda Y, Onaka H et al. Usefulness of serum CA125 measurement for monitoring pericardial effusion. Jpn Circ J 1993; 57(6): 489–494

133. Yücel AE, Calguneri M, Ruacan S. False positive pleural biopsy and high CA125 levels in serum and pleural effusion in systemic lupus erythematosus. Clin Rheumatol 1996; 15(3): 295–297

134. Roy N, Blurton DJ, Azakie A, Karl TR. Immature intrapericardial teratoma in a newborn with elevated alpha-fetoprotein. Ann Thorac Surg 2004; 78(1): e6–8

135. Carachi R, Campbell PE, Chow CW, Mee BB. Alpha-fetoprotein-(AFP-)-secreting intra-pericardial teratoma – report of a case diagnosed on CT scanning. Z Kinderchir 1986; 41(6): 369–370

136. Upadhyaya M, Jaffar Sajwany M, Tomas-Smigura E. Recurrent immature mediastinal teratoma with life-threatening respiratory distress in a neonate. Eur J Pediatr Surg 2003; 13(6): 403–406

137. Calick A, Bishop R. Pericardial effusion in rheumatoid arthritis. Chest 1973; 64: 778–779

138. Dogan R, Demircin M, Sarigul A, Ciliv G, Bozer AY. Diagnostic value of adenosine deaminase activity in pericardial fluids. J Cardiovasc Surg (Torino) 1896; 40: 501–504

139. Godfrey-Faussett P, Wilkins EG, Khoo S, Stoker N. Tuberculous pericarditis confirmed by DNA amplification. Lancet 1991; 337: 176–177

140. Shikama N, Terano T, Hirai A. A case of rheumatoid pericarditis with high concentrations of interleukin-6 in pericardial fluid. Heart 2000; 83(6): 711–712

141. Thadani U, Iveson JM, Wright V. Cardiac tamponade, constrictive pericarditis and pericardial resection in rheumatoid arthritis. Medicine (Baltimore) 1975; 54: 261–270

142. Leventhal LJ, DeMarco DM, Zurier RB. Antinuclear antibody in pericardial fluid from a patient with primary cardiac lymphoma. Arch Intern Med 1990; 150: 1113–1115

143. Ng TT, Strang JI, Wilkins EG. Serodiagnosis of pericardial tuberculosis. Q J Med 1995; 88: 317–320

Pericardiosopy: Endoscopic Insight in Pericardial and Epicardial Pathology

Introduction

Percutaneous pericardioscopy is a diagnostic tool for the endoscopic visualization of lesions in both the epicardium and parietal pericardium. It enables safe and efficient targeted epicardial and parietal pericardial biopsy and provides the cardiologist with not only macroscopic but also microscopic evidence of pathologic changes [1].

Pericardial endoscopy was enthusiastically introduced more than 50 years ago by Synitsin [2] and Volkmann [3] (see Chapter 1), and further developed by Santos and Frater [4], Kondos et al. in 1986 [5, 6], Little and Ferguson in 1986 [7], Millaire et al. in 1988 [8] and 1992 [9], Wurtz et al. in 1992 [10], Nugue et al. in 1996 [11], and Porte in 1999 [12]. Since 1991 Maisch et al. have reported in the several publications on the transcutaneous method in local anesthesia [13–20]. The same method was later on modified and also clinically applied by Seferović and Ristić since 1998 [1, 21–24], allowing the increasing use of the procedure in patients with various pericardial diseases. Additional diagnostic progress came from thoracoscopic surgeons [25–39]. The improvement associated with the substitution of rigid to flexible fiberglass instruments and to video documentation instead of photography [18–20, 23, 24] further ameliorated the clinical application of the method.

Refined new methods to access the pericardium such as especially atraumatic Touhy needle, the PerDUCER, and PeriAttacher (see Chapters 5 and 6) have opened the window to very small effusions. However, the technique is at present not widely accepted in clinical practice, still mostly because of its technical complexity. More recently, interest has been focused on immunocytochemistry, immunohistochemistry and molecular biology techniques such as polymerase chain reaction (PCR) to cardiotropic agents which have significantly improved the diagnostic yield of epicardial and pericardial biopsies, therefore offering wider indications for pericardioscopy [15–20, 40–44].

Technical Considerations

Selection of the Endoscope

Despite five decades of world-wide experience with pericardioscopy, no specific device of any endoscope-producing companies has been designed and approved for application in pericardial diseases. The high technical demands that are imposed on the manufacturers include: small outer diameter to allow use in local anesthesia (less than 5 mm), but still large enough to accommodate the working channel for aimed pericardial and epicardial biopsy (minimum

Table 8.1. Rigid endoscopes used for pericardioscopy

Model of endoscope	Author (year of publication)	Reference
Optical system fixed on the thoracic wall (not the true endoscope)	N.P. Synitsin (1955)	2
Encephaloscope (1923) and cystoscope (1930) C.G. Heymann (Leipzig and Munich, Germany)	J. Volkmann (1957)	3
Rigid mediastinoscope	Santos and Frater 1977	4
Rigid mediastinoscope	Little and Ferguson 1986	7
Rigid mediastinoscope	Azorin 1988	25
Rigid mediastinoscope 17 cm (Hesen) or pericardioscope 24 cm long, 2 cm thick Karl Storz 10970B	Porte 1999, Nugue 1996, Millaire 1992, Wurtz 1992	8-12
Rigid urethroscope, Storz	Maisch 1991	13, 14
Video thoracoscope	Mack 1993	26
Rigid mediastinoscope	Houdelette 1993	27
Video thoracoscope	Liu 1994	31
Rigid laparoscope	Staltari 2007	50
Video thoracoscope	Pego-Fernandes 2008	39

Table 8.2. Flexible endoscopes applied for pericardioscopy

Model of endoscope	Author	Reference:
Olympus bronchoscope BF 4B2, D 4.8 mm, working channel 2 mm	Kondos 1986	5, 6
Flexible choledochoscope, Olympus CHF 4B	Wong 1987	51
Flexible urethroscope, Vantec, Baxter, and Storz	Maisch 1991, 1994	13-15
Flexible bronchoscope	Urschel 1993	52
Olympus HYF-1D, 16F, diagnostic hysterosalpingoscope	Rodriguez 1994	53
Olympus HYF-1T, 16F, interventional hysterosalpingoscope	Seferović and Ristić 1998, 2000, 2003	1, 21-24
Karl Storz AF1101B1	Maisch 2001, 2002	17-21
Karl Storz AIDA™ DVD image capture system	Maisch 2003	20

1.2 mm, and preferably more than 2 mm). Furthermore, the device should be flexible in at least two directions, easily steerable and fully immersible for ethylene oxide gas sterilization, or prolonged chemical disinfection. However, for inspection of limited segments of the pericardial surface, rigid endoscopes have also been successfully applied [8–12, 45–50]. They offer good visualization/device diameter ratio, are much less delicate for maintenance and considerably less expensive (Table 8.1).

The clinical assessment and comparison of various endoscopic pericardial approaches remains difficult, due to insufficient data on this aspect in existing publications. In order to enable a reliable

and precise aimed biopsy, the endoscope should give a sharp and high quality image under conditions of a beating heart. Simultaneous image transmission and online video display with magnification facilitate the procedure but also increase the procedural costs.

Besides the improvement of standard fiberoptic flexible endoscopes, in the last several years a new image quality was achieved by the introduction of digital-image transmission from the distal end of the device. The major advantage of these devices is their durability, in contrast to the more sensitive fiberoptic flexible endoscopes. In the latter, vigorous manipulation and forced flexion can result in permanent damage to the expensive instrument. Therefore, meticulous care, strictly controlled storage and sterilization are mandatory.

The electrical safety of the device is extremely important for its clinical application. All the devices used in cardiovascular medicine should be "class A" double insulation systems. Electrical insulation is obligatory and will reduce the probability of an electrical shock to zero. In order to prevent arrhythmias, the procedure should be performed with all electrical devices insulated and supplied from the same electrical source. In addition, an external defibrillator should be on stand-by in the room where the procedure is performed (usually cardiac catheterization laboratory or the operating theater) [1].

No currently available endoscope meets all these criteria. According to published data and personal experience, it seems that the diagnostic possibilities of the device are directly related to its size, while in terms of feasibility smaller instruments are preferable. Therefore, the ideal device is a compromise between efficiency and the safety of the procedure (Table 8.2).

Technique

Depending on the selection of the instrument and the approach to the pericardium, the most suitable setting for pericardioscopy is the cardiac catheterization laboratory. If the procedure is performed after subxiphoid pericardiotomy, the operating theater is the more appropriate surrounding. In the majority of cases the method is applied immediately after pericardiocentesis, and after the drainage of the pericardial fluid. Complete drainage of the effusion is important to provide a clear pericardial space for further endoscopy and biopsies. Either manual aspiration or a suction pump can be applied for the drainage of the effusion.

To improve visualization, sampling efficiency, and the safety of the procedure, several modifications of the pericardioscopical technique have been introduced. A critical step in achieving optimal image quality is routine intrapericardial instillation of 50–300 ml of air after complete drainage of pericardial effusion. The air instillation can be performed prior to the subsequent dilatation and application of the 16-F introducer-dilator set with a peel-off sheath

(Braun-Melsungen) for flexible pericardioscopy. Previously, instead of air the same amount of normal saline has been injected and the pericardioscopy has been performed through the fluid. Both with the instillation of saline or air the manipulation with large dilators and introducer sets were safe. However, the visualization was not optimal, and the instillation of air enabled a significantly better image quality in comparison to the previous approach.

In patients with a hemorrhagic effusion, an additional maneuver may be required. In these cases, it is useful to either repeatedly inject and remove 100–150 ml volumes of saline (37 °C) thus rinsing the pericardial sac until the fluid from the pericardial sac becomes clear, or to postpone pericardioscopy for 1–3 days of active drainage. This results in a considerable improvement of visibility, which is only transiently disturbed by heart motion.

The worldwide experience with pericardioscopy is limited and one of the ways for a new operator to acquire some knowledge about macroscopic pericardial changes is to refer to autopsy descriptions and cardiac surgery experience. Bearing in mind that all these findings are based on "the view through the air" it is easy to recognize the advantage of the air instillation for pericardioscopy, especially in the early phase of the investigator's learning curve. Furthermore, a macroscopic view of larger areas of the pericardial surface is achieved by this technique, which is impossible to visualize through fluid. Better visualization remarkably contributes to the proper selection of the biopsy site and therefore to the diagnostic value of the entire procedure [18, 19, 23, 24].

Rigid Instruments

As far as the quality of visualization is concerned, rigid pericardioscopes in general provided better images when compared to the initially used flexible devices. Figure 8.1 represents images from the early Marburg series, confirming this fact. However, new flexible fiberoptical and digital video endoscopes have considerably improved image quality.

In a large pericardioscopy series from Lille, surgical rigid pericardioscopy was used for more than a decade and demonstrated excellent results, especially in patients with neoplastic pericardial effusions

(21% diagnostic yield). The diagnostic value was also evident for irradiation-induced pericarditis (100% increase in sensitivity) and tuberculous pericarditis (66% increase in sensitivity) [11]. The diagnostic yield of pericardioscopy was more evident due to the low diagnostic value of pericardiocentesis (18.3%), as was reported in some other studies (6–26%) [54, 55]. False negative findings in this study were rare (2/141 patients (1.4%)) [11].

Certain parts of the pericardial cavity cannot be completely explored with the rigid pericardioscope, especially around the lateral wall of the left ventricle. However, because of the size of the working channel, the rigid endoscope allows larger tissue biopsies for pathological studies than a flexible pericardioscope.

A disadvantage of the procedure is not only the limited pericardial surface that can be inspected with the rigid instrument in comparison to the flexible one, but also the size of the instrument which is usually larger than the flexible endoscope. To avoid discomfort during the insertion of a large introducer-set the initial patients in the Lille pericardioscopy series were studied in the general anesthesia. However, this resulted in increased mortality in patients with cardiac tamponade and further patients underwent the pericardioscopy in local anesthesia only.

Video-Assisted Thoracoscopy

Pericardial fenestration by video-assisted thoracoscopy was introduced in order to gain simultaneous access to the pleural and pericardial regions and to treat loculated pericardial effusions under direct vision [26–39, 56]. The technique provides an excellent view of the pleural cavity and the pericardium so that suspicious sites, whether pericardial, pleural, pulmonary, or mediastinal, could be precisely localized for biopsy. Thoracoscopic management of chylopericardium with successful preparation and dissection of the thoracic duct was recently reported by Mitsui et al. [56]. The thoracoscopic surgical approach is less traumatic than anterior thoracotomy, and a more extensive pericardial resection is possible when compared with the subxiphoid route. Furthermore, better visualization is afforded comparing with the classic subxiphoid approach. Loculated effusions, even those located posteriorly, which cannot be reached without open thoracotomy, can be targeted and drained with video-assisted thoracoscopy. It should be noted, however, that video-assisted thoracoscopy is contraindicated for patients with tamponade or altered respiratory function in which one-lung ventilation or the lateral operative position is necessary.

Flexible Pericardioscopy

The application of flexible endoscopes enables the precise visualization of both the visceral and parietal layers of the pericardium and allows safe and targeted epicardial and parietal pericardial biopsy (Fig. 8.2) [16-24]. The mandatory precondition for the introduction of a pericardioscope is a pericardial effusion

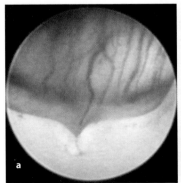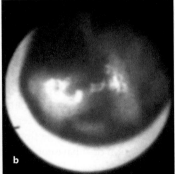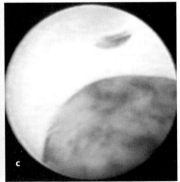

◻ **Fig. 8.1. a** Pericardioscopy images: clear view on the pericardium with some increase in vascularization in autoreactive pericardial effusion. **b** The protrusion on the epicardial surface from a metastasis in breast cancer. **c** Epicardial bleeding in hemorrhagic malignant pericardial effusion due to bronchus carcinoma

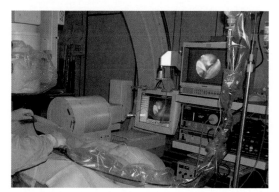

□ **Fig. 8.2.** Pericardioscopy and pericardial and epicardial biopsy using a Stortz AF 110181 flexible endoscope and the AIDA image capture system

large enough to allow a safe entry into pericardium. Therefore, most of the pericardial pathology that has been described by pericardioscopy and given access to pericardial and epicardial biopsies stems from patients with a medium-sized or large pericardial effusion. Both the macroscopic pathological appearance and the extension of various pericardial disorders can be clearly visualized during pericardioscopy. Although various classifications of pericardioscopical findings have been attempted, the clinically most applicable one is outlined by Maisch et al. [15]. Fibrin threads and adhesions, as well as increased vascular injection, hyperemia or neovascularization are seen with various incidence in both inflammatory and neoplastic pericardial disease. Infiltrations, protrusions or protuberances, as well as hemorrhage and areas of infiltrating tissue can also be demonstrated. However, the specificity of these macroscopic findings is rather low and not decisive for the definitive diagnosis, which has to relay on cytology, histology and PCR findings.

Technical Hints in Flexible Pericardioscopy

After the gentle introduction of the flexible instrument through the sheath, a general orientation in the pericardial sac should be made, in order to identify the location and extent of the pathological changes. The pericardial inspection usually starts at the point of entry into the pericardial sac, then selecting the areas where the pericardial lesions are most expressed.

With the contemporary flexible endoscopes, around 70% of the pericardial sac can be examined, the blind spots sometimes being the inferior and apical portions of the pericardium. A sharp and high quality image is essential for the proper selection of the biopsy site, and for the final diagnostic value of the procedure. In order to avoid slipping of the bioptome and to enable a precise aimed biopsy, the pericardioscope prior the biopsy should be bend and directed nearly perpendicular to the lesion. At least three sample should be taken to diminish the sampling error. Biopsies from the marginal parts of the lesion may offer sometimes more specific results than from the central or necrotic area. If lesions with various macroscopic appearances are identified, biopsies should be taken from each of them. If the biopsy is taken from soft or granulomatous lesions prone to hemorrhage, it is mandatory to check pericardioscopically the biopsy site for possible bleeding. It should then be avoided to repeatedly take samples from exactly the same spot.

The distance between the tip of the endoscope and the surface that is inspected and from which the biopsy samples are to be taken is very important. If the tip of the endoscope is to close to the lesion the image will be too large, unclear, and frequently disturbed by the movement of the heart. On the contrary, if the endoscope is to far away from the lesion, the bioptome will have to protrude too much from the working channel and will lose its stability and force. In our experience, the optimal distance between the tip of the endoscope and the pericardial or epicardial surface is 2–3 cm. Additional maneuvers, including bending the flexible tip of the instrument and insufflations of air are often necessary to provide enough space free space for inspection and for biopsies.

Pericardioscopic Appearance of Various Pericardial Pathologies

Macroscopic pathological changes seen during pericardioscopy are similar to the "live" surgical and postmortem autopsy findings. They are rarely specific for a particular pericardial etiology. Usually, macroscopic pathological description of pericardial lesions include: the size of the lesions, their confluence, hyperemia and vascular injections, the presence of the fibrin, hemorrhage, neovascularisation, infiltrations, protrusions and protuberances. The two most frequent pathological lesions of the pericardium are signs of inflammation and neoplastic infiltration.

Macroscopic lesions that are characteristic of pericardial inflammation can be described as:

a) fibrin layers and strands between the epicardium and the parietal pericardium (see pericardioscopic sequences on the cover);

b) vascular injections and neoangiogenesis of the epicardium and parietal pericardium;

c) redness (rubor) of the surface, if not covered by fibrin.

The major features of macroscopic neoplastic pericardial changes are:

a) severe hyperemia and vascular injection on the larger areas,

b) infiltrations and protrusions (see Fig. 8.1b),

c) neovasularisation associated often associated with hemorrhage (see Fig. 8.1a).

Pericardioscopic appearance of "idiopathic" pericarditis is not different from the above mentioned description [15] and comprises fibrinous pericardial and sometimes epicardial inflammation, with a shaggy pericardial surface. The pericardium is diffusely hyperemic with various degrees of fibrin deposition, and areas of intense vascular injections. No infiltrations or protrusions can be identified. The frequently large effusions range from serous to sero-sanguineous. The exudate is rich in fibrin, and due to heart movements the fibrin masses are spread over the pericardium. If the entire surface of the epicardium is covered by the exudate and with fibrin, a cor villosum ("hairy heart") can be diagnosed [57].

Viral pericarditis is also of the fibrinous type, which presents pericardioscopically as a diffuse pericardial inflammation, with a serous or sero-hemorrhagic effusion. The visual findings are almost indistinguishable from "idiopathic" pericarditis. Hyperemia, vascular injections and fibrin deposition may predominate. In the exudate and the epicardial layer, a diffuse lymphocytic infiltration can be found.

In patients with purulent pericarditis, the pericardium is severely hyperemic, edematous and covered by a thick layer of a fibrinopurulent gray-green exudate, consisting predominantly by neutrophils.

The pericardoscopic appearance of tuberculous pericarditis depends on the stage of the disease. In the acute phase a fibrinous pericarditis with the typical shaggy appearance and a serous or serous-sanguineous effusion can be seen. In the subacute stage, pathognomonic morphological features of tuberculosis are visible, characterized by a granulomatous inflammation of the both parietal and visceral pericardium. Histological correlates can be histiocytes and Langhans giant cells frequently surrounding areas of caseation necrosis. Special stains may reveal Mycobacterium tuberculosis in the pericardial effusion. In the chronic phase pericardioscopy is rarely feasible, because of the fibroblastic proliferation, the thickening and the fusion of the pericardial layers.

Neoplastic pericarditis is associated with a hemorrhagic effusion in the majority of the cases. Pericardioscopy reveals the diffuse pericardial inflammation with large areas of hyperemia and vascular injections. The most remarkable findings are infiltrations and protrusions associated with neovascularisation and hemorrhage. Cytology and histology demonstrate malignant cells together with inflammatory cells.

Analyses of Diagnostic Value

Pericardioscopy is a unique method in cardiology. It enables the macroscopic inspection of normal or "near-normal" epicardium and pericardium, but most importantly the detection of pathological changes of the peri- and epicardium. The identification of inflammatory lesions or an infiltration is possible by direct visualization of most parts of the peri- and epicardial surface. However, the specificity of these macroscopic findings is rather low and often not decisive for the diagnosis (Table 8.3) [15, 16].

In the diagnostic algorithm for acute pericarditis in the Guidelines on the diagnosis and management of pericardial disease of the European Society of Cardiology [58] pericardioscopy is considered as final part of the diagnostic pathway. It is indicated in the patients with moderate to large pericardial effusion as optional, or if previous tests were inconclusive (level of evidence B, class IIa indication). The same applies to patients with a chronic pericardial inflammation and large effusions, in order to establish the specific etiology.

⬛ **Table 8.3.** Macroscopic pericardioscopy findings in patients with neoplastic, nonspecific inflammatory pericarditis, and tuberculous pericarditis confirmed by pericardial biopsy. Patients with false negative pericardial biopsy findings are excluded. Reproduced with permission from Seferović et al (2000) [23]

Pericardioscopy macroscopic findings	Neoplastic pericarditis (n = 10)	Nonspecific inflammatory pericarditis (n = 10)	Tuberculous pericarditis (n = 3)
Adhesion strands	4 (40%)	2 (28.6%)	1 (33.3%)
Massive adhesions	2 (20%)	0	1 (33.3%)
Fibrin deposition	2 (20%)	4 (57.1%)	1 (33.3%)
Vascular injections	8 (80%)	7 (100%)	2 (66.7%)
Areas of hyperemia	6 (60%)	6 (85.7%)	2 (66.7%)
Infiltration	7 (70%)	1 (14.3%)	1 (33.3%)
Protrusions	6 (60%)	0	1 (33.3%)

The major advantage of flexible percutaneous pericardioscopy is the possibility to perform a targeted biopsy under direct visualization in real time. These two methods combined are "the winning couple" able to provide the superior diagnostic value, in comparison to the pericardial biopsy guided by fluoroscopy alone. It enables not only the selection of the biopsy site by eye control, but also makes it for the first time feasible and safe to take a very large number of biopsies (18–20 per patient). This aggressive approach, provided by the means of pericardioscopy, certainly diminishes the sampling error inherent to all biopsy procedures.

Both the Marburg and the Belgrade experience with Karl Storz AF1101B1 and the Olympus HYF-1T endoscopes confirm the value of aimed pericardial and epicardial biopsies from targeted areas, with a superior sampling efficiency. Although the detailed data on pericardial biopsy will be reviewed later (see Chapter 9), some important aspects of the combined procedures need to be stressed. In the study by Seferović et al. [24] three different control and sampling modalities were compared: fluoroscopy control (Group 1, 3–6 samples per patients), aimed pericardial biopsy using flexible percutaneous pericardioscopy with standard sampling (Group 2, 4–6 samples per patients) and aggressive sampling (Group 3, 18–20 samples per patients). The sampling efficiency was significantly higher in groups 2 and 3 with a 86.2% and 87.3% yield when compared to group 1 with a yield of only 43.7%. Furthermore, a significantly higher diagnostic yield

was the characteristic feature of biopsies targeted with pericardioscopy and aggressive sampling (Group 3).

In a previous study, in which pericardioscopy preceded the pericardial and epicardial biopsy, which was then only carried out under radiological control the diagnostic value of pericardial biopsy was lower [15]. Only 14% positive diagnostic findings could be attributed from the analysis of the pericardial layer to patients with autoimmune pericardial effusion and only 7% to patients with neoplastic pericardial effusion. This difference between both series from Belgrade and Marburg probably came from the different techniques used. In the first studies of Maisch et al. [13–15] a small sized (8 F) endoscope without a working channel was employed. Interestingly, in the same study the diagnostic value of pericardioscopy and epicardial biopsy was much higher, with 93% positive diagnostic findings for patients with autoimmune pericardial effusion and 80% for patients with neoplastic pericardial effusion. Rodriguez et al. [53], also used a flexible endoscope without a working channel to perform aimed pericardial biopsy in six patients, and reported a feasibility of 66%, but a diagnostic value of only 25% as well. The study was, however, never published as a full peer reviewed article. The advantages of pericardioscopy and guided biopsy were confirmed in a large pericardioscopy series, including 141 patients, 24 patients suffering from neoplastic pericarditis, by Nugue et al. [11].

Millaire et al. [9] analyzed the clinical implications of pericardioscopy and pericardial biopsy findings on the prognosis of patients with malignant disease and pericardial effusion. In a cohort of 40 patients with known malignant disease and pericardial effusion, 37% of the patients' pericardial effusion proved to be malignant (Group 1), while in 63% malignancy in the pericardial sac was not confirmed (Group 2). In Group 1, pericardiosopy and aimed pericardial biopsy yielded a diagnosis of malignant pericardial effusion in 23%. In Group 2, despite confirmed malignancy elsewhere, pericardial effusion was associated with various pericardial disorders (idiopathic, post-irradiation, infectious pericarditis, hemopericardium induced by coagulation disturbances). Mean long-term survival in group 2 was significantly better than in group 1 (one year vs. 42 days) revealing the prognostic value of pericardiosopy and aimed pericardial biopsy in the initial assessment of these patients.

Porte et al. [12] reported a feasibility of surgical pericardiosopy in 98%, corresponding to 112 of the 114 patients with previously proven malignancy. Peri-operative mortality was 3.5%, and post-operative morbidity, 6.1%. In the context of pericardiosopy, pericardial effusions were considered malignant in 43 cases. Only one more case (2.3%) was diagnosed during the follow-up due to a false negative result of pericardiosopy. Overall, 44 of the 114 patients (38.6%) had a proven malignant effusion and 70 (61.4%), a non-malignant effusion according the follow-up. In 10 of the 44 patients with malignant pericardial effusion (22.7%), pericardiosopy and histology corrected the results of a false negative pericardial fluid cytology and pericardial window biopsy. The sensitivities of cytological studies of the pericardial fluid, pathological examinations of a pericardial window biopsy and pericardiosopy with targeted biopsy were 75, 65 and 97%, respectively. One patient with a malignant effusion had a non-symptomatic recurrence 1 month after pericardiosopy (2.3%). The lower diagnostic yield of pericardial biopsy from the pericardial window in comparison to cytology was explained by the presence of patients with non-diffuse malignant pericardial infiltration, e.g. resulting from the invasion of contiguous thoracic tumors.

Little et al. [7] evaluated 17 patients with clinically suspected malignant pericardial effusion and performed pericardiosopy at the time when a subxiphoid pericardial window was created. Peri-cardioscopy with targeted biopsy revealed primary neoplasms or metastases in three patients, while in the remaining 14 the procedure did not disclose malignancy, although in four of them fluid cytology and biopsy findings were both positive.

Safety and Complications

Serious complications have not been encountered during pericardiosopy, apart from the inherent complications related to pericardiocentesis and peri-cardial drainage. The safety of the method was also confirmed in the surgical pericardiosopy series of Nugue et al. [11] with no mortality directly related to pericardiosopy. Furthermore, pericardiosopy did not increase the morbidity or mortality of surgical drainage of pericardial effusion. However, total mortality in this series was 2.1% (3/141) due to the application of general anesthesia in cardiac tamponade. In contrast, no major complications were reported in any of the studies on flexible pericardiosopy apart from the complications related to the pericardial access [1, 13–24].

Minor complications included short-run ventricular tachycardia, pain during dilatation and introduction of the 16.5-F sheath, as well as transient fever. In one patient in whom pericardiosopy was attempted after successful percutaneous balloon pericardiotomy, right ventricular perforation occurred before pericardiosopy as a result of re-advancing the dilator-introducer set over an inappropriately thin guidewire. Perforation was successfully treated by surgery [23]. In addition, the procedure proved safe and no mortality was directly related to pericardiosopy in the studies by Nugue et al. [11] and Millaire et al. [8, 9]. Furthermore, pericardiosopy did not increase the morbidity or mortality of the surgical drainage of pericardial effusions.

Future Perspectives and Recommendations

Recent advances in the study of pericardial disorders have disclosed new diagnostic opportunities in pericardial diseases, mainly due to the development of pericardiosopy and aimed epicardial/pericardial biopsy.

A new direction in the development of pericardioscopy in patients with suspected pericardial malignancy is the application of a combined autofluorescence/fluorescence system for photodynamic early diagnosis (Storz, Germany, K. Haeussinger) [59].

Similar endoscopic systems have already been successfully applied in pulmonology, gastroenterology and urology [60–64]. The advantage of Häussinger`s system is the combination of D-light fluorescence and autofluorescence used subsequently in the same endoscopic view, enabling double demarcation of the pathologic area. When using the autofluorescence mode, light of a spectral composition is emitted by endogenic fluorescent substances in the tissue, causing autofluorescence from normal surfaces. If areas with reduced autofluorescent intensity appear, this may be an indicator of neoplastic tissue alteration. This can be appreciated from Fig. 8.3 below.

Another future development could be the administration of 5-aminolevulinic acid (ALA): In the protoporphyrin IX fluorescence mode after the application of ALA tumor tissue may be differentiated from healthy tissue by a stronger contrast. Tumor-specific fluorescence is caused by endogenic conversion of ALA into fluorescent protoporphyrin IX. Using the special excitation light in the protoporphyrin IX fluorescence mode, tumorous regions fluoresce in red color.

This new method of identifying the neoplastic lesions could serve as additional guidance for directing pericardial biopsy during the pericardioscopy. It could significantly increase its sensitivity. This promising new concept will require further studies.

An additional, potentially interesting field for the application of pericardioscopy is the implantation of epicardial pacemaker electrodes, as reported by Kolesov et al. [45]. Other new applications of pericardioscopy are directed towards assessment of the pericardial space for the guidance of epicardial electrophysiological mapping and ablations, which is currently in the focus of attention of several investigators [65].

An alternative to pericardioscopy is video-assisted thoracoscopy with the creation of a pericardial window. This procedure requires general anesthesia and single-lung ventilation. This is a safe technique in patients without cardiac tamponade and advanced hemodynamic compromise which allows effective pericardial drainage (especially for loculated effusions), and accurate biopsies. It is a more invasive procedure and is indicated in patients with pericardial effusions with concomitant pleural disease.

Future prospective randomized trials are needed to compare video-assisted thoracoscopic pericardiectomy to the results of flexible transcutaneous pericardioscopy.

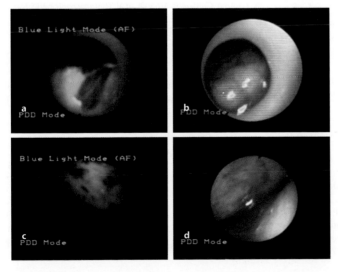

Fig. 8.3. a,c Epicardial metastases of a bronchus carcinoma with biopsy proven oat cell histology in the areas of reduced autoflourescence. **b,d** Metastatic breast cancer was demonstrated in the areas of reduced autoflourescence during pericardioscopy

References

1. Seferović PM, Ristić AD, Maksimović R. New trends in flexible percutaneous pericardioscopy. In: Seferović PM, Spodick DH, Maisch B (eds) Pericardiology: Contemporary answers to continuing challenges. Science, Belgrade, 2000, pp 155–170

2. Sinitsyn NP. Method of implantation of the cannula into the thorax for visual observation of coronary circulation. [Н. П. Синицын. Методика вживления канюли в грудную клетку для визуального наблюдения за коронарным кровообращением] [Russian]. Biull Eksp Biol Med 1955; 39(3): 74–76

3. Volkmann J. Pericardioscopy and contast imaging of the pericardium including essentials of its anatomy. [Perikardioskopie und Kontrastdarstellung des Herzbeutels mit anatomischen Grundlagen] [German]. Z Aerztliche Fortb 1957; 24: 1105–1108

4. Santos GH, Frater RWM. The subxiphoid approach in the treatment of pericardial effusion. Ann Thorac Surg 1977; 23: 467–470

5. Kondos G, Rich S, Levitsky S. Flexible fiberoptic pericardioscopy for the diagnosis of pericardial disease. J Am Coll Cardiol 1986; 7: 432–434

6. Kondos G, Rich S, Levitsky S. Flexible fiberoptic pericardioscopy. Chest 1986; 90(5): 787–788

7. Little AG, Ferguson MK. Pericardioscopy as adjunct to pericardial window. Chest 1986; 89(1): 53–55

8. Millaire A, Wurtza A, Brullard B, et al. Value of pericardioscopy in pericardial effusion. Arch Mal Coeur 1988; 81: 1071–1076

9. Millaire A, Wurtz A, de Groote P, Saudemont A, Chambon A, Ducloux G. Malignant pericardial effusions: usefulness of pericardioscopy. Am Heart J 1992; 124(4): 1030–1034

10. Wurtz A, Chambon JP, Millaire A, Saudemont A, Ducloux G. Pericardioscopy: techniques, indications and results. Apropos of an experience with 70 cases. Ann Chir 1992; 46(2): 188–193

11. Nugue O, Millaire A, Porte H, et al. Pericardioscopy in the etiologic diagnosis of pericardial effusion in 141 consecutive patients. Circulation 1996; 94(7): 1635–1641

12. Porte HL, Janecki-Delebecq TJ, Finzi L, Metois DG, Millaire A, Wurtz AJ. Pericardoscopy for primary management of pericardial effusion in cancer patients. Eur J Cardiothorac Surg 1999; 16(3): 287–291

13. Maisch B, Drude L. Pericardioscopy – a new diagnostic tool in inflammatory diseases of the pericardium. Eur Heart J 1991; 12(Suppl. D): 2–6

14. Maisch B, Drude L. Pericardioscopy – a new window to the heart in inflammatory cardiac diseases. Herz 1992; 17: 71–78

15. Maisch B, Bethge C, Drude L, Hufnagel G, Herzum M, Schönian U. Pericardioscopy and epicardial biopsy – new diagnostic tools in pericardial and perimyocardial disease. Eur Heart J 1994; 15 (Suppl. C): 68–73

16. Maisch B, Pankuweit S, Brilla C, et al. Intrapericardial treatment of inflammatory and neoplastic pericarditis guided by pericardioscopy and epicardial biopsy – results from a pilot study. Clin Cardiol 1999; 22 (Suppl 1): I17–22

17. Maisch B, Ristić AD, Rupp H, Spodick DH. Pericardial access using the PerDUCER and flexible percutaneous pericardioscopy. Am J Cardiol 2001; 88(11): 1323–1326

18. Maisch B, Ristić AD, Pankuweit S. Intrapericardial treatment of autoreactive pericardial effusion with triamcinolone: the way to avoid side effects of systemic corticosteroid therapy. Eur Heart J 2002; 23: 1503–1508

19. Maisch B, Ristić AD, Pankuweit S, Neubauer A, Moll R. Neoplastic pericardial effusion: efficacy and safety of intrapericardial treatment with cisplatin. Eur Heart J 2002; 23: 1625–1631

20. Maisch B, Karatolius K. New possibilities of diagnostics and therapy of pericarditis. Internist (Berl) 2008; 49(1): 17–26

21. Seferović PM, Ristić AD, Petrović P, et al. Flexible video pericardioscopy and aimed pericardial biopsy: a new approach with improved visualization, sampling efficiency and safety. J Am Coll Cardiol 1998; (Suppl. A): 462A–463A

22. Ristić AD. Clinical and hemodynamical assessment and management of pericardial diseases. Master Thesis, Belgrade University School of Medicine, Belgrade, 1998

23. Seferović PM, Ristić AD, Maksimović R, et al. Flexible percutaneous pericardioscopy: Inherent drawbacks and recent advances. Herz 2000; 25(8): 741–747

24. Seferović PM, Ristić AD, Maksimović R, Tatić V, Ostojić M, Kanjuh V. Diagnostic value of pericardial biopsy: improvement with extensive sampling enabled by pericardioscopy. Circulation 2003; 107: 978–983

25. Azorin J, Lamour A, Destable MD, Morere F, de Saint Florent G. Pericardioscopy: definition, value and results. Apropos of a case. Ann Chir 1988; 42(2): 137–140

26. Mack MJ, Aronoff RJ, Acuff TE, Douthit MB, Bowman RT, Ryan WH. Present role of thoracoscopy in the diagnosis and treatment of diseases of the chest. Ann Thorac Surg 1992; 54(3): 403–408

27. Houdelette P, Dussarat G, Talard P, Stephanazzi J, Dumotier J, Espagne P. Subxiphoid pericardiostomy and pericardioscopy. Value and indications apropos of a series of 25 cases. J Chir Paris 1993; 130(1): 23–26

28. Canto A, Guijarro R, Arnau A, et al. Thoracoscopic pericardial fenestration: diagnostic and therapeutic aspects. Thorax 1993; 48: 1178–1180

29. Hazelrigg SR, Mack MJ, Landreneau RJ, Acuff TE, Seifert PE, Auer JE. Thoracoscopic pericardiectomy for effusive pericardial disease. Ann Thorac Surg 1993; 56: 792–795

30. Gossot D, Mourey F, Roland E, Celerier M. Thoracoscopic approach of pericardial effusion. Presse Med 1994; 23(32): 1480–1482

31. Liu HP, Chang CH, Lin PJ, Hsieh HC, Chang JP, Hsieh MJ. Thoracoscopic management of effusive pericardial disease: indications and technique. Ann Thorac Surg 1994; 58(6): 1695–1697

32. Furrer M, Hopi M, Ris HB. Isolated primary chylopericardium: treatment by thoracoscopic duct ligation and pericardial fenestration. J Thorac Cardiovasc Surg 1996; 112: 1120–1121

33. Nataf P, Cacoub P, Regan M, et al. Video-thoracoscopic pericardial window in the diagnosis and treatment of pericardial effusions. Am J Cardiol 1998; 82: 125–126

34. Robles R, Pinero A, Lujan JA, et al. Thoracoscopic partial pericardiectomy in the diagnosis and management of pericardial effusion. Surg Endosc 1997; 11: 253–256

35. Geissbühler K, Leiser A, Fuhrer J, Ris HB. Video-assisted thorascopic pericardial fenestration for loculated or recurrent effusions. Eur J Cardiothorac Surg 1998; 14: 403–408

36. Ohno K, Utsumi T, Sasaki Y, Suzuki Y. Videopericardioscopy using endothoracic sonography for lung cancer staging. Ann Thorac Surg 2005; 79(5): 1780–1782

37. Karthik S, Milton R, Papagiannopoulos K. Simultaneous double video mediastinoscopy and video mediastinotomy – a step forward. Eur J Cardiothorac Surg 2005; 27(5): 920–922

38. Georghiou GP, Stamler A, Sharoni E, et al. Video-assisted thoracoscopic pericardial window for diagnosis and management of pericardial effusions. Ann Thorac Surg 2005; 80: 607–610

39. Pego-Fernandes PM, Mariani AW, Fernandez F, Ianni BM, Stolf NG, Jatene FB. The role of videopericardioscopy in evaluating indeterminate pericardial effusions. Heart Surg Forum 2008; 11(1): E62–65

40. Lidang-Jensen M, Johansen P. Immunocytochemical staining of serous effusions: an additional method in the routine cytology practice? Cytopathology 1994; 5(2): 93–103

41. Satoh T, Kojima M, Ohshima K. Demonstration of the Epstein-Barr genome by the polymerase chain reaction and In situ hybridisation in a patient with viral pericarditis. Br Heart J 1993; 69(6): 563–564

42. Cegielski JP, Devlin BH, Morris AJ, et al. Comparison of PCR, culture, and histopathology for diagnosis of tuberculous pericarditis. J Clin Microbiol 1997; 35(12): 3254–3257

43. Lee JH, Lee CW, Lee SG, et al. Comparison of polymerase chain reaction with adenosine deaminase activity in pericardial fluid for the diagnosis of tuberculous pericarditis. Am J Med 2002; 113(6): 519–521

44. Szymanski M, Petric M, Saunders FE, Tellier R. Mycoplasma pneumoniae pericarditis demonstrated by polymerase chain reaction and electron microscopy. Clin Infect Dis 2002; 34(1): E16–17

45. Kolesov EV, Lukashev SN, Gaiduk AI. Pericardioscopic implantation of electrodes for myocardial electrocardiostimulation. Endosc Surg Allied Technol 1993; 1: 275–276

46. Ready A, Black J, Lewis R, Roscoe B. Laparoscopic pericardial fenestration for malignant pericardial effusion. Lancet 1992; 339(8809): 1609

47. Frank MW, Prystowsky J, Soper W. Laparoscopic pericardiotomy, biopsy, and external drainage. J Laparoendosc Surg 1995; 5(2): 113–117

48. Picardi EJ, Bedingfield J, Statz M, Mullins R. Laparoscopic pericardial window. Surg Laparosc Endosc 1997; 7(4): 320–323

49. Pataki N, Szelig L, Horvath OP, Biki B, Molnar TF. Pericardial drainage using the transdiaphragmatic route: refinement of the laparoscopic technique. Surg Endosc 2002; 16(7): 1105

50. Staltari D, Diaz A, Capellino P, et al. Laparoscopic pericardioperitoneal window: an alternative approach in the treatment of recurrent pericardial effusion, in-hospital evolution and survival. Surg Laparosc Endosc Percutan Tech 2007; 17): 116–119

51. Wong KKS, Li AKC. Use of flexible choledochoscope for pericardioscopy and drainage of a loculated pericardial effusion. Thorax 1987; 42: 637–638

52. Urschel JD, Horan TA. Pericardioscopy and biopsy. Surg Endosc 1993; 7(2): 100–101

53. Rodriguez S, Lemmon CC, Burstein S, Ziskind AA. Feasibility and utility of percutaneous pericardial biopsy and pericardioscopy as an adjunct to balloon pericardiotomy or pericardiocentesis for the diagnosis and treatment of pericardial disease [abstract]. J Am Coll Cardiol 1994; 24(Suppl. A): P1175

54. Permanyer-Miralda G, Sagrista-Sauleda J, Soler-Soler J. Primary acute pericardial disease: a prospective series of 231 consecutive patients. Am J Cardiol 1985; 56: 623–630

55. Zayas R, Anguita M, Torres F, et al. Incidence of specific etiology and role of methods for specific etiologic diagnosis of primary acute pericarditis. Am J Cardiol 1995; 75(5): 378–382

56. Mitsui K, Namiki K, Matsumoto H, Konno F, Yoshida R, Miura S. Thoracoscopic treatment for primary chylopericardium: report of a case. Surg Today 2005; 35: 76–79

57. Roberts WC. Pericardial heart disease: its morphologic features and its causes. Proc Bayl Univ Med Cent 2005; 18(1): 38–55

58. Maisch B, Seferović PM, Ristić AD, et al. Task Force on the Diagnosis and Management of Pericardial Diseases of the European Society of Cardiology. European Society of Cardiology Guidelines: Diagnosis and management of the pericardial diseases. Executive summary. Eur Heart J 2004; 25(7): 587–610

59. Ristic AD, Maisch B. New frontiers of percutaneous flexible pericardioscopy: Detection of neoplastic pericardial involvement by autofluorescence phenomena [abstract]. Eur Heart J 2000; 21(Suppl. August/September): P2223

60. Marcon NE. Is light-induced fluorescence better than the endoscopist's eye? Can J Gastroenterol 1999; 13(5): 417–421

61. Filbeck T, Roessler W, Knuechel R, Straub M, Kiel HJ, Wieland WF. Clinical results of the transurethreal resection and evaluation of superficial bladder carcinomas by means of fluorescence diagnosis after intravesical instillation of 5-aminolevulinic acid. J Endourol 1999; 13(2): 117–121

62. Lam S, Kennedy T, Unger M, et al. Localization of bronchial intraepithelial neoplastic lesions by fluorescence bronchoscopy. Chest 1998; 113(3): 696–702

63. Svanberg K, Wang I, Colleen S, et al. Clinical multi-colour fluorescence imaging of malignant tumours – initial experience. Acta Radiol 1998; 39(1): 2–9

64. Häussinger K, Becker H, Stanzel F, et al. Autofluorescence bronchoscopy with white light bronchoscopy compared with white light bronchoscopy alone for the detection of precancerous lesions: a European randomised controlled multicentre trial. Thorax 2005; 60(6): 496–503

65. Zenati MA, Shalaby A, Eisenman G, Nosbisch J, McGarvey J, Ota T. Epicardial left ventricular mapping using subxiphoid video pericardioscopy. Ann Thorac Surg 2007; 84(6): 2106–2107

Epicardial and Pericardial Biopsy

Introduction

The application of pericardioscopy, targeted pericardial and epicardial biopsy as well as the analyses of the respective tissues, has certainly improved our understanding of the pathophysiology of the pericardial diseases. Most instruments used in the procedure such as endoscope, biopsy forceps and catheters were originally not designed for the application in the pericardium but for the use in other organs for endoscopic inspection or tissue acquisition. Informed consent of this circumstance from patient is recommended. Further progress has been achieved through the implementation of contemporary pathology (immunocytochemistry, immunohistochemistry) and molecular biology techniques (PCR to cardiotropic microbial agents) in the analysis of pericardial and epicardial biopsy samples.

Techniques

Pericardial biopsy, performed by the excision of a small portion of parietal pericardium, is an inherent part of surgical pericardiotomy or the subxiphoid pericardial window procedure. Percutaneous approach for the acquisition of biopsy samples by means of a forceps (bioptome) from either the visceral or the parietal pericardial layer is less invasive and applicable to a larger patient population. To ensure a safe and successful procedure most institutions with clinical and research interest in pericardial diseases, use either fluoroscopy or an optical control during pericardioscopy. Echocardiography-guided bedside pericardial biopsy was attempted but visualization of the biopsy forceps was too poor to enable safe tissue sampling [1].

Pericardial Biopsy Guided by Fluoroscopy

Pericardial biopsy using fluoroscopy control was investigated in studies by Ziskind, Mehan, Endrys, Maisch, Nugue, and Seferović [2–8]. In the majority of institutions, the procedure is performed in the cardiac catheterization laboratory. After pericardiocentesis, a standard 0.038" J-tip guidewire is employed to enter the pericardium. Subsequently, over the guidewire, a 5–7 F drainage catheter (preferably pigtail catheter) is placed in the pericardium. An apical or inferior position of the drainage would enable the most efficient evacuation of the pericardial effusion. After the drainage is almost completed, the same 0.038" J-tip guidewire is reinserted and over the guidewire additional dilatations are performed, and a 7-F or 9-F long sheath-introducer set is advanced and po-

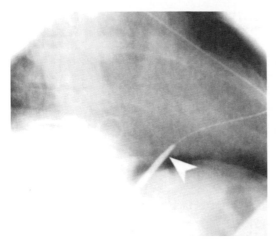

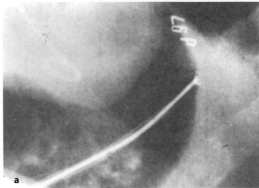

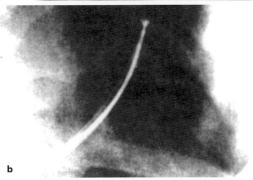

☐ **Fig. 9.1.** Pericardial dilatation. Frontal view. The dilator has entered pericardium (*arrow*), while the J-tip guidewire is positioned deeply in the pericardial sac

sitioned on the lateral surface of the pericardium (Fig. 9.1). For the proper orientation at the beginning and during the pericardial biopsy procedure, intrapericardial injection of contrast media can be used.

Fluoroscopic guidance is mandatory to perform pericardial biopsy. Using a fenestrated forceps with a central needle at least 3–6 samples can be taken mainly from the lateral surface of the parietal pericardium (Fig. 9.2).

After the pericardial biopsies are taken, the sheath should be exchanged for a drainage catheter, to allow further evacuation of the pericardial effusion. The drainage catheter should remain in the pericardial space until the results of the pericardial fluid and tissue analyses are completed and/or pericardial drainage decreased to less than 50 ml/day.

In contrast to this approach, Ziskind et al. [2] developed a special 8F aggressive biopsy forceps, while Mehan et al. [3] implemented a 9-F right Judkins coronary guiding catheter, passed through a 9-F Hemaquet sheath, as a guide for 1.8 mm Byceps (Mansfield Scientific) biopsy forceps. In the studies by Maisch et al. [5, 6, 9–12] a 7-F Schikumed endomyocardial biopsy forceps and later on Cordis 7F and Pilling bioptomes were utilized for taking samples from both the parietal and the visceral pericardial layers. Endrys et al. [4] also applied a 7-F endomyocardial biopsy forceps for pericardial biopsies, through

☐ **Fig. 9.2a,b.** Pericardial biopsy using fluoroscopy control. Frontal view with magnification. The Olympus FB43-ST fenestrated forceps with the central needle is protruding from the long sheath. Biopsy is just about to be taken from the inferolateral parietal pericardium (**a**). By modifying the bioptome position, samples from the superior part of the lateral pericardium can also be taken (**b**)

the 8-F, 40 cm long curved tip sheath. Pericardial biopsy guided by echocardiography, reported by Selig et al. [1], was performed with 6-F Olympus FB18 fenestrated forceps.

Pericardial and Epicardial Biopsy Targeted by Pericardioscopy

The cardiac catheterization laboratory is an optimal setting for pericardioscopy and aimed pericardial biopsy. Pericardioscopy enables targeted pericardial and epicardial biopsies. Since the biopsies are taken under pericardioscopic control the forceps can be directed to the observed lesions and be therefore more selective in sampling specific pathological changes (Fig. 9.3). A sequence of an epicardial biopsy proce-

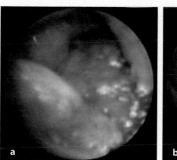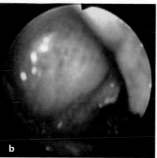

□ **Fig. 9.3a,b.** Flexible percutaneous pericardioscopy with aimed pericardial biopsy in a patient with neoplastic pericarditis using an Olympus endoscope

dure in fibrinous, non-malignant pericardial effusion and epicarditis is depicted on the cover page of this book.

For pericardioscopy a 16.5 F peel-off introducer set (B. Braun, Melsungen) can be used, which is exchanged via a guidewire. Sufficient local anesthetics and i.v. se-dation with midazolam 5–15 mg or propofol 1% (until optimal sedation is reached) together with analgesia (e.g. morphine 10 mg/ml i.v. combined with paspertin 10 mg/ml) are used. The percutaneous subxyphiodal entry can be dilated stepwise from 7 to 16 F by dilators in different sizes over the guidewire under radiographic control until the 16.5 F introducer is set in place.

The ideal position of the guidewire for the subsequent pericardioscopy is at the apex or the inferior wall close to the diaphragm thus performing an U-loop along the pericardial sac first cranially, then along the lateral to the inferior wall. The fiberglass pericardioscope (e.g. originally 16 F instruments for bronchoscopy or urethroscopy with 2 working channels e.g. from Storz or Olympus have been used frequently) can easily ride on the guidewire to different areas of the epi- and pericardium. The 2nd channel can be used for the bioptome.

In order to improve the visibility during pericardioscopy, if pericardial effusion is hemorrhagic, rinsing of pericardial space with 100–150 ml volumes of saline (37 °C) is necessary. A useful hint in achieving optimal image quality is the intrapericardial instillation of 50–300 ml of air, after complete drainage of the pericardial effusion. The amount of air to be instilled should always be much less than the amount of fluid, which has been evacuated to avoid tamponade by a pneumopericardium.

An additional option is a staged procedure, when pericardioscopy is performed two or three days after pericardiocentesis, allowing for the pericardial fluid to drain. Using this approach the pericardium can be inspected under direct eye control, with no fluid interference, which guarantees superior visualization [13].

Sampling Efficiency and Histological Findings

Due to the elastic properties of the pericardial surface, the low sampling efficiency represents a major technical issue in pericardial biopsy. It is reported to differ considerably depending on the biopsy forceps [2, 7]. To highlight this important clinical issue, we used a German shepherd dog as an experimental model to test the biopsy sample size, sampling efficiency and safety of the following bioptomes: Olympus FB-41ST ("alligator jaws"), FB-42ST ("rat tooth"), FB-43ST (fenestrated, with the central needle) and Cordis Bipal endomyocardial biopsy forceps (all 5.4 F) [13]. Sampling efficiency was defined as the percentage of successful biopsies out of the total number of attempts. The results are presented in Table 9.1.

As the above-listed data demonstrate, the most successful device was the FB-43ST, and it was the forceps type selected for clinical application. The design of our pericardial biopsy study included three different technical approaches applied to a population of 41 patients with large pericardial effusions scheduled for pericardiocentesis [8]. Those were:

1. pericardial biopsy using fluoroscopy control only (Group 1: 12 patients, 66.7% male, mean age 46.7 ± 12.2 years, 3–6 samples per patient, mean 5.2),

Table 9.1. Biopsy sample size, sampling efficiency, and safety of various pericardial biopsy forcepses - experimental study on a German shepherd dog. Reproduced with permission from Seferović et al. (2000) [13]

Forceps	Number of samples	Sample size (mg)	Sampling efficiency	Safety
FB-41ST	7	1.68	42.8%	100%
FB-42ST	8	1.45	50.0%	100%
FB-43ST	8	1.73	87.5%	100%
Bipal 5.4F	6	1.94	33.3%	100%

Table 9.2. Pericardial biopsy sampling efficiency in the clinical study. Reproduced with permission from Seferović et al. (2000) [13]

Olympus FB-43ST biopsy forceps	Group 1 (n = 12 pts) Fluoroscopy 3–6 samples	Group 2 (n = 19 pts) Pericardioscopy 4–6 samples	Group 3 (n = 10 pts) Pericardioscopy 18–20 samples
Total number of samples	62	112	192
Mean sample number	5.2	5.9	19.2
Total number of biopsy attempts	142	130	220
Mean number of biopsy attempts	11.8	6.8	22
Sampling efficiency	43.7%	86.2%	87.3%

2. aimed pericardial biopsy using flexible percutaneous pericardioscopy with the standard number of samples (Group 2: 19 patients, 52.6% male, mean age 52.3 ± 11.2 years, 4–6 samples per patient, mean 5.9), and

3. aimed pericardial biopsy using flexible percutaneous pericardioscopy and aggressive sampling (Group 3: 10 patients, 60% male, mean age 42.3 ± 14.6 years, 18–20 samples per patient, mean 19.2).

Prior to aimed pericardial biopsy all patients underwent pericardiocentesis, via the subxiphoid approach, for the drainage of a significant pericardial effusion or imminent tamponade. In Group 1, biopsy of the left lateral portion of the pericardium was performed using a 9-F sheath and Olympus FB-43ST forceps. In Groups 2 and 3 all patients underwent aimed pericardial biopsy guided by pericardioscopy with an Olympus HYF-1T flexible endoscope and the same type of forceps as in Group 1. This modified approach to pericardioscopy, performed through the air, after active pericardial drainage, made it possible to take a very large number of samples in Group 3.

The advantage of optical control during the biopsy resulted in significantly higher sampling efficiency in Groups 2 and 3 compared to Group 1 (86.2%, 87.3% and 43.7%, respectively, $p < 0.01$; Table 9.2). With the larger number of biopsies taken, the difference in sampling efficiency was insignificant (pericardioscopy in Group 2 vs. Group 3). Therefore, in our experience, sampling efficiency for pericardial biopsies was not only affected by the selection of the bioptome, but also by the possibility of performing the biopsy under direct eye control. Both the pericardial biopsy approaches applied and the number of samples taken had a significant impact on the pathohistologic findings in this study, as summarized in Table 9.3.

The distribution of pathohistologic findings was homogenous among all three groups, with predominant neoplastic etiology, probably a characteristic of the study population.

Sensitivity of Pericardial Biopsy: a Key Issue for the Successful Clinical Application

In order to be widely accepted for specific clinical indications, a diagnostic test must demonstrate sufficient sensitivity and specificity compared to other

Table 9.3. Pathohistologic findings from the pericardial biopsy samples obtained by fluoroscopy-guided biopsy (Group 1), and pericardioscopy-guided biopsy (Groups 2 and 3). Reproduced with permission from Seferović et al. (2003) [8]

Pathohistology	Group 1 (n = 12) Fluoroscopy 3–6 samples	Group 2 (n = 19) Pericardioscopy 4–6 samples	Group 3 (n = 10) Pericardioscopy 18–20 samples
Planocellular carcinoma	8.4%	10.5%	10%
Adeno carcinoma	0	15.7%	0
Mesothelioma	0	0	10%
Plasmocytoma	0	5.3%	0
M. Hodgkin	0	5.3%	10%
Tuberculosis	0	5.3%	20%
Nonspecific inflammation	33.3%	15.7%	40%

methods used in similar indications. This, however, is not completely true for pericardial biopsy. The major problem in the diagnosis of pericardial diseases is the lack of a single as reference or "gold standard". Consequently, the final diagnosis and evaluation of any new test has to be made in reference to a "jigsaw puzzle" of comprehensive diagnostic methods. When such a comparison was made with the pathohistologic results depicted in Table 9.3, the sensitivity (ratio of true-positive tests to the number of all patients with the disease) of the histological findings [8] was 41.7% in Group 1, 57.9% in Group 2 and 90% in Group 3. One can appreciate from Fig. 9.4 that the sensitivity of the aggressive approach to pericardial

biopsy was significantly better compared to Group 1 ($p < 0.01$), but not significantly different from standard pericardioscopy-Group 2.

Another problem in interpreting pericardial biopsy results is calculating the procedure's specificity (ratio of true-negative tests to the number of all patients without the disease). Since the described methodology was applied only on patients with significant pericardial effusion, no "true negative" pericardial biopsy could be expected. Possible exceptions for calculating the specificity of pericardial biopsy in revealing the presence of inflammatory or neoplastic infiltration could be patients with uremic and metabolic large pericardial effusions. In such patients, however, the diagnosis can be established by less invasive methods, so they were not included in our study. Similar issues also apply to targeted epicardial biopsy, which is predominantly carried out in the Marburg setting. Protrusions and hemorrhagic imbibitions of the epicardial surface are the landmarks to which the bioptome is directed.

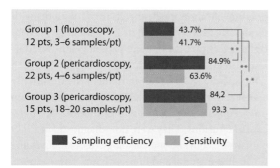

Fig. 9.4. Sampling efficiency and sensitivity of pericardial biopsies performed with different techniques: Group 1 – pericardial biopsy using only fluoroscopy control; Group 2 – aimed pericardial biopsy using flexible percutaneous pericardioscopy with standard sampling; Group 3 –aimed pericardial biopsy using flexible percutaneous pericardioscopy with aggressive sampling (**p < 0.01). Adapted from Seferović et al. (2003) [8]

Diagnostic Value

In the guidelines on the diagnosis and management of pericardial disease of the European Society of Cardiology [14], pericardial and epicardial biopsy guided by pericardioscopy is a decisive part of the diagnostic algorithm for acute and chronic pericarditis with moderate to large pericardial effusions. The procedure is considered the final segment of

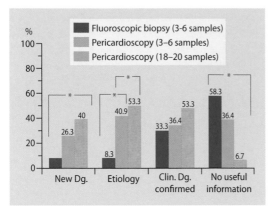

■ **Fig. 9.5.** The diagnostic value of pericardial biopsy expressed as a percentage of: a) new diagnosis discovered, b) etiology revealed, c) clinical diagnosis confirmed, d) no useful information obtained (false negative). Group 1-pericardial biopsy using only fluoroscopy control; Group 2-aimed pericardial biopsy using flexible percutaneous pericardioscopy with standard sampling; Group 3-aimed pericardial biopsy using flexible percutaneous pericardioscopy with aggressive sampling. (*-p < 0.05; **-p < 0.01). Reproduced with permission from Seferović et al. (2003) [8]

the diagnostic pathway and it is frequently reserved for the tertiary institutions. In the majority of cases pericardial and epicardial biopsy may uncover the specific etiology of a pericardial effusion and, according to the guidelines, is indicated in the patients as an optional method, or if previous tests were inconclusive (level of evidence B, class IIa indication).

The diagnostic value of aimed pericardial and epicardial biopsy can be defined, analogous to the diagnostic value of endomyocardial biopsy [15], as the influence of biopsy findings on the final (discharge) diagnosis. According to the impact of this procedure on establishing the correct diagnosis, the following categories can be distinguished:
a) new diagnosis discovered,
b) etiology revealed,
c) clinical diagnosis confirmed,
d) no useful information obtained (false negative).

The obtained diagnostic values of the different pericardial biopsy approaches applied in our study are depicted in Fig. 9.5 [8].

Due to the superiority of aimed pericardial biopsy, the etiology of pericardial disease was established significantly more often in both pericardioscopy groups

when compared to Group 1 (Group 3 vs. Group 1: p < 0.01; Group 2 vs. Group 1: p < 0.05). However, only the aggressive sampling approach (18–20 biopsy samples per patient), enabled by pericardioscopy (Group 3), was proven to be significantly more accurate regarding both the establishment of a new diagnosis (p < 0.05) and the false negative findings (p < 0.05) compared to non-targeted biopsy controlled only by fluoroscopy (Group 1). A new diagnosis in the pericardioscopy group with aggressive sampling was established in 40%, etiology was revealed in 50%, clinical diagnosis was confirmed in 30%, while the procedure provided no useful information (false negative) in only 10% of patients. Such extensive pericardial sampling, not previously reported, provides diagnostic value comparable to the results of surgical pericardioscopy (general anesthesia, larger sized instrument) in the study of Nugue et al. [7] (sensitivity 92%, false negative findings 1.4%). The pericardial biopsy results were also comparable to the epicardial biopsy findings reported in the study by Maisch et al. [10] (sensitivity of 80 % in neoplastic disease, and 93% in inflammatory disease). Pericardial biopsy results in the experience of the same authors had much lower diagnostic value (the probability of diagnosing an infiltrate was 7% in neoplastic disease and 14% in inflammatory disease) [10].

In the initial study, Maisch et al. [9] investigated the diagnostic value of aimed epicardial biopsy in 36 patients with inflammatory pericardial effusion. Pathohistologic findings revealed lymphocytes and polymorphomononuclear cells in 5/7 patients with viral pericarditis (71.4%), in 2/5 patients with bacterial infection (40%), in all patients with tuberculous infection (100%), and in 14/16 patients with lymphocytic (87.5%) but in none of the humorally autoreactive forms. Pericardial biopsies were taken only from 19/36 patients with inflammatory pericardial effusions. They were non-diagnostic in 12/19 patients on conventional histology (63.1%), revealing fibrin-like material and fibrous tissue. These reports are comparable to our findings for false negative results (58.3%) taken under fluoroscopy control only (Group 1).

In the subsequent study published by the same group (11) the probability of diagnosing an infiltrate was also significantly higher in epicardial than in parietal pericardial biopsy (80% vs. 7% in neoplastic disease, and 93% vs. 14% in inflammatory disease) [10]. In addition, epicardial biopsy demonstrated higher sensitivity for identifying neoplastic disorders in the pericardium than cytology alone (80% vs. 71%). In ten patients with perimyocarditis, in which epicardial and endomyocardial biopsy were simultaneously performed epicardial biopsy was shown to be superior to endomyocardial biopsy in revealing a lympho-monocytic infiltrate (60% vs. 20% of patients respectively; p < 0.05), as well as in revealing a CD3+ positive infiltrate (80% of epimyocardial biopsies vs. 40% of endomyocardial biopsies; p < 0.05).

The diagnostic advantages of epimyocardial in comparison with endomyocardial biopsy are prominent in both neoplastic and inflammatory pericardial disease. Epicardial biopsy enables not only pathohistological analyses, (e.g. lymphocytic infiltration in perimyocarditis), but also, immunohistological and molecular virological analysis (Fig. 9.6).

It appears that the sensitivity and specificity of epimyocardial biopsies examined by light microscopy may not be subject to the same degree of sampling error as in endomyocardial biopsies [9–12]. Therefore, the probability of diagnosing an infiltrate is significantly higher in epicardial biopsies [16]. Immunoglobulin binding, class I and class II de novo expression, and PCR for viral RNA or DNA are comparable with both techniques. Immunocytochemistry (IgG-, IgA-, IgM- and C3-fixation to the autologous biopsy specimen) is a more sensitive measure of inflammatory lymphocytic or humoral autoreactive processes than endomyocardial biopsy in myocarditis and perimyocarditis [17]. With adequate sampling, the specificity of the method is almost 100% for immunoglobulin fixation in autoreactive and lymphocytic effusions.

Due to the focal character of inflammatory heart muscle disease, sensitivity and specificity of the histological examination in this condition largely depends on the number of endomyocardial biopsies and the

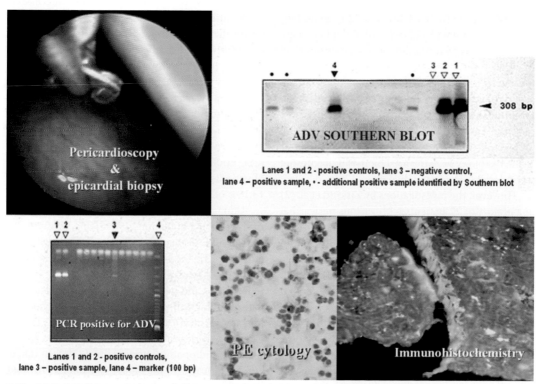

Fig. 9.6. Pericardioscopy and epicardial biopsy revealing adenovirus (ADV) positive epicarditis confirmed by polymerase chain reaction (PCR) and Southern blot (Marburg Pericardial Disease Registry)

histological criteria. In perimyocarditis, epicardial biopsies taken under pericardioscopic control establish specific diagnosis comparable to endomyocardial biopsy, and since they can be targeted, they may be more selective for sites of abnormal structure and pathohistology.

Fernandes et al. [18] reported the results obtained from 38 patients who underwent pericardial biopsy using the subxiphoid approach. Biopsy identified the etiology of pericardial disease in 10.5% (tuberculosis and malignancy in 2 cases each), while in 89.5% of patients biopsy findings demonstrated non-specific chronic pericarditis. PCR for cardiotropic viruses and immunohistochemistry for autoreactive pericarditis were not performed, however. So it remains unclear, to which extend the non-specific cohort was comprised in reality of viral or autoimmune forms of pericardial effusions or of underdiagnosed malignant effusions. Remarkably the pericardial biopsy experience of the same institution published earlier, which included 12 patients with neoplastic disease, demonstrated a higher diagnostic yield, revealing the diagnosis in 41% of patients [19].

In the study by Bardales et al. [20], including 96 patients, a total of 112 pericardial fluid cytology specimens and 61 surgical pericardial biopsies were analyzed. After reviewing cytological and histological specimens, seven discrepant cases were observed, six of which had a positive cytology for malignancy. The sampling error of pericardial biopsy was believed to be the cause of such inconsistency. According to these results fluid cytology was shown to be superior to the histology of pericardial biopsy in diagnosing secondary pericardial malignancies [20].

However, the investigations by Ziskind et al. [2] in a cohort of 27 patients with various pericardial disorders indicated a 46% to 62% increase in the diagnostic yield of pericardial biopsy for patients with malignancies, compared to pericardial fluid cytology and a 7% to 29% increase in the diagnostic yield in patients without malignant disease. It was stated that the larger sample volume (8-F bioptome) and more aggressive sampling (6–8 samples from each patient) may have resulted in an improved diagnostic value.

Mehan et al. [3] applied a modified percutaneous technique for pericardial sampling with the use of angioplasty guiding catheters. Four to nine samples

were taken from each patient, with a mean number of six. In a group of 25 patients, the histological diagnosis of tuberculous pericarditis was established in 44%, purulent pericarditis in 8%, while non-specific inflammatory changes were confirmed in 48% of patients.

An early contribution by Endrys et al. [4] reported on transcatheter pericardial biopsies in 18 patients with pericardial effusion. Pericardial biopsy produced the definitive diagnosis in 50% of patients: tuberculosis in six, mesothelioma in one and carcinoma in two patients.

Aimed pericardial biopsy during pericardioscopy was shown to be particularly useful in the diagnosis of neoplastic pericarditis. In the large pericardioscopy series published by Nugue et al. [7] including 141 patients (24 with malignant pericarditis), the diagnostic sensitivity of pericardiocentesis, subxiphoid window biopsy, and pericardioscopy with aimed pericardial biopsy was found to be 54%, 71% and 92%, respectively. The improvement in diagnostic sensitivity of 21% had a remarkable clinical impact on the further treatment and outcome of these patients. Diagnostic benefit was also evident for irradiation-induced pericarditis (100% increase in sensitivity) and tuberculous pericarditis (66% increase in sensitivity). False negative findings in this study were rare (1.4%).

Similarly, pericardioscopy targeted pericardial biopsy provided the definitive diagnosis in 33 out of 91 patients (36.26%) with pericardial diseases of unknown origin studied by Pêgo-Fernandes et al. [21]. Etiology could be revealed in the same series of patients by pericardial effusion analyses in only 13.18% of the patients.

Uthman et al. [22] implemented pericardial biopsy in a pediatric population (19 patients, aged 2 to 20 years) for the evaluation and treatment of pericardial effusion. The biopsy findings rendered a specific etiological diagnosis in 63% of the cases, and excluded tuberculosis and malignancy in 37%. The details of pathohistologic diagnoses were as follows: tuberculous pericarditis (37%), uremic pericarditis (16%), irradiation pericarditis (5%), connective tissue disease (5%) and "idiopathic" pericarditis (37%). In tuberculous pericarditis, the biopsy specimens provided immediate pathohistologic diagnosis and higher culture positivity (71%) than pericardial fluid (29%).

The Analyses of the Epicardial and Pericardial Biopsy Samples

Processing Techniques

The epicardial and pericardial biopsies are fixed and processed in the usual manner, embedded in paraffin and cut into 4 µm serial sections by a microtome. Further processing includes staining with hematoxylin-eosin for routine histology and a Ziehl-Neelsen stain for mycobacteria. For immunocytochemistry and immunohistochemistry, biopsy samples are separately processed: They were frozen immediately in liquid nitrogen. These biopsy specimens can also undergo the characterization of infiltrating cells with monoclonal antibodies, immunohistochemistry for bound immunoglobulin and complement fixation when the cryostat sections are analyzed under the microscope with the respective marker antibodies. Polymerase chain reaction (PCR) for enteroviral RNA, cytomegalovirus-, adenoviral, Epstein Barr , herpes simplex viruses, parvo B 19, HHV 6, chlamydia- and Borrelia burgdorferi DNA can also be carried out in the obtained frozen samples [9–12]. For scientific purposes isolation and expansion of the cells can be carried out from native tissue specimens.

Molecular Biology Techniques

PCR and in-situ hybridization techniques can identify minute amounts of viral nucleic acid (Coxsackie B and A groups, adenovirus, rhinovirus, echovirus type 8, influenza, cytomegalovirus, Parvo B 19, hepatitis virus, herpes simplex and herpes humanus 6 virus). Studying epicardial biopsy samples, Maisch et al. [5, 9, 10] established the specific diagnosis of viral pericarditis in 7/36 patients: two were positive for cytomegalovirus by in situ hybridization, and five were positive for coxsackie virus, either by microneutralization (n = 4) or virus isolation (n = 1).

Similar to the demonstration of cytomegalovirus DNA in the epicardium, Satoh [23] used PCR and in situ hybridization to verify the presence of the Epstein-Barr genome in the resected pericardium of a patient with viral pericarditis. Andreoletti et al. [24] described a rapid detection method for enteroviruses using PCR and microwell capture hybridization assay in cerebrospinal fluid, broncho-pulmonary lavage, pericardial effusion, throat swabs, stools, sera, muscular and myocardial biopsies. PCR products were labeled directly by digoxigenin-dUTP during the amplification step. The hybridized amplicons labeled with digoxigenin were detected using anti-digoxigenin Fab fragments conjugated to peroxidase and automatically measured by colorimetric reaction. Using this method, it was possible to detect enteroviral RNA in 23/35 clinical specimens obtained from 16/17 patients with suspected acute or chronic enteroviral infection. In contrast, the virus was isolated in cell culture in only 8/28 clinical specimens from 6/17 patients. It is suggested that this methodology could be used for the rapid qualitative detection of other RNA viruses also in pericardial diseases.

Immunohistochemistry of Epicardial Biopsies

Immunohistochemistry, especially IgG-, IgM- and IgA- and complement fixation contribute significantly to the diagnostic value of epicardial biopsies. The specificity of immunoglobulin fixation in the autoreactive and lymphocytic pericardial effusion group is 100% [9]. The immunoglobulin fixation of IgG-, IgM- and IgA-classes was observed in the sarcolemmal membrane, capillaries and extracellular matrix in all patients, but complement fixation [25] was found mainly in patients with the autoreactive form and rarely in patients with neoplastic pericardial effusion [11, 12]. Immunohistochemistry anti-surfactant apoprotein, anti-Lewis a and anti-TN antibodies can also be helpful in distinguishing malignant mesothelioma from pulmonary adenocarcinoma, which is a key obstacle in routine pathohistology [25].

Safety and Complications

Complications are a major issue in the clinical use of any invasive procedure, especially in cardiology. However, the introduction of an epicardial biopsy forceps, especially if not optically controlled, could result in heart perforation or laceration of the right ventricle or, most unlikely, of epicardial vessels. Therefore, optical control is essential for the safety of epicardial biopsy in order to avoid damage to the myocardium, coronary vessels, and especially tumor blood vessels. To avoid heart perforation, the jaws of the biopsy forceps should be fully opened immediately after introduction into pericardial space. Additional safety can be provided by the placement of an additional 0.038" J guidewire through the sheath, before the introduction of the biopsy forceps. With this wire placed intrapericardially, even the most serious complications such as bleeding and heart perforation can be treated by the introduction of a pigtail catheter and prompt drainage together with autotransfusion, which is not applicable only in neoplastic effusions.

Using this approach, bleeding can be controlled until spontaneous cessation. Thus surgical intervention was never needed for biopsy complications in both Marburg and Belgrade experience of more than 300 cases.

The procedural risk of parietal pericardial biopsy, especially when performed at the level of the lateral wall is likely to be lower when compared to epicardial biopsy. Theoretically, there is a possibility of pneumothorax through pericardial biopsy, which, however, was not observed in the Belgrade and Marburg experience. However, surgical stand-by during the early learning stage of the investigator can be useful. Epicardial biopsy in the Marburg registry did not lead to any lethal causality. That was also true for the Belgrade experience, including both fluoroscopy guided and aimed pericardial biopsy during pericardioscopy. Minor complications included short runs of ventricular tachycardia (1/41; 2.4%), pain during the placement of a large pericardioscopy sheath (18/29 patients; 75%) and transient fever (12/41 patents; 29.3%) [8, 13]. After this initial experience, we are currently applying more intensive analgetic premedication including intravenous morphine and midazolam.

In the pericardial biopsy study of Mehan et al. [3], including 25 patients who underwent percutaneous pericardial biopsy, also no major complications occurred. Minor complications included: premature ventricular beats in 10/25 patients (40%) and a small subcutaneous hematoma in 1/25 patients (4%). In the study by Ziskind et al. [2] one patient (1/27; 3.7%) with advanced lung cancer died immediately after pericardiocentesis and pericardial biopsy, but autopsy did not identify the cause of death. Hypothetical causes include: postpericardiocentesis pulmonary edema, bleeding from the biopsy site with recurrent tamponade and generalized cardiovascular collapse. Further complications occurred in patients who underwent percutaneous balloon pericardiotomy immediately following pericardial biopsy. In one patient left apical pneumothorax developed after the procedure (3.7%), but resolved itself spontaneously in the next 24 hours. Two patients had bleeding complications (7.4%), one with uremic platelet dysfunction and the other one who was treated with heparin for concomitant disease.

No major complications were related to the procedure in the study by Nugue et al. [7], who utilized both surgical subxiphoid biopsy (4×4 cm window) and aimed pericardioscopic biopsy through a rigid mediastinoscope. Reported mortality in their study was 2.1% (3 patients), and was associated with the induction to anesthesia before pericardiocentesis and drainage in patients with large pericardial effusion. In the remaining patients pericardiocentesis was performed before general anesthesia and no further mortality occurred. Similarly, no biopsy related complications were noted, but one patient (1/101) died due to cardiac tamponade before the pericardioscopy procedure in the series of Pêgo-Fernandes [21]. Minor complications included premature ventricular beats due to irritation from the endoscope. Endrys et al. [4] had no complications in 18 consecutive patients. Only in two patients there was a sensation of "pulling" inside the chest, when the biopsies were taken.

Future Perspectives and Recommendations

Pericardioscopy and aimed pericardial and epicardial biopsy improved not only the diagnostic specificity of pericardial diseases but also helped to define more precisely some therapeutic modalities.

The diagnoses of inflammatory, postinflammatory, autoreactive or neoplastic pericardial disease could be specified with the combined use of pericardioscopy, pericardial and epicardial biopsy with an adequate histological, immunohistological and molecular (PCR) work-up. These altogether improved sensitivity, specificity and diagnostic accuracy.

In perimyocarditis, optically guided epicardial biopsy can give a more disease-specific result than endomyocardial biopsy in the same patient group.

The characterization of lymphocytic cells and anticardiac antibodies in the pericardial effusion and cardiac tissue demonstrated increased immunological reactivity in viral, autoimmune, and neoplastic disorders of the heart and permitted a highly specific diagnosis.

For viral, tuberculous and other forms of bacterial pericarditis, molecular techniques such as PCR and in situ hybridization are available and provide an accurate diagnosis together with the microbiological analysis of the pericardial fluid.

Future potential could lie in the application of the autofluorescence/fluorescence mode which is available in some endoscopy systems [26, 27]. These modes could help to identify neoplastic lesions and direct the pericardial and epicardial biopsies even better.

References

1. Selig MB. Percutaneous pericardial biopsy under echocardiographic guidance. Am Heart J 1991; 122(3 Pt 1): 879–882
2. Ziskind AA, Rodriguez S, Lemmon C, Burstein S. Percutaneous pericardial biopsy as an adjunctive technique for the diagnosis of pericardial disease. Am J Cardiol 1994; 74(3): 288–291
3. Mehan VK, Dalvi BV, Lokhandwala YY, Kale PA. Use of guiding catheters to target pericardial and endomyocardial biopsy sites. Am Heart J 1991; 121: 882–883
4. Endrys J, Simo M, Shafie MZ, et al. New nonsurgical technique for multiple pericardial biopsies. Cathet Cardiovasc Diag 1988; 15: 92–94
5. Maisch B, Drude L. Pericardioscopy – a new diagnostic tool in inflammatory diseases of the pericardium. Eur Heart J 1991; 12(Suppl. D): 2–6
6. Maisch B, Drude L. Pericardioscopy – a new window to the heart in inflammatory cardiac diseases. Herz 1992; 17: 71–78
7. Nugue O, Millaire A, Porte H, et al. Pericardioscopy in the etiologic diagnosis of pericardial effusion in 141 consecutive patients. Circulation 1996; 94(7): 1635–1641
8. Seferović PM, Ristić AD, Maksimović R, Tatić V, Ostojić M, Kanjuh V. Diagnostic value of pericardial biopsy: improvement with extensive sampling enabled by pericardioscopy. Circulation 2003; 107(7): 978–983
9. Maisch B, Bethge C, Drude L, Hufnagel G, Herzum M, Schönian U. Pericardioscopy and epicardial biopsy – new diagnostic tools in pericardial and perimyocardial disease. Eur Heart J 1994; 15(Suppl. C): 68–73
10. Maisch B, Pankuweit S, Brilla C, et al. Intrapericardial treatment of inflammatory and neoplastic pericarditis guided by pericardioscopy and epicardial biopsy – results from a pilot study. Clin Cardiol 1999; 22(Suppl 1): I17–22
11. Maisch B, Ristić AD, Pankuweit S, Neubauer A, Moll R. Neoplastic pericardial effusion. Efficacy and safety of intrapericardial treatment with cisplatin. Eur Heart J 2002; 23(20): 1625–1631
12. Maisch B, Ristić AD, Pankuweit S. Intrapericardial treatment of autoreactive pericardial effusion with triamcinolone; the way to avoid side effects of systemic corticosteroid therapy. Eur Heart J 2002; 23(19): 1503–1508
13. Seferovic PM, Ristić AD, Maksimovic R, et al. Flexible percutaneous pericardioscopy: inherent drawbacks and recent advances. Herz 2000; 25(8): 741–747
14. Maisch B, Seferović PM, Ristić AD, et al. Task Force on the Diagnosis and Management of Pericardial Diseases of the European Society of Cardiology. Guidelines on the diagnosis and management of pericardial diseases [executive summary]. Eur Heart J 2004; 25(7): 587–610
15. Seferović PM, Maksimović R, Vasiljević JD, et al. Endomyocardial biopsy: a meta analysis of diagnostic value. Postgrad Med J 1994; 70 (Suppl.1): S21–28
16. Andreoletti L, Hober D, Belaich S, Lobert PE, Dewilde A, Wattre P. Rapid detection of enterovirus in clinical specimens using PCR and microwell capture hybridization assay. J Virol Methods 1996; 62(1): 1–10
17. Maisch B, Maisch S, Kochsiek K. Immune reactions in tuberculous and chronic constrictive pericarditis. Am J Cardiol 1982; 50: 1007–1013
18. Fernandes F, Ianni BM, Arteaga E, Benvenutti L, Mady C. Value of pericardial biopsy in the etiologic diagnosis of pericardial diseases. Arq Bras Cardiol 1998; 70(6): 393–395
19. Ianni BM, Barretto AC, Mady C, et al. The biopsy in the diagnosis of pericardial involvement by malignant tumor. Arq Bras Cardiol 1989; 53(3): 157–159
20. Bardales RH, Stanley MW, Schaeffer RF, Liblit RL, Owens RB, Surhland MJ. Secondary pericardial malignancies: a critical appraisal of the role of cytology, pericardial biopsy, and DNA ploidy analysis. Am J Clin Pathol 1996; 106(1): 29–34
21. Pêgo-Fernandes PM, Mariani AW, Fernandes F, Ianni BM, Stolf NG, Jatene FB. The role of videopericardioscopy in evaluating indeterminate pericardial effusions. Heart Surg Forum 2008; 11(1): E62–65
22. Uthaman B, Endrys J, Abushaban L, Khan S, Anim JT. Percutaneous pericardial biopsy: technique, efficacy, safety, and value in the management of pericardial effusion in children and adolescents. Pediatr Cardiol 1997; 18(6): 414–418
23. Satoh T. Demonstration of the Epstein-Barr genome by the polymerase chain reaction and in situ hybridization in a patient with viral pericarditis. Br Heart J 1993; 69: 563–564

24. Andreoletti L, Hober D, Belaich S, Lobert PE, Dewilde A, Wattre P. Rapid detection of enterovirus in clinical specimens using PCR and microwell capture hybridization assay. J Virol Methods 1996; 62(1): 1–10
25. Noguchi M, Nakajima T, Hirohashi S, Akiba T, Shimosato Y. Immunohistochemical distinction of malignant mesothelioma from pulmonary adenocarcinoma with anti-surfactant apoprotein, anti-Lewis a, and anti-Tn antibodies. Hum Pathol 1989; 20(1): 53–57
26. Ristic AD, Maisch B. New frontiers of percutaneous flexible pericardioscopy: Detection of neoplastic pericardial involvement by autofluorescence phenomena [abstract]. Eur Heart J 2000; 21 (Suppl. Aug/Sept): P2223
27. Häussinger K, Becker H, Stanzel F, et al. Autofluorescence bronchoscopy with white light bronchoscopy compared with white light bronchoscopy alone for the detection of precancerous lesions: a European randomised controlled multicentre trial. Thorax 2005; 60(6): 496–503

Intrapericardial Treatment in Pericardial Disease

Introduction

Independent of the etiology of the underlying disease the intrapericardial application of drugs offers the advantage that a high local dose can be applied with little systemic side effects. The pericardial sac is, similarly as the pleural space, a nearly ideal compartment for such an application with a very limited exchange of its content to the systemic circulation or other organs.

In patients with chronic autoreactive pericardial effusions as well as in uremic pericarditis intrapericardial instillation of glucocorticoids has effectively prevented recurrences and at the same time avoided many of their systemic side effects. A similar treatment concept with cytostatic agents has been applied in chronic and recurrent neoplastic pericardial effusion. Finally, intrapericardial application of fibrinolytic agents in purulent pericarditis has also been beneficial for these often critically ill patients since it enabled complete drainage of the purulent content from the pericardium without a need for sternotomy and pericardiotomy.

Intrapericardial Treatment of Neoplastic Pericarditis

Malignant invasion of the heart and pericardium occurs in one tenth of all patients with a neoplastic disease, and one third of these will die as a consequence of such involvement [1–3]. Some of these patients may be misdiagnosed ante mortem because malignant disease was not suspected or clinically occult. Conversely, symptomatic pericardial effusion and even cardiac tamponade may be the first clinical manifestation of an occult malignancy [2, 4]. Signs of pericardial effusion, with or without tamponade, pericardial constriction, impaired coronary circulation, and disorders of cardiac innervation may occur during the course of disease.

Primary tumors of the pericardium are extremely rare. Secondary or metastatic malignant pericardial disease is much more common and arises in the majority of cases from lung and breast tumors, less frequently from gastrointestinal, hematological malignancies, and melanoma (Fig. 10.1) [1, 4, 5].

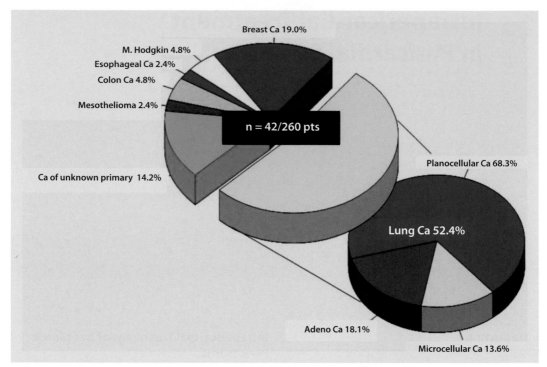

□ **Fig. 10.1.** Pathological spectrum of pericardial malignancies from the Marburg Pericardial Disease Registry (tertiary referral center; n = 42 patients)

Although pericardiocentesis alone can occasionally provide prolonged relief, other measures usually have to be used to prevent recurrences. The management of the initial neoplastic effusion or of relapses include [5]: pericardial sclerosing therapy, intrapericardial and systemic chemotherapy, radiotherapy, surgical creation of a pleuropericardial or pleuroperitoneal window and, most recently, percutaneous balloon pericardiotomy [6, 7]. Since there are no randomized trials in this area, the management of large and recurring malignant pericardial effusions is mainly based on local technical possibilities and experience.

The advantage of intrapericardial antineoplastic treatment, as a locoregional approach, should be seen in addition to systemic tumor treatment. The pathophysiological principle of this adjunctive effect relies on the antineoplastic property of the specific drug used and its additional non-specific sclerosing effect. A number of different intrapericardial treatment regimens have been applied in recent years: radionuclides e.g. 32 Phosphor, the antimetabolite

5-Fluorouracil for breast, colorectal, esophageal, and gastric tumors, the plant alkaloid Vinblastin for breast and lung carcinoma, Hodgkin's and Non-Hodgkin's lymphoma. The antitumor antibiotics Bleomycin and Mitomycin C have been used for the same indications. Anthracyclines such as mitoxantrone have been utilized for lung and breast cancer, acute myeloid leukemia, as well as the non-Hodgkin's lymphoma, whereas the anthracycline Adriamycin has been avoided because of its well-known cardiotoxicity. Alkylating agents, which have been used for intrapericardial therapy were Cispalatin and Carboplatin for ovarian cancer, tumors of the head and neck area, osteosarcoma and carcinoma of the bladder [8-27].

There is also a limited experience with intrapericardial instillation of interferon alpha, -beta, and interleukin-2 [28] as well as with OK-432 [29]. In addition, nitrogen mustard and quinacrine were used for intrapericardial instillation in the 1970s, but severe pain and bone marrow toxicity occurred [22] (Table 10.1).

Table 10.1. Cumulative analysis of intrapericardial treatment studies in patients with neoplastic pericardial effusion

Intrapericardial treatment	Number of patients treated	Treatment success [%]	Follow-up [months]	Side effects and complications
Cisplatin [3, 8–17, 26]	107	83.3–100	4–24	– Nausea (6.7%) – Atrial arrhythmias (4.4%) – Constriction (1.1%) – Myocardial ischemia (1%)
Thiotepa [18–22, 27]	112	79–83	6–24	– Thrombocytopenia (0.9%) –Leucopenia (0.9%)
Antitumor antibiotics – bleomycin [24, 30–33] – mitomycin C [23, 25, 34, 35] – aclarubicin [23]	74	70–100	3–12	– Constriction (2.4%) in a patient treated with mitomycin C
Tetracycline [30, 36–41]	222	73–75	3–25	– Severe pain (15-70%) – Atrial arrhythmias (9%) – Fever (7.5-9%) – Infection (0.5%)
Mitoxantrone [42–45]	48	60–100	5–15	– Mild leucopenia in 2 patients – Lack of appetite
Radioactive chromic phosphate [36–39]	75	71–95	8–24	– None
Autologous tumor-infiltrating lymphocytes activated with IL-2 [46]	4	100	3–15	– Low grade fever 100% – Tachycardia 25%
OK-432 [29, 47–50]	10	70	1–11	– Fever (60%) – Pain (50%)

IL interleukin, *OK-432* penicillin-treated and heat- treated lyophilized powder of Streptococcus pyogenes A3).

Cisplatin

Cisplatin was selected for intrapericardial application in several studies [3, 8–17, 26] because of its proven clinical efficacy against the most frequent secondary pericardial malignancies, its favorable sclerosant action verified in malignant pleural effusions, and its low incidence of side effects when applied locally.

In our clinical practice the following inclusion criteria are implemented for intrapericardial application of cisplatin:

1. Verification of neoplastic cells in the pericardial fluid or malignant histology in epicardial biopsy.
2. Need for pericardial puncture because of tamponade or large effusion (>200 ml).
3. Age 18–75 years.

In addition the following exclusion criteria were applied:

1. Terminal phase of the malignant disease with life expectancy < 7 days (patients permanently dependent from the active life support).
2. Pericardial constriction.
3. Contraindication for cisplatin.
4. Coagulation disorders.

In our study [3], instillation of cisplatin (30 mg/m^2) in 100 ml of 0.9% NaCl was performed in 42 patients as a single slow injection using a 7-F pigtail catheter introduced after pericardiocentesis. The cisplatin solution was kept intrapericardially for 24 hours and than evacuated. After aspiration of the residual fluid the pigtail catheter was removed.

Intrapericardial therapy with cisplatin was highly successful regarding the immediate result of the procedure. After the drainage of the effusion and cisplatin instillation 41/42 patients could be promptly discharged with only minimal or no residual pericardial effusion.

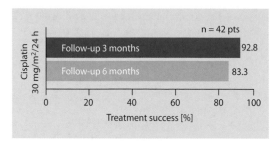

□ Fig. 10.2. Proportion of patients free of symptoms and a hemodynamically relevant pericardial effusion 3- and 6-months after intrapericardial treatment with 30 mg/m2 cisplatin. Reproduced with permission from Maisch et al. (2002) [3]

During the follow-up of 1–12 months (mean follow-up of survivors 8.5 ± 3.2 months) none of the patients treated with cisplatin intrapericardially died due to cardiac tamponade. Intrapericardial administration of cisplatin appeared to prevent recurrence of symptoms and a hemodynamically relevant pericardial effusion during the first 3 months of the follow-up in 92.8% of the patients, and after 6 months in 83.3% of the surviving patients (Fig. 10.2).

Cumulative distribution of pericardial effusion relapses after six months follow-up was 3/8 (37.5%) patients with breast cancers, one patient (100%) with mesothelioma, one patient (50%) with Hodgkin's disease and 1/22 patient with lung cancer (4.5%). Comparing the six-month frequency of relapses between the two largest subgroups in our patient population the results of cisplatin instillation were significantly better in lung cancer in comparison to breast cancer (4.5% vs. 37.5%, p < 0.05).

Similar to our findings Tomkowski and Filipecki reported encouraging results of intrapericardial administration of cisplatin in 16 consecutive patients with malignant pericardial effusion in the course of the adenocarcinoma of the lung [12]. Cisplatin (10 mg in 20 ml normal saline) was instilled into pericardial space over 5 min during 1–5 consecutive days (maximal total dose 50 mg). Positive effect of treatment was achieved in 15/16 cases (93.8%).

In the subsequent publication Tomkowski et al. [14] studied the effectiveness of intrapericardial administration of tetracycline, 5-fluorouracil, and cisplatin in 20 patients with recurrent malignant pericardial effusion. However, good results (no fluid reaccumulation) were observed only after cisplatin therapy.

More recently, Tomkowski et al. [51] reported on the effectiveness and side effects of intrapericardial administration of cisplatin in the prevention of recurrent malignant pericardial effusion in 46 patients. 35 patients underwent pericardiocentesis and 11 patients had video-assisted thoracoscopic surgery (VATS) for drainage of pericardial effusion. Cisplatin was instilled intrapericardially only if daily drainage of pericardial fluid observed during 5–7 days exceeded 50 ml. One of the following three regimens were applied:

1. 10 mg of cisplatin dissolved in 20 ml of normal saline administered over 5 min during 5 consecutive days directly into the pericardial space (39 patients);
2. 50 mg of cisplatin dissolved in 100 ml of normal saline administered during 30 min (six patients)
3. 20 mg of cisplatin dissolved in 40 ml of normal saline administered over 10 min during 5 consecutive days (one patient).

The treatment was considered successful when recurrence of symptoms or no large pericardial effusion was observed in echocardiography and no other interventions directed to the pericardium were required. A positive effect of intrapericardial treatment with cisplatin was achieved in 43 out of 46 patients (93.5%) in the entire investigated group and in 35 out of 38 patients (92%) who survived more than 30 days. In the subgroup of patients with non-small cell lung cancer (NSCLC) and survival longer than 30 days, high efficacy was documented (29 out of 31 cases; 93.5%). Median survival time in the group of 38 patients who survived more than 30 days was 102.5 days. Atrial fibrillation due to cisplatin administration was observed in seven out of 46 patients (15.2%). Sclerosis of the pericardial space without symptoms of constriction occurred in five out of 46 cases (10.9%). In five out of 46 patients, intrapericardial treatment was repeated due to recurrent pericardial effusion initially treated according to the regimen 1 (cisplatin 10 mg daily for five days). In two cases reaccumulation of pericardial fluid stopped after delivery of the second course. In the remaining three cases, treatment with intrapericardial administration of cisplatin was unsuccessful (there were patients with survival longer than 30 days – two with NSCLC and in one with lung angiosarcoma). There were no relapses of significant pericardial effusion in patients treated according to regimens 2 and 3. Symptoms and signs of constrictive pericarditis were not observed in any of the treated patients.

Pavon-Jimenez et al. [10] also performed the intrapericardial administration of cisplatin in 6 patients (breast carcinoma in 2, lung in 1, ovary in 1, mediastinal fibrosarcoma in 1, and unknown in 1). In contrast to our experience with pericardial effusion in the course of breast cancer, there were no recurrences, with a survival of 2 to 18 months (mean 5.6).

Lestuzzi et al. [17] have suggested an interesting concept of "tumor specific" treatment for neoplastic pericardial effusion: 50 mg of cisplatin in pericardial lung carcinoma metastases, and 30 mg of bleomycin in pericardial breast carcinoma metastases. Although the entire study is not yet published, this view could be supported by our findings of a lower efficacy of cisplatin in patients with breast cancer.

Fiorentino et al. [15] have treated intrapericardially six patients affected by malignant pericardial effusion with cisplatin (10 mg in 20 ml of normal saline, instilled over 5 minutes on 5 consecutive days; total cisplatin dose, 50 mg). The median number of courses was two, with a range of one to three courses. Courses were repeated every 2 or 3 weeks in case of fluid reaccumulation. Three patients (50%) achieved complete response without evidence of pericardial recurrence or stricture.

Tondini et al. [16] treated seven patients with lung cancer and two with breast cancer and symptomatic pericardial effusion with cisplatin intrapericardially. A single cycle with 10 mg of cisplatin diluted in 20 ml of normal saline was administered for five consecutive days via an intrapericardial catheter. Control of recurrent effusions was obtained in eight of the nine patients (88.9%).

Thiotepa

Thiotepa (triethylenephosphoramide) is an alkylating agent, used for many years in the treatment of solid tumors [52] and pleural effusions [53], thanks to both sclerosing and cytostatic activities. Experience with intracavitary thiotepa administration was encouraging by means of minimal myelosuppression and absence of infusional pain [19, 20, 27]. Bishiniotis et al. [19] treated 19 women with malignant cardiac tamponade due to advanced breast cancer with subxiphoid pericardiocentesis and local thiotepa instillation (30 mg). The method had no serious side effects, prevented pericardial fluid reaccumulation, and in contrast to any other studies with intrapericardial treatment of neoplastic pericardial effusion, in combination with systemic adjuvant therapy, thioteapa prolonged survival. Fluid reaccumulation was detected in four patients (21%) during the 6-month follow-up period, but the effusions were small (<0.5 cm) and there was no need to repeat pericardiocentesis.

Intrapericardial chemotherapy with thiotepa was also proven to be an effective and well-tolerated regimen in the study of Colleoni et al. [20]. Twenty-three patients with malignant pericardial effusions (9 with breast cancer, 11 with lung cancer, two with an unknown primary tumor, and one with metastatic melanoma) were treated with intracavitary thiotepa (15 mg on days 1, 3, and 5) after evacuation of pericardial fluid on day 0. Nineteen patients (83%) responded to treatment with a rapid improvement of symptoms. The median time to pericardial effusion progression was 8.9 months (range, 1 to 26). No significant side effects were registered. Only one patient had transient grade III thrombocytopenia and leukopenia and one patient had grade I leukopenia. Indeed, a higher risk of myelotoxicity has been described with doses greater than 60 mg, even if the drug is administered via the intracavitary route [54, 55].

The same group reported in 2004 their long-term results with intrapericardial application of Thiotepa in 33 patients [27]. Underlying neoplastic pathology included breast cancer in 11 patients, lung cancer in 16 patients, microcytoma in 4 patients, endometrial cancer in 1 patients, and melanoma also in 1 patient. After pericardiocentesis, drainage of the pericardial effusion and confirmation of malignant cells in the drained fluid intrapericardial treatment with 15 mg thiotepa was administered on days 1, 3, and 5 after pericardiocentesis. No procedure-related complications or side effects were observed. The treatment was successful in 90.9% of cases with no significant pericardial effusion in the follow-up. Three recurrences occurred (9.1%), requiring additional pericardiocentesis and intrapericardial treatment was repeated as well. The median survival time was better than otherwise expected for patients with advanced stage metastatic malignancies: 115 days (range, 22 to 1,108 days) in the overall population, and 272 days in patients with breast cancer.

Girardi et al. [21] have also reported high efficacy of a similar regimen with intrapericardial thiotepa treatment in malignant pericardial effusions. Thiotepa (15 mg in 50 ml 0.9% NaCl) was administered intrapericardially after 37 pericardiocentesis and 4/35 surgical pericardiotomies. During the two years follow-up recurrence rate was 8.1%. Pericardiocentesis was as effective as open surgical drainage as the route of administration of thiotepa for the management of malignant pericardial effusions. The only side effects were SVTs observed in four patients (9.7%).

Intrapericardial treatment with thiotepa was combined with hydrocortisone in the study of Beretta et al. [18]. Sixteen patients were treated by pericardiocentesis and in 10 of these thiotepa and hydrocortisone were instilled intrapericardially (3×15 mg thiotepa + 30 mg hydrocortisone). They reported in 80% (8 out of 10 patients) a long term success and a relapse in 20% whereas in the six patients who underwent only pericardiocentesis without intrapericardial instillation the recurrence rate was 33%.

Alternative Agents

Intrapericardial Treatment with Antitumor Antibiotics (Bleomycin, Mitomycin C, Aclarubicin)

With regard to the mechanism of intrapericardial action of bleomycin, it is difficult to differentiate its cytostatic and sclerosing effect. Yano et al. [32] examined the efficacy of bleomycin on the local control of malignant pericardial effusion in seven patients cardiac tamponade in non-small cell carcinoma of the lung. After the effusions were completely drained, 5 mg of bleomycin were instilled locally via the catheter. In all patients but one, the draining catheter could be successfully removed. The duration of drainage ranged from four to 13 days (mean: 9.2 days). Five of the seven patients achieved a complete remission of pericardial effusions.

Clinical efficacy and toxicity of bleomycin as sclerosing agent in the primary management of malignant pericardial effusion was also compared with doxycycline [30]. Twenty-seven consecutive adult patients were alternately assigned to undergo bleomycin or doxycycline pericardial sclerosis after pericardiocentesis and complete drainage of pericardial effusion. They mainly had lung (70%) and breast cancers (11%), and all had clinical and echocardiography evidence of cardiac tamponade. One patient in each group failed to respond to sclerosis with the initial agent, but both were sclerosed successfully with the other agent. Sclerosis was achieved with a median of two instillations for each agent and total median doses of bleomycin 20 mg or doxycycline 1,250 mg respectively. Seventy percent of doxycycline patients developed significant retrosternal pain, compared with no pain in all bleomycin patients (p = 0.04). Doxycycline patients required a median of 3.5 more days of hospitalization (8.5 vs. 5) and two more days of pericardial drainage (7 vs. 5) compared with bleomycin patients. Tamponade recurred in one bleomycin patient at 253 days, and in no doxycycline patient.

Van Belle et al. [56] treated five patients with pericardial tamponade of neoplastic origin by pericardiocentesis, drainage and local instillation of bleomycin. The pericardial effusion was adequately controlled in all patients and the side effects were minimal. Survival was not influenced by the pericardial involvement.

Intrapericardial instillation of mitomycin C was effective in controlling the malignant pericardial effusion in 70% of 20 patients without causing side effects, except for pericardial constriction seven months later in one subject [104]. Kaira et al. [25] have treated eight patients with cardiac tamponade or symptomatic large pericardial effusion caused by advanced non-small cell lung cancer with pericardiocentesis, pericardial drainage and subsequent instillation of 2 mg of mitomycin C. Only patients with cytologically confirmed neoplastic effusion and no chemotherapy, radiotherapy or surgery at least 1 month prior to the intrapericardial treatment were included in the study. The duration of pericardial drainage ranged from 7 to 14 days (median 10.5 days). Six of the eight patients achieved a complete remission of pericardial effusions without any adverse effects.

In addition, Fukuoka et al. [23] have treated 24 patients with malignant pericardial effusion with pericardial drainage and intrapericardial instillation of Carbazilquinone, Mitomycin-C or ACNU. The range of survival time from the instilllation of anti-cancer drug was 3–365 days. In only 4/24 patients, reaccumulation of pericardial effusion was recognized. There were no serious complications with this procedure.

Experience with the intrapericardial administration of aclarubicin hydrochloride (a sclerosing and cytotoxic agent) is limited to five patients with malignant pericardial effusion and cardiac tamponade. All patients were women, and all were initially treated surgically for breast cancer (two patients), or lung cancer (three patients). All patients received 15 mg of aclarubicin hydrochloride intrapericardially after pericardiocentesis and drainage of pericardial effusion. Two patients (40%) had a complete remission of the malignant pericardial effusion. The other three patients were difficult to evaluate because nonpericardial metastases limited their survival. All patients, however, showed disappearance of malignant cells from the pericardial sac with no cytopathologically demonstrable recurrence [57].

Intrapericardial Instillation of Tetracycline, Oxytetracycline, and Minocycline

Treatment with tetracycline instillation usually requires multiple installations to be effective. Of the 58 patients described, each treated with a mean tetracycline installation of 500 mg per installation, a success of longer than one month was seen in 75%, with a mean of 120 days without recurrence [41]. Complications included mild fever, arrhythmias, and pain.

Davis et al. [37] treated 33 patients with cardiac tamponade secondary to malignant pericardial effusion by intrapericardial instillation of tetracycline hydrochloride. Complete control of the initial signs and symptoms of tamponade was obtained in 30 patients (90.9%) without concomitant chemotherapy or radiotherapy. The procedure did not result in clinically significant complications. None of the successfully treated patients subsequently developed recurrent cardiac tamponade or constrictive pericarditis.

In the experience of Celermajer et al. [58] after intrapericardial sclerotherapy with tetracycline only three of 28 patients with neoplastic pericardial effusion required another pericardiocentesis. However, in four of seven patients in whom sclerotherapy was not performed initially, symptomatic effusions recurred. Median survival following pericardiocentesis in breast cancer patients was 10 months (range, 0–36 months) and in all other malignancies was four months (range, 0–12 months).

In their preliminary study Shepherd et al. [40] reported on 22 patients treated with tetracycline hydrochloride, 500 to 1000 mg, dissolved in 20 ml normal saline. The primary malignancy included lung cancer in 15 patients, breast cancer in two patients, and carcinoma of the stomach, ovary, pleural mesothelioma, chronic granulocytic leukemia, and adenocarcinoma of unknown primary in one patient each. Xylocaine hydrochloride, 100 mg, was first instilled intrapericardially, followed by tetracycline hydrochloride. The catheter was clamped for one to two hours and then allowed to drain. This procedure was repeated every 24 to 48 hours until the net drainage was less than 25 ml/24 hours. Twenty patients received one to five instillations of tetracycline. Minor complications included transient arrhythmia in two patients, postinjection pain in four patients, and self-limited fever greater than 38.5 °C in two patients. Fifteen patients had good control of their malignant pericardial effusion for more than 30 days (median survival, 160 days; range, 38 to 275 days). Three patients died before 30 days without evidence of effusion, and no patient surviving longer than 30 days developed recurrent effusion or pericardial constriction.

In the subsequent study by Shepherd and co-workers [41] 74% of 58 treated patients were free from recurrences of pericardial effusions for more than 30 days (median survival 168 days, range 30 to 1149+). Five patients (9%) died before 30 days without effusion. Eight patients (14%) did not achieve control of the effusion relapses. One declined further therapy after one instillation, and three died within six days due to progressive malignancy. One patient had persistent drainage after three instillations, and three had reaccumulation of fluid two, six, and 27 days after catheter removal. Complications included transient atrial arrhythmias (5 patients), pain after injection (9 patients) and temperature higher than 37.5 °C (five patients). One patient had a cardiac arrest during pericardiocentesis.

The largest study on the intrapericardial management of malignant pericardial effusion included 93 patients from Toronto, treated with 500 to 1000 mg tetracycline or doxycycline hydrochloride [38]. The catheter was clamped for one to two hours and then reopened, and the procedure was repeated daily until the net drainage was less than 25 ml in 24 hours. Eighty-five patients underwent sclerosis and required a median dose of 1500 mg of the sclerosing agent (range 500 to 700 mg), given in a median of three injections (range 1–8). Complications included pain (17 patients), atrial arrhythmias (8 patients), fever with temperature greater than 38.5 °C (7 patients), and infection (1 patient). Two patients had cardiac arrest before sclerosis could be attempted. Sixty-eight patients (73%) had the effusion controlled for longer than 30 days, with an overall control rate of 81%. Seven other patients had no recurrences of the pericardial effusion but died of progressive malignant disease in less than 30 days. The overall median survival was 98 days (range 1 to 1724 days).

Grau et al. [36] treated eleven consecutive patients with malignant pericardial tamponade with intracavitary oxytetracycline, 500–1000 mg/day, administered via an indwelling pericardial cannula after evacuation of pericardial fluid. This procedure was repeated every 24 hours for six consecutive days or until no more fluid could be drained. The primary cancer was located in the breast in seven patients, in the stomach in two patients, and in the lung in two patients. In all cases, systemic chemotherapy or hormonal therapy was started after the pericardial tamponade was resolved. The mean tetracycline dose per patient was 3000 mg (range 1500–6000). All patients responded to the treatment with rapid improvement. Response persisted during a median of nine months with no evidence of pericardial relapse. The main concomitant effects were mild local pain during tetracycline instillation in four patients, and transient fever in three.

Lashevsky et al. [59] evaluated the effectiveness and safety of minocycline hydrochloride intrapericardially in 14 consecutive patients with malignant pericardial effusion. Following percutaneous insertion of a pericardial drain, minocycline was administered at a dosage of 10 mg/kg every 48 h until fluid drainage stopped or until further therapy was deemed necessary. The mean amount of minocycline administered was 1.9 ± 1.0 g given in 2.4 divided doses. The total drainage time was 5.4 ± 2.5 days. Recurrence of malignant pericardial effusion was seen in only one of 14 patients. However, minocycline instillation was associated with severe chest pain in seven patients, and with ECG changes suggesting pericardial or subepicardial injury in two patients. The same group studied the acute effects of intrapericardial instillation of minocyclin in the experimental model and later in humans with malignant pericardial disease [60]. Twenty-three open-chest dogs were divided into four groups according to the solution injected intrapericardially:

1. minocycline, 5 mg/kg;
2. minocycline, 10 mg/kg;
3. normal saline solution, 100 ml, followed by minocycline, 10 mg/kg;
4. a mixture of 50 ml of the dog's own blood mixed ex vivo with minocycline, 10 mg/kg to evaluate the effect of rising on the pH of minocycline solution.

Nine consecutive patients with malignant cardiac tamponade receiving minocycline intrapericardially are evaluated for the appearance of chest pain and ECG changes. Minocycline (5 and 10 mg/kg) caused marked, transient ST-T segment deviation in all dogs, whether or not saline solution was previously injected into the pericardial sac. Prior mixing of minocycline with blood markedly increased the acidic pH of the minocycline solution and significantly reduced the extent of ST-T segment deviation. Four of nine patients had chest pain during minocycline injection. None had ST-T segment changes.

Markiewicz et al. [61] also evaluated in a dog model whether intrapericardial instillation of tetracycline is superior to the effect of drainage alone in causing pericardial adhesions and cavity obliteration. Twelve mongrel dogs were randomly divided into two experimental groups. All dogs received a pericardial drain through a sterile thoracotomy. Group A dogs (n = 6) received minocycline hydrochloride, 20 mg/kg, group B received normal saline. All dogs were sacrificed one month later. Echocardiograms performed one week postsurgery were normal in all dogs. Macroscopic evaluation disclosed that all group

A dogs had over 25% cavity obliteration whereas group B dogs had no adhesions or had obliteration of less than 25% of the cavity area. Microscopic evaluation showed that group A dogs had severe pericardial fibrosis and thickening with slight focal lymphoplasmocytic infiltration. Myocardial damage was not seen.

Intrapericardial Treatment with Mitoxantrone

The antineoplastic anthraquinone mitoxantrone shows a strong dose-response relation in respect to its antiproliferative and cytotoxic properties [62], in particular when regularly high substance levels can be achieved permanently. High local substance levels can be achieved due to the high molecular weight of the substance and its long half-life (long retention time in the place of application). Following their previous positive experiences in the treatment of malignant pleural effusions, Musch et al. [42] applied mitoxantrone $1-3 \times 10-20$ mg for the intrapericardial therapy of malignant pericardial effusions in 16 patients with cytologically verified malignant pericardial effusions (8 with bronchial carcinoma, 7 with carcinoma of the breast, 1 with adenocarcinoma of the stomach). Mitoxantrone was diluted in 30 ml of physiological saline solution and applied after warming-up to the body temperature within 48 h of the initial drainage of the pericardial effusion. This instillation was drained 24 h later. If the volume of the recurrence of the pericardial effusion was greater than 100 ml at that time, a second (3 patients) and, if necessary after a further 24 h, a third instillation (6 patients) was carried out in the same way. In 6 patients, a single application was sufficient without renewed formation of effusion or non-drainage-dependent recurrence. In order to avoid interactions, no further local or systemic cytotoxic chemotherapy was performed within 30 days following mitoxantrone instillation. The total mean dose of mitoxantrone was 27.5 mg (range 10–60 mg) with one patient receiving a total dose of 10 mg, 7 patients 20 mg each, 6 patients receiving a total dose of 30 mg each, one patient 50 mg and another one 60 mg. The average time during which a pigtail catheter was kept intrapericardially was 4.3 days (range 3–8 days). The treatment was successful in 15/16 patients (93.7%). After 30 days 12 of 16 patients were still in complete remission (no recurrence of a detectable effusion), 3 patients had recurrence of a small effusion without need for further treatment. Within the mean follow-up period of 189 days no recurrences occurred. Side effects were mild (World Health Organization grade II–III) and included loss of appetite and leukocytopenia both in one patient (6.3%).

Norum et al. [43] treated five patients (breast cancer – 4 patients, ovarian cancer – 1 patient) with ultrasound-guided pericardiocentesis followed by instillation of Mitoxantrone (10 mg). Evaluation was performed at a median follow-up of 59 days (range 28–294 days): two patients achieved complete remission, and one partial remission. Two patients were alive 213 and 294 days following therapy.

Also in several other studies carried out with smaller patient numbers and case reports, mitoxantrone demonstrated high effectiveness in intracavitary application for palliative therapy of malignant pericardial effusions (96% responses in total) [63–65]. Here, apart from one mild case of transient leucopenia, again no significant side effects were observed.

Intrapericardial Treatment with OK-432

Imamura et al. [29] have treated ten patients with malignant pericardial effusion with intrapericardial injection of OK-432 (penicillin- and heat-treated lyophilized powder of the substrain of Streptococcus pyogenes A3). Five or 10 units of OK-432 diluted in 20 ml of saline were injected into the pericardial space in seven and three patients, respectively. Seven patients were treated only once and the remaining three required a second treatment. Complete control of pericardial effusion was achieved in all patients for an average of 329 days (range 54–790). Fever and chest pain were experienced in six and five patients, respectively, but were controlled with antipyretics. Two of three patients who received 10 units of OK-432 experienced hypotension that was successfully controlled with vasopressor drugs with or without re-aspiration of pericardial fluid.

A follow-up computed tomography scan was performed in seven patients and a thickened pericardium was noticed in five, but no patient had developed constrictive pericarditis.

Radioactive Chromic Phosphate

Martini et al. [38] have treated 28 patients with malignant pericardial effusion by intrapericardial instillation of radioactive chromic phosphate. At the time of diagnosis of pericardial disease, 14 patients had major manifestations of tamponade; the rest had little or no clinical evidence of effusion. Only eight of the 28 patients had further problems with effusion after the initial pericardiocentesis and 32P instillation. Additional aspirations were done on those patients two weeks to five months later. The average survival was nine months; seven patients lived more than one year. Firusian et al. [37] treated 11 patients with malignant pericardial tamponade by instillation of radioactive phosphorus. Only two patients had further problems with effusion after radioisotope therapy. Remarkable long-lasting remission could be observed in the rest of patients. Dempke and Firusian [36] evaluated the efficacy of intrapericardial 32P-colloid in terms of response rates and duration of remissions using 185-370 MBq (5-10 mCi) 32P-colloid in 36 patients with malignant pericardial effusion. This treatment resulted in a complete remission rate of 94.5% (34 patients) whereas two patients did not respond to treatment due to a massive formation of pericardial fluid. The median duration of remission was 8 months (range 3–24 months).

Intrapericardial Immunotherapy in Malignant Pericardial Effusion

It has been shown that the repeated transfer of autologous tumor-stimulated T cells into tumor sites can be effective not only as a local adoptive immunotherapy for the target tumor, but also in spreading the immune response systemically to distant metastatic tumor sites [66, 67]. Toh et al. [46] investigated the presence of cytotoxic T lymphocytes (CTLs) in malignant pericardial effusion and clinical response to intrapericardial administration of IL-2-activated autologous tumor infiltrating lymphocytes (TILs). Four patients were treated: one male with advanced esophageal cancer, one female with recurrent lung cancer, and two females with metastatic breast cancer. Autologous TILs from pericardial effusion were expanded in vitro with IL-2, characterized for CD3, CD4 and

CD8 markers, checked for contamination and then infused into the patient's pericardial space through a catheter. This was repeated biweekly. After treatment, there were no signs of recurrence of pericardial effusion. The only adverse effect was a low-grade fever.

Complications and Side Effects of Intrapericardial Treatment of Neoplastic Pericarditis

In our study one patient with breast cancer (2.4%) developed myocardial ischemia after cisplatin instillation with an increase in plasma concentrations of creatine kinase and lactate dehydrogenase (CK_{max} 894 IU, and LDH_{max} 2346 IU)[3]. There were no other complications of the treatment. In the experience of Tomkowski et al. [12] transient atrial fibrillation was detected in three patients (18.8%) and mild nausea occurred in one case. Sclerosation of the pericardium and constrictive pericarditis were detected after the procedure in one case. With cisplatin, no hypotension and retrosternal pain were observed in contrast to some other agents. Mild or moderate nausea occurred in all patients, but no hematological and renal toxicity and local or infectious complications were observed in the study of Fiorentino et al. [15]. Similarly, no significant side-effects were observed in the study of Tondini et al. [16].

Intracavitary instillation of some antitumor agents can result in severe pain, arrhythmias, and bone marrow toxicity. The instillation of sclerosing agents has the disadvantage of an unpredictable sclerotic process especially for long-term survivors [29, 33, 41]. Although not related to intrapericardial treatment, reports of Tulleken et al. [68] on constrictive pericarditis after high-dose systemic chemotherapy and Kahles et al. [69] on mitoxantrone-induced acute left heart failure after intrapleural administration are indicating the need for a close follow-up of all patients treated with anti-neoplastic agents intrapericardially.

Intrapericardial Treatment of Autoreactive Pericarditis

With the application of standard clinical, biochemical, and cytological methods only, the etiology of the majority of acute and chronic/recurrent pericarditis cases remains unresolved [70, 71]. Many of these idiopathic cases will represent either viral infections or autoreactive pericarditis, however. Autoreactive pericarditis is a newly recognized form of acute pericarditis with an increased number of lymphocytes and mononuclear cells, as well as the presence of antisarcolemmal antibodies in the pericardial fluid, signs of myocarditis on epicardial or endomyocardial biopsies and the exclusion of any other specific etiology of pericardial disease. Identification of this form of pericarditis was enabled by a comprehensive diagnostic evaluation of patients, including early pericardiocentesis, pericardioscopy, epicardial biopsy as well as molecular and immunological evaluation of obtained fluid and tissue samples. These patients might have constituted part of the patients with "idiopathic" pericarditis in the study of other investigators.

The diagnosis of chronic autoreactive pericarditis can be established using the same criteria in patients with a longer duration of the effusion or recurrence of symptoms[3, 72, 73]:

1. increased number of lymphocytes and mononuclear cells, as well as the presence of antibodies against heart muscle tissue (primarily antisarcolemmal antibodies) in the pericardial fluid;
2. signs of myocarditis on epicardial or endomyocardial biopsies by >14 infiltrating cells/mm^2;
3. exclusion of active viral infection both in pericardial effusion and endomyocardial/epimyocardial biopsies (no virus isolation, no IgM-titer against cardiotropic viruses in pericardial effusion, and negative polymerase chain reaction (PCR) for major cardiotropic viruses;
4. tuberculosis, Borrelia burgdorferi, Chlamydia pneumoniae, and other bacterial infection excluded by PCR and/or cultures;
5. neoplastic cells absent in the cytological of pericardial effusion and no neoplastic changes in the biopsy samples;
6. exclusion of systemic and metabolic disorders, as well as uremia.

In virus-positive effusions corticosteroid treatment is not recommended. In autoreactive and "idiopathic" effusions therapeutic efficacy has been shown for the treatment with colchicine [75–77]. However, a substantial number of patients with chronic forms are resistant to either non-steroid anti-inflammatory treatment or colchicine. Remaining classic treatment options such as systemic glucocorticoid treatment has almost always considerable side effects. Pericardiectomy must be considered as the last treatment option due to its potential risks and discomfort caused for the patients by sternotomy and the hemodynamic consequences for the cardiac stiffness.

In patients with chronic or recurring autoreactive pericardial effusions intrapericardial instillation of crystalloid glucocorticoids can avoid systemic side effects, still allowing a high local dose application. This concept has proven its long-term efficacy in our experience and in the studies of other investigators [72–74, 78–82].

In the study of Maisch et al. [74] the intrapericardial instillation of triamcinolone was applied in 84 patients with autoreactive pericardial effusion in two different regimens (group 1: 54 patients, 600 mg/m^2/24 h; group 2: 30 patients, 300 mg/m^2/24 h). Colchicine 0.5 mg tid was used as adjuvant oral treatment for the first six months of follow-up.

The instillation of crystalloid suspension of triamcinolone in 100 ml of 0.9% NaCl was performed as a single slow injection over a 7-F pigtail catheter introduced after pericardiocentesis. The instillation may be painful and analgesic premedication may be given (morphine 5 mg i.v.). The triamcinolone solution was kept intrapericardially for at least 24 hours but most of the time left in place, if in the follow-up no further evacuation was needed. After aspiration of excessive residual fluid the pigtail catheter was removed within 24 to 48 hours.

Both therapeutic regimens (triamcinolone 300 mg/m^2/24 h and 600 mg/m^2/24 h) were successful in all patients regarding the immediate result of the procedure – i.e. after the drainage of the effusion and triamcinolone instillation all patients could be promptly discharged with only minimal or no residual effusion.

During the follow-up of 12 months there was no cardiovascular mortality in either group. The intrapericardial administration of crystalloid triamcinolone resulted in symptomatic improvement and prevented effusion recurrence in 92.6% vs. 86.7% of the patients after 3 months and in 86.0% vs. 82.1% after one year in the group 1 (high dose) and group 2 (lower dose) respectively (p > 0.05 for both compari-

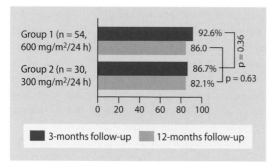

⬛ Fig. 10.3. Proportion of patients free of pericardial effusion three and twelve months after intrapericardial treatment with 600 mg/m²/24 h or 300 mg/m²/24 h of triamcinolone. Both regimens are highly efficient, without significant advantage for the higher dosage (p > 0.05). Reproduced with permission from Maisch et al. (2002) [74]

sons; Fig. 10.3). Patients with relapses of pericardial effusion in group 1 were asymptomatic in 100% (4/4) and 71.4% (5/7) after 3 and 12 months of follow-up, respectively. Patients with effusion relapses in group 2 were asymptomatic in 75% (3/4) and 60% (3/5) after 3 and 12 months of follow-up, respectively (mean time to relapse 4.9 ± 3.8 vs. 3.0 ± 2.9 months in group 1 vs. group 2, respectively; p>0.05). The higher dose of triamcinolone was successfully instilled for the treatment of symptomatic recurrences in two patients and also in two patients in group 2. For the recurrences of small, asymptomatic pericardial effusions intrapericardial treatment was not repeated.

There were no treatment-related acute complications in both groups. However, during the follow-up, a significantly larger proportion of the patients developed transitory iatrogenic Cushing syndrome in group 1 (29.6%) in contrast to 13.3% in group 2 (p<0.05). Six patients in group 1 and four patients in group 2 had gastrointestinal side effects of colchicine treatment, which were promptly relieved after discontinuation of the medication. In none of them either pericardial effusion or relapses of symptoms were noted during the follow-up. None of the patients have developed signs of constriction and none had to undergo surgical pericardiectomy.

The application of intrapericardial steroids was for the first time proposed by Spodick in 1964 [83] for the prevention of constriction after tuberculous pericarditis and later on by Zeman and Scovern [84] in 1977 for the treatment of rheumatoid pericardial

tamponade. Further application was, however, mostly dedicated to uremic and dialysis-associated pericardial effusion (see next section).

In our experience, as well as in most of the published reports in uremic pericarditis, there were no major complications. It must be, however, kept in mind that in the setting of high-dose glucocorticoid treatment an increased risk of infection and development of purulent pericarditis certainly exists. We therefore treat all patients undergoing intrapericardial triamcinolone therapy with i.v. antibiotics as long as the pigtail catheter is in the pericardium and the patients are treated in hospital and experienced no infection of the puncture site and the pericardium. However, an infection with Staphylococcus aureus complicating intrapericardial steroid instillation in uremic pericarditis that lead to purulent pericarditis requiring pericardiectomy was described by Feinroth et al. [85]. Even a more serious warning is coming from a report on staphylococcal purulent pericarditis requiring pericardiectomy and prolonged intubation developed in a 17-months old girl even after a single application of steroid cream on the skin for varicella lesions [86]. Asymptomatic iatrogenic arteriovenous fistula of the mammary artery and vein was noted in two patients [78, 87].

An important detail in the application of intrapericardial triamcinolone is that it can be painful. Therefore, the instillation must be covered by proper analgesia, carried out slowly, with using 37 °C warm normal saline solution. Hemodynamic monitoring during the application of the intrapericardial treatment is a useful precaution measure for any side effect.

Intrapericardial application of corticosteroid therapy avoids major side effects of systemic treatment as well as compliance problems. However, the systemic absorption and an iatrogenic Cushing's syndrome cannot be completely avoided as noted in the report by Grubb et al. [88]. However, our experience has shown that the effect is dose-dependent and that side effects could be significantly diminished with the application of a lower dose of traimcinolone as applied in most of the studies in uremic pericarditis [78–82] and in our pilot trials [72, 73]. Further clinical studies are necessary to investigate if the same therapeutic effect could be achieved with even a lower dose than 300 mg/m².

Intrapericardial Treatment of Uremic Pericarditis

Renal failure is producing large pericardial effusions in approximately 20% of patients [89, 90]. It results from inflammation of the visceral and parietal pericardium and correlates with the degree of azotemia (BUN >60 mg/dl). Two forms have been described:

1. Uremic pericarditis: 6–10% of patients with advanced renal failure before dialysis has been instituted or shortly thereafter.
2. Dialysis-associated pericarditis: in up to 13% of patients on maintenance hemodialysis, and occasionally with chronic peritoneal dialysis due to inadequate dialysis and/or fluid overload.

Adhesions between the thickened pericardial membranes make a "bread and butter" appearance. Fever, pleuritic chest pain, and pericardial rubs may be noticed regardless of the size of the effusion. Autonomic impairment may occur in some uremic patients, causing that heart rate remains 60–80 beats/min despite tamponade. Anemia, due to erythropoietin resistance worsens the symptoms [91]. The ECG does not show the typical diffuse ST/T wave elevations due to the lack of the myocardial inflammation. Otherwise, intercurrent infection should be suspected [90].

Most patients with uremic pericarditis respond to hemodialysis (heparin-free to avoid hemopericardium) with the resolution of chest pain and of the pericardial effusion within 1–2 weeks. Peritoneal dialysis may be therapeutic in pericarditis resistant to hemodialysis, or if heparin-free hemodialysis cannot be performed. NSAIDs and systemic corticosteroids have limited success when intensive dialysis is ineffective. Cardiac tamponade and large effusions resistant to dialysis must be treated with pericardiocentesis. Large, non-resolving symptomatic effusions can be treated with intrapericardial instillation of corticosteroids (triamcinolone hexacetonide 50 mg every 6 hours for 2 to 3 days). Pericardiectomy is indicated only in refractory, severely symptomatic patients. Colchicine may worsen the impaired renal function, but benefit was also noted in a resistant case of uremic pericarditis [92].

Peraino et al. [93] emphasized that in patients with large uremic pericardial effusion elective pericardial drainage with instillation of triamcinolone hexacetonide is the treatment of choice according to their experience in 22 patients. However, for small pericardial effusions they recommended a trial of nonsteroid anti-inflammatory drugs and/or intensive dialysis.

Buselmeier et al. [78] have treated 45 patients with uremic pericardial effusion instillating 200 mg of methylprednisolone and 80–1250 mg of triamcinolone intrapericardially for an average of 50 hours. Triamcinolone doses were administered in 4–6 hours intervals until the pericardial drainage was stopped. Before the removal of the catheter a final dose of 50 mg of triamcinolone was instilled. The procedure had an immediate success rate of 97.8% regarding both pericardial pain and effusion production. During the mean follow-up 14 months (range 1–54 months) there was no recurrence of symptoms or pericardial effusion in 95.6% of patients. However, one patient developed an unusual complication – an asymptomatic internal mammary artery fistula. Notably, our treatment regimen in autoreactive pericarditis had similar efficacy despite its single administration of triamcinolone and its shorter duration of treatment [74].

Reversal of intractable uremic pericarditis by triamcinolone hexacetonide was also achieved in small group of patients by Fuller et al. [79] and Quigg et al. [80]. In all patients a prompt hemodynamic and symptomatic improvement was maintained during the long-time follow-up (six months to six years). The successful use of intrapericardial triamcinolone in a 10-year anephric boy on chronic dialysis was reported by Medani et al. [94].

Instillation of triamcinolone after surgical pericardiotomy in uremic patients was also highly efficient [81, 95] with only one recurrence in 16 patients during the median follow-up of 4.2 years [95].

Intrapericardial Treatment of Purulent Pericarditis

Purulent pericarditis is a rare, acute, fulminate infectious illness, always fatal if untreated. Predisposing conditions include previous pericardial effusion, immunosuppression, chronic diseases (alcohol abuse, rheumatoid arthritis, etc.), cardiac surgery, and chest trauma. The pericardial infection (or superinfection) can arise by direct infection during trauma, thoracic surgery, or catheter drainage, by spread from an intrathoracic, myocardial or subdiaphragmatic focus, and by hematogenous dissemination. The most frequent causes are Staphylococcus, Pneumococcus, Streptococcus, Haemophilus, and Mycobacterium tuberculosis. Less common are anaerobic isolates such as Prevotella species, Peptostreptococcus species, and Propionibacterium acnes [96]. The incidence of purulent pericarditis has declined since the introduction of broad-spectrum antibiotics [97] but it remains an important differential diagnosis, especially with concomitant chronic diseases or immunosuppression, because if left untreated, the combination of tamponade and sepsis results in a mortality rate approaching 100% [98]. Even in patients who underwent combined maximal antibiotic treatment with early complete surgical drainage survival was not better than 50% [99]. Moreover, acute constrictive pericarditis can develop, which may necessitate emergency pericardiectomy [100, 101].

The mortality rate in treated patients is 40%, mostly due to cardiac tamponade, toxicity, and constriction [102, 103]. Percutaneous pericardiocentesis must be promptly performed. The pericardial fluid should undergo Gram, acid-fast, and fungal staining, followed by cultures of the pericardial and body fluids. Rinsing of the pericardial cavity, combined with an effective systemic antibiotic therapy is mandatory (antistaphylococcal antibiotic plus aminoglycoside, tailored according to pericardial fluid and blood cultures) [104]. Intrapericardial instillation of antibiotics (e.g. gentamycin) is useful but not sufficient. Open surgical drainage and pericardiectomy are required in patients with dense adhesions, loculated and thick purulent effusion, recurrence of tamponade, persistent infection, and progression to constriction [104, 105]. However, surgical mortality is up to 8% or even more. More recently, surgical management of purulent pericarditis using thoracoscopic pericardiectomy was reported in 21 children, with no intraoperative or postoperative complications during 4–15 months follow-up [106].

Instead of surgery, pericardiocentesis and frequent irrigation of the pericardial cavity with urokinase or streptokinase was applied in a small series of patients and several case reports since 1951 when it was applied for the first time by Wright et al. [98–100, 107–121]. Streptokinase has been previously used intrapleurally for over 30 years to aid the drainage of loculated empyema, without inducing any systemic fibrinolytic effects [122, 123]. More recently, tissue plasminogen activator was applied for the management of two complex patients with fibropurulent pericarditis [124, 125]. Importantly, if intrapericardial fibrinolytic therapy is selected for the management of these difficult patients, it should be started as soon as fibrin deposits are detected and before fibrocytes can invade and organize exudate. Intrapericardial streptokinase helps to dissolve the fibrinous components of these exudates and is also used to prevent drainage failure caused by the fibrin clots and loculation.

Ekim et al. [121] have treated nine children (five boys, mean age of 6.7 ± 2.9 years, range 3–13 years) with purulent pericarditis by pericardial drainage followed by the streptokinase instillation and antibiotics. Streptokinase regimen included instillation of 15000–18000 IU/kg dissolved in 50 ml of isotonic solution warmed to body temperature to prevent arrhythmias. The catheters remained clamped for 2 h after instillation. Instillation was done twice daily until the drainage had ceased. None of the patients had systemic bleeding, arrhythmias, or hypotension suggesting an anaphylactic reaction. Drainage was required for 3–9 days (mean 5.2 ± 2.2 days). The average daily drainage volume was 45 ± 15 ml. The amount of drainage decreased continuously and catheters were removed when fluid production had stopped. All patients have survived. During the follow-up ranging from 6 months to 5 years after the treatment none experienced a recurrence of the effusion and none developed pericardial constriction.

Schafer et al. [116] reported on the successful treatment of a non-resolving fibrino-purulent pericardial effusion in a 39-year-old man by combined intrapericardial irrigation of fibrinolytics and systemic corticosteroids administration as an alternative to pericardiectomy.

Ustunsoy et al. [115] have treated six children and three adult purulent pericarditis patients with intrapericardial fibrinolysis by streptokinase (2000 U/kg/day diluted in 50 ml of saline). No patients had systemic bleeding, arrhythmias, or hypotension. However, despite this treatment, one patient died due to sepsis and progression of congestive heart failure. In the remaining eight patients repeat echocardiograms showed neither reaccumulation of the pericardial effusion, nor pericardial thickening nor constrictions after six months follow-up.

To investigate whether intrapericardial urokinase irrigation along with pericardiocentesis could prevent pericardial constriction in patients with infectious exudative pericarditis Cui et al. performed a randomized study in 34 patients with purulent pericarditis and in 60 patients with tuberculous pericarditis [100]. Patients were randomized to receive either intrapericardial urokinase along with conventional treatment in the study group, or conventional treatment alone (including pericardiocentesis and drainage) in the control group. The dosage of urokinase ranged from 200,000 to 600,000 U (mean 320,000 ± 70,000 U). During the mean follow-up of 56.8 ± 29.0 months, there were no cardiac deaths, and pericardial constriction was observed less frequently in 9 (19.1%) patients in the study group treated with urokinase when compared to 27 patients (57.4%) of the control group (p < 0.0001).

There are several adverse effects of fibrinolytic therapy including allergic reactions, yet systemic side effects have been very rarely reported after pleural or pericardial application of fibrinolytic therapy [126]. Juneja et al. [112] reported a case of a right atrial thrombus and a submitral aneurysm after intrapericardial streptokinase. Other reported complications of staphylococcal pericarditis include the development of a mycotic aneurysm of the proximal aorta and metastatic septic emboli [127]. Streptokinase stimulates interstitial collagen breakdown [128] and it is possible that a high local concentration of streptokinase caused the aneurysm. Furthermore, Huang et al. [109] described a hyperacute cardiac tamponade that complicated thrombolytic therapy in a patient with purulent pericarditis. Importantly, Cui et al. [100] reported on intrapericardial bleeding in 6/47 patients treated with urokinase (mean dose 320,000 ± 70,000 U). Finally, Bridgman et al. [113] reported on a failure of intrapericardial treatment with 100,000 IJ of streptokinase given every 8 hours in a 61-years old woman with purulent pericarditis. After 24 hours of this treatment, no sufficient drainage was possible and the patient had to undergo open surgical drainage and pericardiectomy.

Future Perspectives and Recommendations

The ultimate outcome for patients with malignant pericardial disease depends on the clinical status of the patient, the presence and extension of the metastatic disease, the efficacy of adjuvant systemic therapy, and the local management of the pericardial effusion for the long-term abolition of tamponade. Up to now there are no prospective randomized trials comparing different methods and drugs of local therapy to evaluate long-term effectiveness or survival.

Intrapericardial treatment of neoplastic pericarditis with cisplatin in addition to the systemic chemotherapy successfully prevents recurrences of symptoms and pericardial effusion. The treatment was more successful in lung than in breast cancer patients. Instillation of thiotepa, colloid 32P and other agents was also confirmed as beneficial by other authors. Double-blind randomized trials are necessary to prove the final clinical value of intrapericardial treatment of neoplastic pericardial effusion and to verify the selection of the most efficient agent for the specific tumors.

The current findings of all intrapericardial treatment studies are however limited by the lack of control groups as well as by the possible combined effect of different systemic chemotherapeutic agents with the intrapericardial treatment. However, the high incidence of recurrences of large neoplastic pericardial effusion treated only with pericardiocentesis and systemic chemotherapy is well known and from the ethical reasons it would be difficult to define an appropriate control group receiving no treatment or placebo.

Furthermore, it would be even more unethical to deprive patients from the systemic chemotherapy in order to see the "pure" effect of intrapericardial cisplatin or thiotepa.

A final limitation could be the effect of previous radiotherapy, or concomitant infection, or lymphatic obstruction, which could be a cause of non-malignant pericardial effusion in patients with known malignancies. Therefore, intrapericardial application of antineoplastic agents should be performed in patients with proven neoplastic involvement of the pericardium either by cytology or by histology.

References

1. Mukai K, Shinkai T, Tominaga K, Shimosatto Y. The incidence of secondary tumors of the heart and pericardium: A 10 year study. Jpn J Clin Oncol 1988; 18(3): 195–201

2. Posner MR, Cohen GI, Skarin AT. Pericardial disease in patients with cancer. Am J Med 1981; 71(3): 407–413

3. Maisch B, Ristić AD, Pankuweit S, Neubauer A, Moll R. Neoplastic pericardial effusion. Efficacy and safety of intrapericardial treatment with cisplatin. Eur Heart J 2002; 23(20): 1625–1631

4. Wilding G, Green HL, Longo DL, Urba WJ. Tumors of the heart and pericardium. Cancer Treat Rev 1988; 15: 165–181

5. Spodick DH. Pericardial diseases. In: Braunwald E, Zipes DP, Libby P (eds) Heart Disease, 6th ed. W.B. Saunders, Philadelphia, PA, 2001, pp 1823–1876

6. Ziskind AA, Palacios IF. Percutaneous balloon pericardiotomy for patients with pericardial effusion and tamponade. In: Topol EJ (ed) Textbook of Interventional Cardiology, 3rd edn. W.B. Saunders, Philadelphia, PA, 1999, pp 869–877

7. Ristić AD, Seferović PM, Maksimović R, Ostojić M. Percutaneous balloon pericardiotomy in neoplastic pericardial effusion. In: Seferović PM, Spodick DH, Maisch B. (eds) Pericardiology: Contemporary answers to continuing challenges. Science, Belgrade, 2000, pp 427–438

8. Aitini E, Cavazzini G, Pasquini E, et al. Treatment of primary or metastatic pleural effusion with intracavitary cytosine arabinoside and cisplatin. A phase II study. Acta Oncol 1994; 33(2): 191–194

9. Bindi M, Trusso M, Tucci E. Intracavitary cisplatin in malignant cardiac tamponade. Tumori 1987; 73(2): 163–165

10. Pavon-Jimenez R, Garcia-Rubira JC, Garcia-Martinez JT, Sanchez-Escribano R, Calvo-Jambrina R, Cruz-Fernandez JM. Intrapericardial cisplatin for malignant tamponade. Rev Esp Cardiol 2000; 53(4): 587–589

11. Tomkowski W, Szturmowicz M, Fijalkowska A, Filipecki S, Figura-Chojak E. Intrapericardial cisplatin for the management of patients with large malignant pericardial effusion. J Cancer Res Clin Oncol 1994; 120(7): 434–436

12. Tomkowski WZ, Filipecki S. Intrapericardial cisplatin for the management of patients with large malignant pericardial effusion in the course of the lung cancer. Lung Cancer 1997; 16(2-3): 215–222

13. Tomkowski WZ, Filipecki S. Intrapericardial administration of cisplatin in treatment of metastatic pericardial involvement in adenocarcinoma of the lung. Arch Chest Dis 1997; 52: 221–224

14. Tomkowski W, Szturmowicz M, Fijalkowska A, Burakowski J, Filipecki S. New approaches to the management and treatment of malignant pericardial effusion. Support Care Cancer 1997; 5(1): 64–66

15. Fiorentino MV, Daniele O, Morandi P, et al. Intrapericardial instillation of platin in malignant pericardial effusion. Cancer 1988; 62(9): 1904–1906

16. Tondini M, Rocco G, Bianchi C, Severi C, Corbellini D. Intracavitary cisplatin (CDDP) in the treatment of metastatic pericardial involvement from breast and lung cancer. Monaldi Arch Chest Dis 1995; 50(2): 86–88

17. Lestuzzi Ch, Viel E, Sorio R, Meneguzzo N. Local chemotherapy for neoplastic pericardial effusion [letter]. Am J Cardiol 2000; 86: 1292

18. Beretta F, Martinelli G, Cavalli F, Marone C. Pericardial effusion in patients with malignant neoplasms. Schweiz Med Wochenschr 1992; 122: 1517–1524

19. Bishiniotis TS, Antoniadou S, Katseas G, Mouratidou D, Litos AG, Balamoutsos N. Malignant cardiac tamponade in women with breast cancer treated by pericardiocentesis and intrapericardial administration of triethylenethiophosphoramide (thiotepa). Am J Cardiol 2000; 86(3): 362–364

20. Colleoni M, Martinelli G, Beretta F, et al. Intracavitary chemotherapy with thiotepa in malignant pericardial effusions: an active and well-tolerated regimen. J Clin Oncol 1998; 16: 2371–2376

21. Girardi LN, Ginsberg RJ, Burt ME. Pericardiocentesis and intrapericardial sclerosis: effective therapy for malignant pericardial effusions. Ann Thorac Surg 1997; 64(5): 1422–1447

22. Martinoni A, Cipolla CM, Civelli M, et al. Intrapericardial treatment of neoplastic pericardial effusions. Herz 2000; 25(8): 787–793

23. Fukuoka M, Takada M, Tamai S, et al. Local application of anti-cancer drugs for the treatment of malignant pleural and pericardial effusion. Gan To Kagaku Ryoho 1984; 11(8): 1543–1549

24. Thai V, Oneschuk D. Malignant pericardial effusion treated with intrapericardial bleomycin. J Palliat Med 2007; 10(2): 281–282

25. Kaira K, Mori M. Intrapericardial instillation of mitomycin C in recurrent cardiac tamponade due to malignant pericardial effusion. Clin Oncol (R Coll Radiol) 2006; 18(6): 506

26. Bischiniotis TS, Lafaras CT, Platogiannis DN, Moldovan L, Barbetakis NG, Katseas GP. Intrapericardial cisplatin administration after pericardiocentesis in patients with lung adenocarcinoma and malignant cardiac tamponade. Hellenic J Cardiol 2005; 46(5): 324–329

27. Martinoni A, Cipolla CM, Cardinale D, Civelli M, Lamantia G, Colleoni M, Fiorentini C. Long-term results of intrapericardial chemotherapeutic treatment of malignant pericardial effusions with thiotepa. Chest 2004; 126(5): 1412–1416

28. Lissoni P, Barni S, Tancini G, et al. Intracavitary therapy of neoplastic effusions with cytokines: comparison among interferon alpha, beta and interleukin-2. Support Care Cancer 1995; 3(1): 78–80

29. Imamura T, Tamura K, Takenaga M, Nagamoto Y, Ishikawa T, Nakagawa S. Intrapericardial OK-432 instillation for the management of malignant pericardial effusion. Cancer 1991; 68: 259–263

30. Liu G, Crump M, Goss PE, Dancey J, Shepherd FA. Prospective comparison of the sclerosing agents doxycycline and bleomycin for the primary management of malignant pericardial effusion and cardiac tamponade. J Clin Oncol 1996; 14(12): 3141–3147

31. van der Gaast A, Kok TC, van der Linden NH, Splinter TA. Intrapericardial instillation of bleomycin in the management of malignant pericardial effusion. Eur J Cancer Clin Oncol 1989; 25(10): 1505–1506

32. Yano T, Yokoyama H, Inoue T, Takanashi N, Asoh H, Ichinose Y. A simple technique to manage malignant pericardial effusion with a local instillation of bleomycin in non-small cell carcinoma of the lung. Oncology 1994; 51(6): 507–509

33. Cormican MC, Nyman CR. Intrapericardial bleomycin for the management of cardiac tamponade secondary to malignant pericardial effusion. Br Heart J 1990; 63: 61–62

34. Kohnoe S, Maehara Y, Takahashi I, et al. Intrapericardial mitomycin C for the management of malignant pericardial effusion secondary to gastric cancer: case report and review. Chemotherapy 1994; 40: 57–60

35. Lee LN, Yang PC, Chang DB, et al. Ultrasound guided pericardial drainage and intrapericardial instillation of mitomycin C for malignant pericardial effusion. Thorax 1994; 49(6): 594–595

36. Grau JJ, Estape J, Palombo H, et al. Intracavitary oxytetracycline in malignant pericardial tamponade. Oncology 1992; 49: 489–491

37. Davis S, Rambotti P, Grignani F. Intrapericardial tetracycline sclerosis in the treatment of malignant pericardial effusion: an analysis of thirty-three cases. J Clin Oncol 1984; 2(6): 631–636

38. Maher EA, Shepherd FA, Todd TJ. Pericardial sclerosis as the primary management of malignant pericardial effusion and cardiac tamponade. J Thorac Cardiovasc Surg 1996; 112(3): 637–643

39. Salamon P, Berliner S, Shachner A, Pinkhas J. Tetracycline treatment for malignant pericardial effusion. Med Interne 1989; 27(1): 73–74

40. Shepherd FA, Ginsberg JS, Evans WK, Scott JG, Oleksiuk F. Tetracycline sclerosis in the management of malignant pericardial effusion. J Clin Oncol 1985; 3(12): 1678–1682

41. Shepherd FA, Morgan C, Evans WK, Ginsberg JF, Watt D, Murphy K. Medical management of malignant pericardial effusion by tetracycline sclerosis. Am J Cardiol 1987; 60: 1161–1166

42. Musch E, Gremmler B, Nitsch J, Rieger J, Malek M, Chrissafidou A. Intrapericardial instillation of mitoxantrone in palliative therapy of malignant pericardial effusion. Onkologie 2003; 26: 135–139

43. Norum J, Lunde P, Aasebo U, Himmelmann A. Mitoxantrone in malignant pericardial effusion. J Chemother 1998; 10(5): 399–404

44. Ammon A, Eiffert H, Reil S, Beyer JH, Droese M, Hiddemann W. Tumor-associated antigens in effusions of malignant and benign origin. Clin Investig 1993; 71(6): 437–444

45. Kuhn K, Purea H, Selbach J, Westerhausen M. Treatment with locally applied mitoxantrone. Acta Med Austriaca 1989; 16(3-4): 87–90

46. Toh U, Fujii T, Seki N, Niiya F, Shirouzu K, Yamana H. Characterization of IL-2-activated TILs and their use in intrapericardial immunotherapy in malignant pericardial effusion. Cancer Immunol Immunother 2006; 55(10): 1219–1227

47. Nanjo T. Intracavitary injection of OK-432 for malignant pericardial effusion, a case report. Radiat Med 1990; 8(4): 155–158

48. Imamura T, Tamura K, Taguchi T, Makino S, Seita M. Intrapericardial instillation of OK-432 for the management of malignant pericardial effusion: report of three cases. Jpn J Med 1989; 28(1): 62–66

49. Wakiyama S, Shirabe K, Nagaie T. A case of carcinomatous cardiac tamponade due to breast cancer treated with OK-432 and mitomycin C. Gan To Kagaku Ryoho 2007; 34(3): 439–441

50. Furukawa A, Itoh A, Nakamura T, et al. Efficacy of percutaneous balloon pericardiotomy and intrapericardial instillation for the management of refractory pericardial effusion: a case report. J Cardiol 2007; 50(6): 389–395

51. Tomkowski W7, Wiśniewska J, Szturmowicz M, et al. Evaluation of intrapericardial cisplatin administration in cases with recurrent malignant pericardial effusion and cardiac tamponade. Support Care Cancer 2004; 12(1): 53–57

52. Ultmann JE, Hyman GA, Grandall C, et al. Triethylenethiophosphoramide (thiotepa) in the treatment of neoplastic disease. Cancer 1957; 19: 902–910

53. Anderson CB, Philpott GW, Ferguson TB. The treatment of malignant pleural effusions. Cancer 1974; 33: 916–922

54. Koontz WW, Prout GR, Smith W, et al. The use of intravesical thiotepa in the management of non-invasive carcinoma of the bladder. J Urol 1981; 125: 307–312

55. De Kock mIS, Breytenbach IH. Local excision and topical thiotepa in the treatment of transitional cell carcinoma of the renal perlvis: a case report. J Urol 1986; 135: 566–567

56. van Belle SJ, Volckaert A, Taeymans Y, Spapen H, Block P. Treatment of malignant pericardial tamponade with sclerosis induced by instillation of bleomycin. Int J Cardiol 1987; 16(2): 155–160

57. Kawashima O, Kurihara T, Kamiyoshihara M, Sakata S, Ishikawa S, Morishita Y. Management of malignant pericardial effusion resulting from recurrent cancer with local instillation of aclarubicin hydrochloride. Am J Clin Oncol 1999; 22(4): 396–398

58. Celermajer DS, Boyer MJ, Bailey BP, Tattersall MH. Pericardiocentesis for symptomatic malignant pericardial effusion: a study of 36 patients. Med J Aust 1991; 154(1): 19–22

59. Lashevsky I, Ben Yosef R, Rinkevich D, Reisner S, Markiewicz W. Intrapericardial minocycline sclerosis for malignant pericardial effusion. Chest 1996; 109(6): 1452–1454

60. Markiewicz W, Lashevsky I, Rinkevich D, Teitelman U, Reisner SA. The acute effect of minocycline on the pericardium: experimental and clinical findings. Chest 1998; 113(4): 861–866

61. Markiewicz W, Ben-Arieh Y, Best L, et al. The effect of Minocin on the pericardium. Oncology 1993; 50: 478–482

62. Ehninger G, Proksch B, Heinzel G, Schiller E, Weible KH, Woodward DL. The pharmacokinetics and metabolism of mitoxantrone in man. Invest New Drugs 1985; 3: 109–116

63. Lentsch S, Reichardt P, Gürtler R, Dörken B. Intrapericardial application of mitoxantrone for treatment of malignant pericardial effusion. Onkologie 1994; 17: 504–507

64. Hoffmann W, Reichel H, Schiebe M, Bültmann B, Bamberg M. Intrapericardial instillation of mitoxantrone in malignant pericarditis: Histomorphological appearance. Reg Cancer Treat 1993; 2: 91–93

65. Ammon J, Icking D, Sigmund M, Zimmermann U. Intraperikardiale Instillation von Mitoxantron bei malignen Perikardergüssen. In: Musch E, Dietel M, Schenk S (Hrsg) Aktuelle Onkologie 54. Zuckschwerdt, München, 1990, S 70–84

66. Toh U, Yamana H, Sueyoshi S, et al. Locoregional cellular immunotherapy for patients with advanced esophageal cancer. Clin Cancer Res 2000; 6: 4663–4673

67. Toh U, Sudo T, Kido K, et al. Locoregional adoptive immunotherapy resulted in regression in distant metastases of a recurrent esophageal cancer. Int J Clin Oncol 2002; 7: 372–375

68. Tulleken JE, Kooiman CG, van der Werf TS, Zijlstra JG, de Vries EG. Constrictive pericarditis after high-dose chemotherapy. Lancet 1997; 350(9091): 1601

69. Kahles H, Bastian HJ, Schiffmann O, Geck M, Helmke FR, Golz N. Mitoxantrone-induced acute left heart failure after intrapleural administration. Herz 1997; 22(4): 217–220

70. Permanyer-Miralda G, Sagrista-Sauleda J, Soler-Soler J. Primary acute pericardial disease: A prospective series of 231 consecutive patients. Am J Cardiol 1985; 56: 623–630

71. Sagrista-Sauleda J, Angel J, Permanyer-Miralda G, Soler-Soler J. Long-term follow-up of idiopathic chronic pericardial effusion. N Engl J Med 1999; 341: 2054–2059

72. Maisch B, Pankuweit S, Brilla C, et al. Intrapericardial treatment of inflammatory and neoplastic pericarditis guided by pericardioscopy and epicardial biopsy - results from a pilot study. Clin Cardiol 1999; 22(suppl 1): I17–22

73. Maisch B, Bethge C, Drude L, Hufnagel G, Herzum M, Schönian U. Pericardioscopy and epicardial biopsy-new diagnostic tools in pericardial and perimyocardial disease. Eur Heart J 1994; 15 (Suppl C): 68–73

74. Maisch B, Ristic AD, Pankuweit S. Intrapericardial treatment of autoreactive pericardial effusion with triamcinolone: the way to avoid side effects of systemic corticosteroid therapy. Eur Heart J 2002; 23: 1503–1508

75. Adler Y, Finkelstein Y, Guindo J, et al. Colchicine treatment for recurrent pericarditis. A decade of experience. Circulation 1998; 97: 2183–2185

76. Markel G, Imazio M, Brucato A, Adler Y. Colchicine for the prevention of recurrent pericarditis. Isr Med Assoc J 2008; 10(1): 69–72

77. Imazio M, Bobbio M, Cecchi E, et al. Colchicine as first-choice therapy for recurrent pericarditis: results of the CORE (COlchicine for REcurrent pericarditis) trial. Arch Intern Med 2005; 165(17): 1987–1991

78. Buselmeier TJ, Davin TD, Simmons RL, Najarian JS, Kjellstrand CM. Treatment of intractable uremic pericardial effusion. Avoidance of pericardiectomy with local steroid instillation. JAMA 1978; 240(13): 1358–1359

79. Fuller TJ, Knochel JP, Brennan JP, Fetner CD, White mg. Reversal of intractable uremic pericarditis by triamcinolone hexacetonide. Arch Intern Med 1976; 136(9): 979–982

80. Quigg RJ Jr, Idelson BA, Yoburn DC, Hymes JL, Schick EC, Bernard DB. Local steroids in dialysis-associated pericardial effusion. A single intrapericardial administration of triamcinolone. Arch Intern Med 1985; 145(12): 2249–2250

81. Popli S, Ing TS, Daugirdas JT, et al. Treatment of uremic pericardial effusion by local steroid instillation via subxiphoid pericardiotomy. J Dial 1980; 4(2-3): 83–89

82. Kristal B, Shasha SM, Mahmoud H, Stamler B. Management of uremic pericarditis. Isr J Med Sci 1986; 22(6): 442–444

83. Spodick DH. Chronic tuberculous and other granulomatous pericariditis. In: Spodick DH. Chronic and constrictive pericarditis. Grune & Stratton, New York, 1964, p 34

84. Zeman RK, Scovern H. Intrapericardial steroids in treatment of rheumatoid pericardial tamponade [letter]. Arthritis Rheum 1977; 20(6): 1289–1290

85. Feinroth MV, Goldstein EJ, Josephson A, Friedman EA. Infection complicating intrapericardial steroid instillation in uremic pericarditis. Clin Nephrol 1981; 15(6): 331–333

86. Brumund MR, Truemper EJ, Lutin WA, Pearson-Shaver AL. Disseminated varicella and staphylococcal pericarditis after topical steroids. J Pediatr 1997; 131(1): 162–163

87. Silverstein R, Crumbo D, Long DL, Kokko JP, Hull AR, Vergne-Marini P. Iatrogenic arteriovenous fistula. An unusual complication of indwelling pericardial catheter and intrapericardial steroid instillation for the treatment of uremic pericarditis. Arch Intern Med 1978; 138(2): 308–310

88. Grubb SR, Cantley LK, Jones DL, Carter WH. Iatrogenic Cushing's syndrome after intrapericardial corticosteroid therapy. Ann Intern Med 1981; 95(6): 706–707

89. Rostand SG, Rutsky EA. Pericarditis in end-stage renal disease. Cardiol Clin 1990; 8: 701–706

90. Gunukula SR, Spodick DH. Pericardial disease in renal patients. Semin Nephrol 2001; 21: 52–57

91. Tarng DC, Huang TP. Uraemic pericarditis: a reversible inflammatory state of resistance to recombinant human erythropoietin in haemodialysis patients. Nephrol Dial Transplant 1997; 12: 1051–1057

92. Spaia S, Patsalas S, Agelou A, et al. Managing refractory uraemic pericarditis with colchicine. Nephrol Dial Transplant 2004; 19(9): 2422–2423

93. Peraino RA. Pericardial effusion in patients treated with maintenance dialysis. Am J Nephrol 1983; 3(6): 319–322

94. Medani CR, Ringel RE. Intrapericardial triamcinolone hexacetonide in the treatment of intractable uremic pericarditis in a child. Pediatr Nephrol 1988; 2(1): 32–33

95. Daugirdas JT, Leehey DJ, Popli S, et al. Subxiphoid pericardiostomy for hemodialysis-associated pericardial effusion. Arch Intern Med 1986; 146(6): 1113–1115

96. Pankuweit S, Ristić AD, Seferović PM, Maisch B. Bacterial pericarditis: diagnosis and management. Am J Cardiovasc Drugs 2005; 5(2): 103–112

97. Klacsmann PG, Bulkley BH, Hutchins GM. The changed spectrum of purulent pericarditis. Am J Med 1977; 63: 666–673

98. Mann-Segal DDM, Shanahan EA, Jones B, Ramasamy D. Purulent pericarditis: rediscovery of an old remedy. J Thorac Cardiovasc Surg 1996; 111: 487–488

99. Defoullloy C, Meyer G, Slama M, et al. Intrapericardial fibrinolysis: a useful treatment in the management of purulent pericarditis. Intensive Care Med 1997; 23(1): 117–118

100. Cui HB, Chen XY, Cui CC, et al. Prevention of pericardial constriction by transcatheter intrapericardial fibrinolysis with urokinase. Chin Med Sci J 2005; 20(1): 5–10

101. Allaria A, Michelli D, Capelli H, Berri G, Gutierrez D. Transient cardiac constriction following purulent pericarditis. Eur J Pediatr 1992; 151(4): 250–251

102. Leoncini G, Iurilli L, Queirolo A, Catrambone G. Primary and secondary purulent pericarditis in otherwise healthy adults. Interact Cardiovasc Thorac Surg 2006; 5(5): 652–654

103. Sagrista-Sauleda J, Barrabes JA, Permanyer-Miralda G, et al. Purulent pericarditis: review of a 20-year experience in a general hospital. J Am Coll Cardiol 1993; 22: 1661–1665

104. Maisch B, Seferovic PM, Ristic AD, et al. Task Force on the Diagnosis and Management of Pericardial Diseases of the European Society of Cardiology. Guidelines on the diagnosis and management of pericardial diseases. Executive summary. Eur Heart J 2004; 25(7): 587–610

105. Kennedy C, McEvoy S. Purulent pericarditis. Ir J Med Sci. 2009; 178 (1): 97–99

106. Liem NT, Tuan T, Dung le A. Thoracoscopic pericardiectomy for purulent pericarditis: experience with 21 cases. J Laparoendosc Adv Surg Tech A 2006; 16(5): 518–521

107. Wright LT, Smith DH, Rothman M, Metzger WI, Quash ET. Use of streptokinase-dornase in certain surgical conditions. J Int Coll Surg 1951; 15: 286–299

108. Pierret R, Lorriaux A, Ratel J, Graillot M, Mesmacque R. Purulent pericarditis treated with streptokinase. Echo Med Nord 1953; 24(7): 232–233

109. Huang CH, Wu CC, Lee YT. Thrombolytic therapy complicated hyperacute cardiac tamponade in a patient with purulent pericarditis. Int J Cardiol 1996; 55(2): 209–210

110. Maynar J, Corral E, Manzano A, et al. Intrapericardial streptokinase fibrinolysis in the management of purulent pneumococcal pericarditis. Intensive Care Med 1997; 23(8): 925–926

111. Mann-Segal DD. The use of fibrinolytics in purulent pericarditis. Intensive Care Med 1999; 25(3): 338–339

112. Juneja R, Kothari SS, Saxena A, Sharma R, Joshi A. Intrapericardial streptokinase in purulent pericarditis. Arch Dis Child 1999; 80: 275–277

113. Bridgman PG. Failure of intrapericardial streptokinase in purulent pericarditis. Intensive Care Med 2001; 27(5): 942

114. Cakir O, Gurkan F, Balci AE, Eren N, Dikici B. Purulent pericarditis in childhood: ten years of experience. J Pediatr Surg 2002; 37(10): 1404–1408

115. Ustunsoy H, Celkan MA, Sivrikoz MC, et al. Intrapericardial fibrinolytic therapy in purulent pericarditis. Eur J Cardiothorac Surg 2002; 22(3): 373–376

116. Schafer M, Lepori M, Delabays A, Ruchat P, Schaller MD, Broccard AF. Intrapericardial urokinase irrigation and systemic corticosteroids: an alternative to pericardectomy for persistent fibrino-purulent pericarditis. Cardiovasc Surg 2002; 10(5): 508–511

117. Kamimura M, Suzuki T, Kudo K. Intrapericardial infusion of urokinase for the treatment of purulent pericarditis. Intern Med 2002; 41(5): 412–413

118. Tomkowski WZ, Kuca P, Gralec R, et al. Management of purulent pericarditis. Monaldi Arch Chest Dis 2003; 59(4): 308–309

119. Zimmermann C, Braun B, Hust MH. Intrapericardial fibrinolysis as a therapeutic option in a case of purulent pericarditis. Dtsch Med Wochenschr 2003; 128(43): 2248–2250

120. Tomkowski WZ, Gralec R, Kuca P, Burakowski J, Orłowski T, Kurzyna M. Effectiveness of intrapericardial administration of streptokinase in purulent pericarditis. Herz 2004; 29(8): 802–805

121. Ekim H, Demirbağ R. Intrapericardial streptokinase for purulent pericarditis. Surg Today 2004; 34: 569–572

122. Tillet WS, Sherry S, Read T. The use of Streptokinase- Streptodornase in the treatment of post pneumonic empyema. J Thorac Cardiovasc Surg 1951; 21: 275–297

123. Fraedrich G, Hofmann D, Efferhauser P, Jarder R. Instillation of fibrynolytic enzymes in the treatment of pleural empyema. Thorac Cardiovasc Surg 1982; 30: 36–38

124. Reznikoff CP, Fish JT, Coursin DB. Pericardial infusion of tissue plasminogen activator in fibropurulent pericarditis. J Intensive Care Med 2003; 18(1): 47–51

125. Bigham MT, Brady PW, Manning PB, Jacobs BR, Kimball TR, Wong HR. Therapeutic application of intrapericardial tissue plasminogen activator in a 4-month-old child with complex fibropurulent pericarditis. Pediatr Crit Care Med 2008; 9(1): e1–4

126. Aye RW, Froese DP, Hill LD. Use of purified streptokinase in empyema and hemothorax. Am J Surg 1991; 161: 560–562

127. Rubin RH, Moellering RC Jr. Clinical microbiologic and therapeutic aspects of purulent pericarditis. Am J Med 1975; 59: 68–78

128. Peuhkurinen K, Risteli L, Jounela A, Risteli J. Changes in interstitial collagen metabolism during acute myocardial infarction treated with streptokinase or tissue plasminogen activator. Am Heart J 1996; 131: 7–13

Percutaneous Balloon Pericardiotomy

Introduction

The management of hemodynamic instability caused by a growing pericardial effusion and cardiac tamponade requires the prompt evacuation of the effusion. This can be done either by pericardiocentesis or a surgical procedure. However, long-term prognosis of the patient and the risk for recurrences are not determined by the type of the initial procedure selected, but rather by the underlying etiology and the physician's ability to treat the causal disease. Percutaneous balloon pericardiotomy is a palliative, alternative approach for the management of recurring pericardial effusion, applied so far mainly for recurrences of the neoplastic pericardial effusion [1]. The procedure is more complex than pericardiocentesis. It requires the availability of a cardiac catheterization laboratory with experience in this approach and special balloon catheters. Therefore, the percutaneous balloon pericardiotomy it is currently performed in a few specialized centers only.

Indications and Contraindications

The major indication for percutaneous balloon pericardiotomy is a large, recurrent neoplastic pericardial effusion or imminent tamponade [2, 3]. In the "Guidelines for Management of Pericardial Disease of the European Society of Cardiology (ESC)" the procedure is listed as a treatment of choice in most patients with large, recurrent neoplastic pericardial effusion (level of evidence B, class IIa indication) [2]. The clinical rationale beyond this indication is that percutaneous balloon pericardiotomy in patients with neoplastic pericardial effusion can decrease the risk of the effusion to relapse, which can be as high as 62% [4]. However, the success rate of this procedure is low in patients with malignant mesothelioma, so this malignancy can also be considered as contraindication [5]. As noted in the published studies, the spread of neoplastic cells from pericardial space to the pleural cavity or to the peritoneum remains a principal concern after percutaneous balloon pericardiotomy and is one of the reason why this procedure is not widely applied. Apart from neoplastic disease, the procedure has also been performed in non-malignant, non-infectious large pericardial effusion/cardiac tamponade in whom prolonged pericardial drainage after pericardiocentesis has not been successful [1, 6]. According to the ESC Guidelines [2], percutaneous balloon pericardiotomy may also be indicated in the patients with chronic persistent or recurrent large pericardial effusion (level of evidence B, class IIa indication), if an infectious etiology of the inflammation can be excluded.

So far, no randomized studies comparing percutaneous balloon pericardiotomy with other procedures are available (e.g. pericardiocentesis, prolonged drainage of pericardial effusion, the intrapericardial instillation of cytostatics). In addition to repeated pericardiocentesis with prolonged pericardial drainage [7] and percutaneous balloon pericardiotomy [1, 3, 5, 8–32], the armamentarium for the management of the relapses of neoplastic pericardial effusions includes the instillation of cytostatics, of radioactive or sclerosing drugs (see Chapter 10), the surgical creation of a pleuropericardial or pleuroperitoneal window (see Chapter 4), systemic chemotherapy, and radiotherapy. The surgical subxiphoid pericardiotomy is much more invasive than balloon pericardiotomy. It increases the patient's discomfort and the risk of secondary infections, with a mortality of 1.2% [33].

Randomized trials comparing the feasibility, safety, the short and long-term efficacy of the different procedures, and the overall cost/benefit as well as the degree of discomfort for the individual patient are yet to be done.

The successful application of percutaneous balloon pericardiotomy in a patient with purulent effusion was also reported. The procedure was performed in a septic patient who was too ill to undergo surgery [29]. However, most authors consider the infectious etiology of pericardial effusion as a relative contraindication, being concerned about the risk of the spread of infection [1, 14]. Other generally accepted contraindications include major coagulation disorders, effusive-constrictive pericarditis, a large left pleural effusion, an advanced respiratory insufficiency, and a history of pneumonectomy [1, 14]. In addition, patients with loculated effusions are not considered as good candidates. The procedure is not limited to the tertiary care centers, but it can also be carried out in institutions and by the operators who perform pericardiocentesis routinely.

Methodological Considerations

Fluoroscopy guidance is necessary for the successful and safe performance of percutaneous balloon pericardiotomy in the cardiac catheterization laboratory.

The procedure is performed under local anesthesia and mild sedation. The first step of the procedure is pericardiocentesis. The percutaneous balloon pericardiotomy can than be carried out in the same or in the next session, depending on the condition of the patient. If balloon pericardiotomy is performed in the same session with pericardiocentesis, at least 50% of the initial effusion should be evacuated.

Then, the pericardium is gradually dilated with a set of fascial dilators (7–11 F), depending on the size of the balloon catheter. Finally, a corresponding sheath is introduced into the pericardial cavity. In order to visualize the pericardial margin it is useful to inject 20–30 ml of angiographic contrast medium intrapericardially, and to perform the positioning of the balloon in left anterior oblique positions with caudal or cranial angulations and in a left lateral view. Care should be taken to advance the distal end of the balloon beyond the level of the skin and subcutaneous tissue.

The balloon is partially inflated and using a "countertraction technique" the subcutaneous tissue is released [1]. Afterwards, the balloon is fully inflated until the central indentation disappears (Fig. 11.1).

The use of fluoroscopy is mandatory since neither transthoracic nor transesophageal echocardiography can visualize position of the balloon on the pericardial margins. Usually, up to 3 inflations of 1–2 minutes each, applied at 6 atmospheres of pressure are sufficient. Inflations are painful for the patients and proper analgesia is necessary.

Double balloon pericardiotomy is performed with two balloons used simultaneously (one long, and one short) [15, 25, 32]. Two balloons inflated at the same time lying adjacent to each other are creating a stronger tension, are more rectangular in shape, and tend to be more securely located in the pericardial border (Fig. 11.2).

After the procedure, a pigtail catheter is reintroduced for the drainage of the residual fluid. The final result can be confirmed with 20 ml injection of contrast medium. Endoscopic confirmation of the pericardial window using flexible percutaneous pericardioscopy is also feasible (see Fig. 11.1) [3]. A prophylactic administration of antibiotics is usually performed (e.g. gentamycin 80 mg i.v. bid

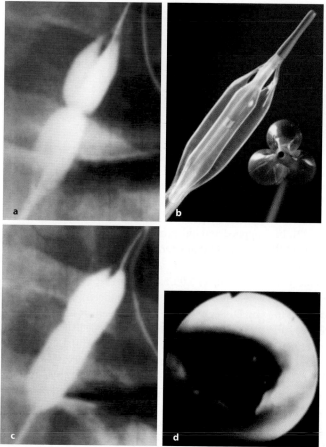

■ **Fig. 11.1a–d.** Percutaneous balloon pericardiotomy using a triangular Schneider Trefoil-Meier balloon catheter. **a** Inflated balloon with indentation, **b** formation of the triple balloon catheter, **c** fully inflated balloon (indentation disappears), **d** post procedural pericardioscopy verifying successful triangular balloon pericardiotomy

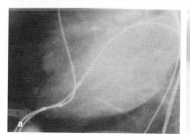
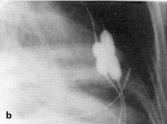
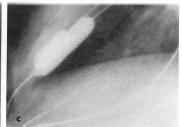

■ **Fig. 11.2.** Double balloon pericardiotomy. Reproduced with permission from Wang et al. (2002) [32]

and ampicillin 500 mg orally qid), which should start six hours before the procedure. The outcome of the procedure should be closely followed with standard radiography and echocardiography, especially for the potential formation of a large, usually spontaneously resolving, pleural effusion (Fig. 11.3).

Mechanism of Action

Multiple inflations of the balloon create a window at the parietal pericardium and either a pericardio-peritoneal or a pericardio-pleural shunt. The creation and shape of the pericardial window was verified by pericardioscopy in Ziskind's report [1]

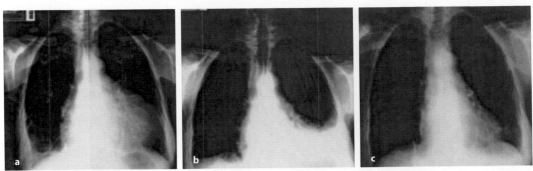

◘ **Fig. 11.3a–c.** Pleural effusion after percutaneous balloon pericardiotomy: **a** before the procedure, **b** one day after the procedure, and **c** one week after the procedure. Reproduced with permission from Navarro del Amo et al. (2002) [34]

as well as in the study by Seferović et al. [3, 22]. In the experimental autopsy work of Chow et al. [12] percutaneous balloon pericardiotomy was found to create a fragmentation of the fibroelastic connective tissue of the parietal pericardium. In the first days after the procedure, pericardial fluid is drained to the left pleural, or to the peritoneal space [14, 20]. Since both the pleural and peritoneal cavities have much larger surfaces and better resorptive capacities than the pericardium, it would be logical to accept this mechanism as a therapeutic effect of the procedure.

However, according to data from the American registry [1], there was no significant difference in the success rate of the procedures in patients in whom pericardio-pleural or pericardio-peritoneal shunts were or were not created. Therefore, the suggestion of Sugimoto et al. [23] seems valid that the long-term effect of percutaneous balloon pericardiotomy results from the inflammatory fusion of the pericardial layers which significantly decreases or brings the production of pericardial effusion to the standstill.

Balloon Catheter Selection

Good feasibility and therapeutic value was shown with several types of large, round balloons for percutaneous balloon pericardiotomy [8–21]. The type of balloon catheter is a major technical factor that influences the feasibility and success rate of the procedure. In the largest study so far, the American registry for percutaneous balloon pericardiotomy, Ziskind et al.

applied a round-profiled Mansfield balloon catheter 20 mm in diameter, in 130 patients, with 96.2% of immediate success, and 85% success during the mean follow-up of 5.0 ± 5.8 months [1, 14].

The Mansfield balloon catheter was also applied by Di Segni et al. [16] and Galli et al. [18] with a 100% long-term success. An Inoue balloon catheter was used by Chow et al. [12] and Bahl et al. [24] with an 85–91% success rate. However, in 44% of patients in the initial report of Ziskind et al. [14], the procedure had to be repeated at different sites, and in two patients the procedure needed to be re-done with two balloons at the same place, due to pericardial resistance.

In the study by Iaffaldano et al. [15] double balloon pericardiotomy was also performed in patients with significant pericardial stiffness. Hsu et al. [25] implemented under these conditions the double balloon technique with one longer and one shorter balloon.

Encouraged by the results of double balloon pericardiotomy techniques Seferović et al. [3, 22] used a balloon catheter with a triangular profile (Schneider Trefoil-Meier, 3×5 or 3×7 mm). The triangular profile of this balloon ensured improved feasibility of the procedure with a comparable effect to the other balloon catheters. Importantly, due to its smaller size, the application of this balloon catheter was less traumatic for the patients. This concept was further developed by Sochman et al. [26] who successfully used a cutting pericardiotome for the similar procedure. However, with this device great care has to be taken to avoid epicardial trauma.

Table 11.1. Catheters used for percutaneous balloon pericardiotomy			
Catheter type	Diameter [mm]	Length [mm]	Pressure [ATM]
Mansfield	18–25	30–40	3–5
Inoue	20	–	8
Crystal	25	40	4
Schneider Trefoil-Meier	3´5/3´7	40	6

Analysis of Feasibility and Long-Term Results

The final report of the US Percutaneous Balloon Pericardiotomy Registry [1] included 110 patients with malignant diseases (55 lung cancers, 21 breast cancers) out of the total of 130 patients. During the mean follow-up of 5.0 ± 5.8 months recurrence of pericardial effusion occurred in 13 patients, with a mean time to recurrence of 54 ± 65 days. Mean survival of patients with malignant pericardial effusion was 3.8 ± 3.3 months and was not influenced by the procedure. In 12/13 patients with recurrences a surgical pericardial window was created, but in six patients a large pericardial effusion reappeared. There was no significant difference in the long-term outcome considering the timing of percutaneous balloon pericardiotomy from the initial pericardiocentesis (single or two-step procedure).

Di Segni et al. [16] could successfully create a pericardial window in all patients (seven patients with malignant effusion and one with chronic renal failure) with no recurrences of cardiac tamponade during the follow-up of 32–342 days. Two patients died, from the primary disease, on the 3rd and 14th day after the procedure. Galli et al. [18] also report a 100% long-term success in ten high-risk patients with malignant cardiac tamponade. Chow et al. [21] implemented the Inoue balloon catheter in 11 patients with recurrent pericardial effusion of various etiologies. The procedure was successful in 91% of patients, with no recurrent effusion during the mean follow-up of 4.2 months. Despite symptomatic improvement, 82% of patients died due to the underlying disease with a mean survival of 1.4 months after the procedure. In comparison to these findings, the long-term results of their study can be regarded as comparable, although the balloon catheters were smaller.

Seferović et al. [3, 22] were the first to investigate feasibility, safety and long-term results of triangular percutaneous balloon pericardiotomy using a Schneider-Meier triple balloon catheter in comparison with prolonged pericardial drainage after pericardiocentesis in patients with recurrent large neoplastic pericardial effusions. The percutaneous balloon pericardiotomy procedure was feasible in 70% of patients using 3×5mm balloon catheter. In the remaining 30% of patients the procedure could be also successfully performed using a larger 3×7 mm balloon catheter and repeated inflations. In 5/20 patients percutaneous flexible pericardioscopy was performed simultaneously with percutaneous balloon pericardiotomy and in all cases the triangular shape of pericardial window was confirmed (see Fig. 11.1). During the mean follow-up of 121.2 ± 119.2 days this triangular percutaneous balloon pericardiotomy significantly reduced the recurrence rate of large pericardial effusion and cardiac tamponade. It decreased the need for a new pericardiocentesis in comparison to the previous disease history as well as in comparison to group of patients undergoing prolonged pericardial drainage after pericardiocentesis. Only in two patients (10%), both with end stage lung carcinoma, the procedure failed during the follow-up. In one of them percutaneous balloon pericardiotomy was successfully repeated and the other one had to undergo surgical pericardiectomy.

In the US registry on percutaneous balloon pericardiotomy [1] 12.8% (11/86) of patients had non-malignant pericardial effusion (4 idiopathic, 1 uremic, 3 AIDS, 1 viral, 1 hypothyroidism, 1 posttraumatic). During the follow-up of 5.1 ± 5.3 months, no significant constriction was observed. However, one patient with AIDS died.

Furthermore, Thanopoulos et al. [6] were the first to apply percutaneous balloon pericardiotomy in the treatment of large, nonmalignant pericardial effusions in children aged 5–12 years, with the excellent result of 9 successful out of performed 10 procedures. During the follow-up of 14.6 months effusion recurred only in the patient in whom the procedure was incomplete due to balloon rupture.

Jalisi et al. [31] utilized this procedure as the initial treatment for 17 patients with cardiac tamponade who had a high likelihood of recurrence of their pericardial effusion. Primary pericardiotomy was successful after the initial procedure in 82% (n = 14) of these patients, being significantly less costly than pericardiocentesis followed by the creation of a surgical pericardial window.

Safety

In the US percutaneous balloon pericardiotomy registry [1] major complications such as coronary artery laceration (2%) and prolonged bleeding due to a preexisting coagulation disorder (3.5%) were noted. Both complications were successfully treated surgically. There was no procedure-related mortality. Other complications included fever in 13%, apical pneumothorax in 2.3%, and large left pleural effusion requiring pleural puncture and drainage in 15% and 9.3% of patients with and without previous left pleural effusion, respectively.

Neither Galli [18] nor Chow [21] reported any complications or recurrences during the follow-up. Bleeding from the entry site was the only complication observed in one patient in the study by Di Segni et al. [16]. Thanopoulos et al. [6] had a case (1/10) with rupture of the balloon and entrapment of its distal part within the pericardium. In addition, Wang et al. [32] have reported a case of post-pericardiotomy syndrome after percutaneous balloon pericardiotomy.

Similar as in the majority of others studies, only minor complications, including pain during the balloon inflation (12/22) and transient fever (8/22), occurred in the study of Seferović et al. [3, 22]. Two patients developed a large pleural effusion and pleural drainage had to be performed (10%). There were no additional risks of the procedure above the intrinsic risk of pericardiocentesis. In this, as well as in none of the published studies, percutaneous balloon peri-

cardiotomy did not increase the dissemination of the neoplastic process, which was one of the major concerns of some investigators.

Pericardial injury during percutaneous balloon pericardiotomy produces a sterile inflammatory reaction with thickening of the pericardial layers and obliteration of pericardial space [1, 12]. However, the proportion of patients who can progress to clinically significant constriction after the procedure is unknown. In the majority of the patients with neoplastic pericardial effusion this was not an issue due to the progression of the underlying neoplastic disease and limited survival. However, no significant constriction was reported in other studies involving patients with non-malignant effusions.

Future Perspectives and Recommendations

In patients with neoplastic pericardial effusion percutaneous balloon pericardiotomy did not influence the survival of patients, which was poor, as it could be expected in the disseminated malignant disease. However, importantly enough, the procedure prevented mortality due to cardiac tamponade and avoided the risks of repeated pericardial punctures in these terminally ill patients. The therapeutic value of percutaneous balloon pericardiotomy was better in comparison with pericardiocentesis followed by prolonged pericardial drainage. However, no study provided a direct comparison of percutaneous balloon pericardiotomy with surgical subxiphoid window and/or intrapericardial cytostatic therapy or sclerosation. Some of the agents for intrapericardial treatment of neoplastic pericardial effusions were shown to be safe and highly efficient such as cisplatin, thiotepa, and P32-colloid. Randomized studies comparing effects of these agents with the percutaneous balloon pericardiotomy would be valuable.

References

1. Ziskind AA, Palacios IF. Percutaneous balloon pericardiotomy for patients with pericardial effusion and tamponade. In: Topol EJ (ed) Textbook of Interventional Cardiology, 5th Edition. W.B. Saunders, Philadelphia, 2007, pp 977–985

2. Maisch B, Seferović PM, Ristić AD, et al. Task Force on the Diagnosis and Management of Pericardial Diseases of the European Society of Cardiology. European Society of Cardiology Guidelines: Diagnosis and management of the pericardial diseases. Executive summary. Eur Heart J 2004; 25: 587–610

3. Ristić AD, Seferović PM, Maksimović R, Ostojić M. Percutaneous balloon pericardiotomy in neoplastic pericardial effusion. In: Seferović PM, Spodick DH, Maisch B. (eds) Pericardiology: Contemporary answers to continuing challenges. Science, Belgrade 2000, pp 427–438

4. Laham RJ, Cohen DJ, Kuntz RE, Baim DS, Lorell BH, Simons M. Pericardial effusion in patients with cancer: outcome with contemporary management strategies. Heart 1996; 75: 67–71

5. Ovunc K, Aytemir K, Ozer N, et al. Percutaneous balloon pericardiotomy for patients with malignant pericardial effusion including three malignant pleural mesotheliomas. Angiology 2001; 52(5): 323–329

6. Thanopoulos BD, Georgakopoulos D, Tsaousis GS, Triposkiadis F, Paphitis CA. Percutaneous balloon pericardiotomy for the treatment of large, nonmalignant pericardial effusions in children: immediate and medium-term results. Cathet Cardiovasc Diagn 1997; 40: 97–100

7. Tsang TS, Enriquez-Sarano M, Freeman WK, et al. Consecutive 1127 therapeutic echocardiographically guided pericardiocenteses: clinical profile, practice patterns, and outcomes spanning 21 years. Mayo Clin Proc 2002; 77: 429–436

8. Palacios IF, Tuzcu EM, Ziskind AA, Younger J, Block PC. Percutaneous balloon pericardial window for patients with malignant pericardial effusion and tamponade. Cathet Cardiovasc Diag 1991; 22: 244–249

9. Hajduczok ZD, Ferguson DW. Percutaneous balloon pericardiostomy for non surgical management of recurrent pericardial tamponade: a case report. Intensive Care Med 1991; 17: 299–301

10. Jackson G, Keane D, Mishra B. Percutaneous balloon pericardiotomy in the management of recurrent malignant pericardial effusions. Br Heart J 1992; 68: 613–615

11. Deb B, Crean P, Graham I. Percutaneous balloon pericardiotomy in the treatment of malignant pericardial effusion. Ir J Med Sci 1993; 162: 456–457

12. Chow LT, Chow WH. Mechanism of pericardial window creation by balloon pericardiotomy. Am J Cardiol 1993; 72: 1321–1322

13. Jackson G. Cardiology update. Balloon pericardiotomy. Nurs Stand 1994; 8: 52–53

14. Ziskind AA, Pearce AC, Lemmon CC, et al. Percutaneous balloon pericardiotomy for the treatment of cardiac tamponade and large pericardial effusions: description of technique and report of the first 50 cases. J Am Coll Cardiol 1993; 21: 1–5

15. Iaffaldano RA, Jones P, Lewis BE et al. Percutaneous balloon pericardiotomy: a double balloon technique. Cathet Cardiovasc Diagn 1995; 36: 79–81

16. Di Segni E, Lavee J, Kaplinsky E, Vered Z. Percutaneous balloon pericardiostomy for treatment of cardiac tamponade. Eur Heart J 1995; 16: 184–187

17. Fakiolas CN, Beldekos DI, Foussas SG, et al. Percutaneous balloon pericardiotomy as a therapeutic alternative for cardiac tamponade and recurrent pericardial effusion. Acta Cardiol 1995; 50: 65–70

18. Galli M, Politi A, Pedretti F, Castiglioni B, Zerboni S. Percutaneous balloon pericardiotomy for malignant pericardial tamponade. Chest 1995; 108: 1499–1501

19. Devlin GP, Smyth D, Charleson HA, Heaven DJ, McAlister HF. Balloon pericardiostomy: a new therapeutic option for malignant pericardial effusion. Aust N Z J Med 1996; 26: 556–558

20. Bertrand O, Legrand V, Kulbertus H. Percutaneous balloon pericardiotomy: a case report and analysis of mechanism of action. Cathet Cardiovasc Diagn 1996; 38: 180–182

21. Chow WH, Chow TC, Yip AS, Cheung KL. Inoue balloon pericardiotomy for patients with recurrent pericardial effusion. Angiology 1996; 47: 57–60

22. Seferović PM, Ristić AD, Petrović P, et al. Percutaneous balloon pericardiotomy – a novel interventional technique in clinical cardiology. Kardiologija (Yu) 1998; 3: 13–20

23. Sugimoto JT, Little AG, Ferguson MK, et al. Pericardial window: mechanisms of efficacy. Ann Thorac Surg 1990; 50: 442–445

24. Bahl VK, Chandra S, Goel A, Goswami KC, Wasir HS. Versatility of Inoue balloon catheter. Int J Cardiol 1997; 59: 75–83

25. Hsu KL, Tsai CH, Chiang FT, et al. Percutaneous balloon pericardiotomy for patients with recurrent pericardial effusion: using a novel double-balloon technique with one long and one short balloon. Am J Cardiol 1997; 80: 1635–1637

26. Sochman J, Peregrin J, Pavcnik D. The cutting pericardiotome: another option for pericardiopleural draining in recurrent pericardial effusion. Initial experience. Int J Cardiol 2001; 77(1): 69–74

27. Grumbach IM, Werner GS, Figulla HR. Percutaneous balloon pericardiotomy for the treatment of a malignant pericardial tamponade. Dtsch Med Wochenschr 1998; 123(23): 726–729

28. Furukawa A, Itoh A, Nakamura T, et al. Efficacy of percutaneous balloon pericardiotomy and intrapericardial instillation for the management of refractory pericardial effusion: a case report. J Cardiol 2007; 50(6): 389–395

29. Aqel R, Mehta D, Zoghbi GJ. Percutaneous balloon pericardiotomy for the treatment of infected pericardial effusion with tamponade. J Invasive Cardiol 2006; 18(7): E194–197

30. Marcy PY, Bondiau PY, Brunner P. Percutaneous treatment in patients presenting with malignant cardiac tamponade. Eur Radiol 2005; 15(9): 2000–2009

31. Jalisi FM, Morise AP, Haque R, Jain AC. Primary percutaneous balloon pericardiotomy. W V Med J 2004; 100(3): 102–105

32. Wang HJ, Hsu KL, Chiang FT, Tseng CD, Tseng YZ, Liau CS. Technical and prognostic outcomes of double-balloon pericardiotomy for large malignancy-related pericardial effusions. Chest 2002; 122(3): 893–899

33. Vaitkus PT, Herrmann HC, LeWinter MM. Treatment of malignant pericardial effusion. JAMA 1994; 272(1): 59–64

34. Navarro Del Amo LF, Cordoba Polo M, et al. Percutaneous balloon pericardiotomy in patients with recurrent pericardial effusion. Rev Esp Cardiol 2002; 55(1): 25–28

Frontiers and Emerging Procedures

Introduction

The ability to access the normal pericardium in the absence of any effusion induced increasing interest in the pericardial space as a location of and novel approach for various cardiac and intrapericardial applications. Intrapericardial drug delivery may be superior to other routes in special indications. Medication applied intrapericardially will maintain the effective concentration for a longer time. Drugs given in the pericardial space may access the vessel wall and the myocardial tissue directly for a much longer time, but also more predictably and consistently than by an intracoronary or intravenous injection [1]. The intrapericardial route might have additional important advantages for the application of pharmacological agents like an easier access to perivascular tissue. The delivery into a low-turnover reservoir with a minimum loss of the respective agent into circulation, and the perfusion of atrial and ventricular epicardial tissue can increase efficacy with little or no side-effects. The delivery of drugs, mediators such as growth factors to the adventitial rather than to the luminal surface of the vasculature bypasses the endothelial layer. It might improve efficacy [2] and reduce the risk of intimal hyperplasia, which could complicate intravenous or intracoronary injection for some substances [2–4]. Another advantage is the low clearance of compounds by intrapericardial application. It thus maximizes the concentration and the contact time of drugs with a high coronary and myocardial tissue deposition while minimizing the potential for systemic toxicity and side effects [2–6].

Several authors have reported that the intrapericardial administration of neuroactive medications can completely block the transmission of both afferent and efferent cardiac nerves [7–13]. It was documented by intravascular ultrasound that an intrapericardial nitroglycerin injection results in marked vasodilatation of the epicardial coronary vessels [14]. Therefore, the pericardial space might be the more appropriate route for the administration of some cardioactive pharmacological agents than their systemic application, especially if concentrations are needed that would not be tolerated systemically. However, the long-term stay of a drainage catheter in the pericardium for the purpose of intrapericardial instillation of several doses or a prolonged therapy could slowly induce fibrosis imposing the risk of pericardial constriction. The extent of this risk and its correlation with application of specific agents and duration of therapy warrants further investigation.

Intrapericardial therapy is potentially advantageous for the clinical application of gene and stem cell therapy. It offers the advantage of a regional application in a defined compartment with high concentration. The amount of cells or vectors could be much less than by systemic or intracoronary application.

In addition, epicardial electrophysiological mapping and ablation of malignant arrhythmias have been made available to the cardiologist by the pericardial approach even in the absence of any effusion. Furthermore, intrapericardial echocardiography has become possible, whereby its potential clinical benefit remains to be established.

Intrapericardial Echocardiography

The development of intracardiac echocardiography and epicardial electrophysiology and ablation has motivated various investigators to apply intracardiac echocardiography systems also to the pericardial space [15–17]. The underlying idea of intrapericardial positioning of the echocardiography probe was to enhance efficacy and safety and save fluoroscopic exposure time during complex electrophysiology procedures. Intrapericardial echocardiography has been successfully used to help with the guidance of catheter ablation and electrophysiological procedures in animal experiments (goats) [15]. A phased-array ultrasound transducer was placed into the pericardial space via a subxiphoidally introduced 10-F steerable catheter (Fig. 12.1).

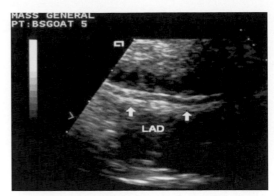

◘ **Fig. 12.2.** Visualization of the left anterior descending branch of the left coronary artery by intrapericardial echocardiography. Reproduced with permission from Rodrigues et al. [15]

Pericardial access was obtained via the subxiphoid approach with a 17-gauge Tuohy needle, guided by fluoroscopy as described by Sosa et al. [18–20] (see previous chapter). The needle angle was adjusted to the medial third of the right ventricle (by fluoroscopy) to avoid the laceration of major coronary vessels.

In all seven animals images of cardiac structures and of intracardiac ablation catheters were successfully obtained using an AcuNav 10-F steerable catheter (2D imaging and Doppler, tissue penetration up to 12 cm; Acuson/Siemens, Mountain View, California, USA) which was connected to a standard echocardiography system. Longitudinal and short-axis views of right- and left-sided chambers and valves were obtained in all cases. The images were similar to those obtained transesophageal echocardiography. Atrial appendages (6/7), pulmonary veins (6/7), coronary arteries (6/7), and the coronary sinus (3/6) were also visualized in most cases. Intracardiac transvalvular and venous blood flow were assessed by spectral and color flow Doppler. The ablation catheter could be clearly visualized inside the cardiac chambers. No arrhythmias were induced with the manipulation of the intrapericardial echocardiography probe and no epicardial lesions resulting from the echocardiography procedure were observed.

The potential of intrapericardial echocardiography lies in the identification of landmarks for the placement of endocardial or epicardial radiofrequency ablation catheters. Their proper placement could prevent energy delivery to inappropriate sites, and also monitor acute cardiac changes following

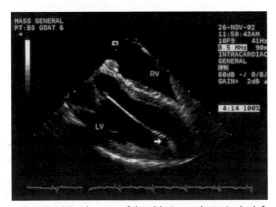

◘ **Fig. 12.1.** Visualization of the ablation catheter in the left ventricle (*LV*) by intrapericardial echocardiography. The tip of the ablation catheter (*arrow*) is adjacent to apex of the left ventricle. The position of the AcuNav ultrasound probe is in front of the base of the right ventricle. Reproduced with permission from Rodrigues et al. [15]

the ablation procedure. It could guide the ablation procedure in patients with atrial fibrillation or ventricular tachycardia. In patients undergoing pericardiocentesis intrapericardial echocardiography could be performed for evaluations requiring a high resolution transducer such as in infective endocarditis for endocarditic vegetations and suspected abscess formation. Recently, ultrasound-imaging catheters have been introduced into the mediastinal position after open heart surgery for cardiac imaging, a term coined substernal epicardial echocardiography [21]. But the potential of intrapericardial echocardiography is even better, because it enables an even wider exposure to imaging planes and in contrast to the mediastinal approach the placement of a chest tube is not required. Nevertheless, the indications for accessing of the normal pericardium are yet to be established. It is currently unlikely that the procedure will be used as the sole reason for pericardiocentesis in the absence of the pericardial effusion. On the other hand, if pericardial access is already necessary for epicardial cardiac mapping and ablation intrapericardial echocardiography might prove to provide useful additional information.

Intrapericardial Treatment in Non-Pericardial Diseases

Potential Advantages of Intrapericardial Approach for the Treatment of Non-Pericardial Diseases

Injecting drugs into the pericardial space may offer several advantages in comparison with systemically delivered medications, e.g. tissue specific application, increased efficacy, prolonged duration of action, lower doses, and less toxicity.

Intrapericardial treatment is cardiospecific; the agents are targeted to those structures from which the therapeutic effect is expected: the epicardial coronary vessels, the intracardiac nerves, the atrial and ventricular myocardium. Several studies have indicated that the intrapericardial administration of procainamide or esmolol have a potent antiarrhythmic effect. In addition, the intrapericardial instillation of neuroactive agents can completely block the transmission of both afferent and efferent cardiac

nerves. The intrapericardial injection of nitroglycerin results in coronary vessel dilatation, as measured by intravascular ultrasound [22].

An important advantage of intrapericardial treatment is also the maximal efficacy by delivering a high concentration of drug at or very near to the target tissue in a small volume. Its release into a low-turnover reservoir results in a minimum loss of the agent into the circulation. Local delivery can combine the benefits of very low therapeutic doses of a drug, and its prolonged duration of action in a compartment with slow pharmacokinetics.

The intrapericardial application of a therapeutic agent reduces its exposure to degradative enzymes, notably those contained in erythrocytes, permitting a high efficacy and longer duration of action. The local action of a drug has minimal or absent systemic effects. This issue is very important if the compound is toxic and has a multiple serious side effects, or is in the investigational phase. Intrapericardial drug delivery offers an opportunity for specific drugs to directly target cells, receptors, channels, and the myocardium, which remains an essential step in the initial assessment of drug efficacy.

Possible Drawbacks of Intrapericardial Pharmacokinetics

Pericardial drug delivery is primarily directed toward epicardial structures. In order to reach subendocardial ventricular tissue, however, a considerable diffusion distance must be crossed. In addition, densely arranged blood vessels within the epicardial ventricular tissue can serve as a drug clearing mechanism, particularly for small, water-soluble compounds. This may wash the highly concentrated drug from the epicardial surface into a larger blood pool and prevent its penetration into the endocardial layer. Due to this effect one can hypothesize that drugs delivered to pericardium will penetrate preferably the thin atrial structure with low blood flow and the coronary, vasculature, rather than the myocardial ventricular tissue. By the intrapericardial application of antiarrhythmic drugs such as esmolol and procainamide the atrial effects may predominant (e.g. decrease in heart rate, but no changes in ventricular inotropy). This would contrast to the intravenous administration of this drug. Little is known at present about the pharmacokinetics of the water-soluble compounds delivered into pericardial space. Staying with anti-arhythmic agents, animal experiments suggest that intrapericardial procainamide delivery produces more pronounced effects in the thin superficial atrial tissue structures when compared to its intravenous delivery. On the other hand we are concerned about the possible proarrhythmic effect of procainamide on the ventricular myocardium.

The physical size and long-acting formulations of drugs delivered into pericardium can strongly influence their residence time as depot therapy. If these agents exert a very low systemic effect, the transmural concentrations gradient will be steep. Therefore, their further investigations are is needed to define the optimal molecular size, the penetration and dissolution properties.

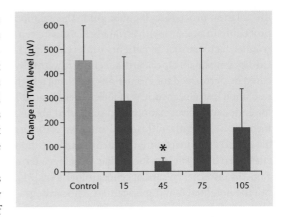

◘ **Fig. 12.3.** Intrapericardial nitroglycerin significantly attenuated the magnitude of the ischemia-induced T-wave alternans (TWA) in the intracoronary lead at 45 min after delivery (*p < 0.05), in parallel with the agent's effect on arrhythmias; TWA recovered to pre-drug levels by 75 min after intrapericardial nitroglycerin. Reproduced with permission from Kumar et al. [24]

Intrapericardial Application of Coronary Vasodilators

Nitroglycerin is acting at multiple levels in the heart including the coronary vessels, the cardiac autonomic nerves, and the myocytes themselves. In comparison to its intracoronary administration, the coronary vasodilator effect is more intensive and lasts longer, if nitroglycerin is delivered intrapericardially. The hypotensive response or the elevations in heart rate owed to a reflex mechanism was, however, minimal [14]. The NO donor sodium nitroprusside was more effective in the prevention platelet aggregation in stenosed and injured coronary arteries when administered intrapericardially than intravenously [23].

Kumar et al. [24] investigated the effect of the local delivery of nitroglycerin into the pericardial space on ischemia-induced arrhythmias. In 29 closed-chest pigs, myocardial ischemia was induced by intra-luminal balloon occlusion of the left anterior descending coronary artery. Intrapericardial nitroglycerin suppressed the occurrence of ventricular fibrillation and reduced the T-wave alternans (Fig. 12.3). The antifibrillatory effect occurred as early as 15 min and persisted for up to 75 min.

Intrapericardial nitroglycerin can also blunt the positive inotropic effect of an intracoronary injection of dobutamine (Fig. 12.4).

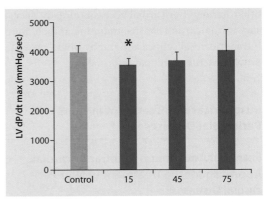

◘ **Fig. 12.4.** Effect of intrapericardial nitroglycerin on the rise in contractility in response to intracoronary bolus injections of dobutamine. At 15 min after intrapericardial nitroglycerin, the rise in contractility induced by intracoronary dobutamine was significantly blunted (*p < 0.05). Thereafter, nitroglycerin's effect did not achieve statistical significance. LV dP/dt max = maximum of the first time derivative of left ventricular pressure. Reproduced with permission from Kumar et al. [24]

Baek et al. [25] demonstrated a prolonged vaso-dilatory effect by the NO donor diazeniumdiolated bovine serum albumin. It has a 22-h intrapericar-dial residence time and it has been suggested that it could protect particularly well against restenosis after angioplasty. As an additional benefit from its vasodilatory effect, the antiarrhythmic efficacy of

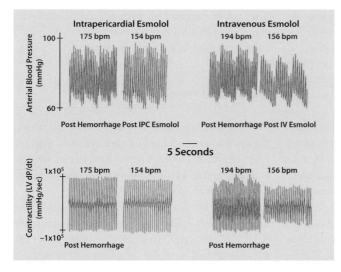

intravenous nitroglycerin has been established both experimentally [26–29] and clinically [30–33]. Its systemic administration, however, can decrease antiarrhythmic efficacy [29].

From these data the functional half-life of intrapericardial nitroglycerin can be inferred as 15 to 45 min, whereas intravenous nitroglycerin has a half-life of 3 to 5 min [34], with cardiovascular effects lasting 10 to 15 min. The prolongation of its effect can be attributed to the absence of erythrocytes from the pericardial fluid and their degradative enzymes. The slow, gradual onset of the described hemodynamic effects of intrapericardial nitroglycerin also confirms the minimum leakage of nitroglycerin from the pericardial space.

Fei et al. [35] found that the intrapericardial application of L-arginine, which is also a NO-donor, reduced the extent of the sympathetically induced shortening of the ventricular effective refractory period as well as the severity of ventricular arrhythmias produced during coronary occlusions.

Intrapericardial Antiarrhythmic Therapy

Beta-Blocking Agents

Several intrapericardially-administered drugs have been also proven capable of suppressing atrial and ventricular arrhythmias [35–39]. So does the in-

trapericardial administration of muscarinic and β-adrenergic blocking agents, which can significantly alter the heart rate response to baroreceptor reflex activation [10, 40]. A controversial question is whether an intrapericardially administered agent could selectively influence the activity of the sinus node without altering cardiac contractility. Theoretically, this could be possible because of the relatively superficial location of the sinus node. Thus an agent could act in this region without penetrating fully across the ventricular wall. Such an action could be useful in treating hyperadrenergic states of various causes that could lead to tachycardia. Accordingly, it could be possible to administer a β-adrenergic blocking agent to reduce excessively elevated heart rates without compromising contractility.

Moreno et al. [39] applied esmolol in a concentration of 1 mg/kg intrapericardially, which exerted a significant and persistent effect on the hemorrhage-induced tachycardia that lasted for more than 10 min (Fig. 12.5). The drug decreased heart rate from 192 ± 9 beats/min at baseline to 164 ± 5 beats/min within 3 min ($p< 0.05$), with a further decrease after 5 min to 159 ± 8 beats/min ($p < 0.05$), which was sustained for > 5 min at 159 ± 10 beats/min ($p<0.05$). Intrapericardial esmolol did not induce a concomitant effect on arterial blood pressure or LV dP/dt max.

Although intravenous esmolol reduced heart rate to a similar degree when compared to intrapericardial application, LV dP/dt max and in arterial blood pressure were diminished as well, which was not the case after intrapericardial instillation. Likewise, Lew et al. [40] found that plasma levels of propranolol and atenolol were 7- to 40-fold lower, respectively, at 30 min after intrapericardial administration when compared with the levels produced by the usual intravenous dose.

Intrapericardially applied antiarrhythmic drugs exert their effect on the sympathetic nerve fibers mainly at the cardiac neuroeffector junction, thus influencing the function of the sinus and atrioventricular nodes and reducing sympathetically mediated tachycardia. In addition to esmolol, baroreceptor-mediated increases in heart rate can be also reduced by intrapericardial blockade with propranolol [10] or atenolol [40]. Therefore, two explanations are likely to account for the relatively persistent action of esmolol when administered intrapericardially, in contrast to its short half-life when applied intravenously:

1. The pericardium is a low-turnover space. Agents can be eliminated from the pericardial sac only by passive diffusion across the microvilli of visceral and parietal layers into the capillary network, by lymphatic drainage, or by penetration through the myocardium into the plasma.
2. The degradation of esmolol depends on the hydrolysis of the methylester by an arylesterase contained in erythrocytes [41]. The relative absence of this esterase from the pericardial fluid would account for the prolonged action of this agent when administered intrapericardially.

Lidocaine

Pericardial injection of lidocaine significantly decreased heart rate without a change in stroke volume in the study of Takada et al. [42] in anaesthetized, mechanically ventilated dogs. Whereas under pericardial lidocaine the tachycardia response to isoproterenol was similar to that observed without pericardial lidocaine, the response to atropine was significantly reduced. Pericardial lidocaine increased the voltage thresholds for inducing arrhythmias and ventricular fibrillation. Intravenous injection of lidocaine elevated the plasma concentration of lidocaine immediately, whereas the plasma concentration peaked much later at 10 minutes after pericardial administration.

These data suggest that pericardial lidocaine can control heart rate during conventional or off-pump coronary artery bypass graft surgery.

Digoxin and Procainamide

The intrapericardial administration of digoxin in pig experiments resulted in a reduction of the QTc interval, which was evident 8 h after administration and returned to baseline values by 24 h in the study of Kolettis et al. [43].

In contrast to the intravenous application, the intrapericardial administration of procainamide (Class IA antiarrhythmic agent) did not affect the RR interval, but increased the duration of ventricular depolarization by significant increase in the QRS duration, an effect that is also seen with very high plasma concentrations of procainamide, however [44].

Similarly, in the study of Ujhelyi et al. [45] the single 2 mg/kg and 3.5 mg/kg cumulative pericardial procainamide doses prolonged the atrial refractoriness and raised the atrial fibrillation threshold similar to the 26 mg/kg cumulative intravenous dose. However, the duration of this effect was similar between both delivery methods. Pericardial procainamide did not affect global or endocardial ventricular electrophysiology nor was it associated with ventricular proarrhythmia.

Hence, intrapericardial delivery may enhance the electrophysiological actions of digoxin and procainamide, while minimizing their extracardiac effects. This effect may be useful in the management of persistent arrhythmic emergencies such as an electrical storm [46].

Intrapericardial Prevention of Restenosis

Hou et al. [47] have demonstrates that the instillation of a single dose of paclitaxel into the pericardial space is associated with a significant reduction of restenosis after porcine coronary balloon injury. The effect was comparable to the widely applied paclitaxel coated coronary stents [48, 49]. The reduced restenosis rates were based on a significant increment in vessel circumference and a reduction in the neointimal mass. This dual effect of paclitaxel on the remodeling and the proliferation is encouraging because both mechanisms contribute to the more favorable restenosis rates after angioplasty, whereas other therapeutic agents affecting predominantly smooth muscle cell proliferation have been found insufficient to prevent vessel renarrowing [47]. Importantly, the intrapericardial instillation of paclitaxel did cause overt damage to neither the endothelial nor the medial layers. As stated by the authors as well, an obvious limitation of this study was the absence of data about the pericardial reaction at later time points after the paclitaxel instillation. Experimental studies with an extended follow-up after the intrapericardial treatment would be necessary to support the safety of this approach before it is applied in a clinical setting.

In an another study Hou et al. [50] were able to confirm that a single-dose intrapericardial injection of 10 ml 30% ethanol could also significantly reduce neointimal proliferation in the porcine balloon-overstretch model. The calculated luminal stenosis decreased in the group, which was treated intrapericardially with ethanol, by 16.1% in contrast to 25.3% in the control group.

Intrapericardial Gene Therapy

Several studies have demonstrated the potential of a direct injection of genes into the myocardium [51–54]. However, intramyocardial injection results in gene expression over a limited area of the heart only at the cost of local tissue damage. The efficiency of intracoronary gene transfer is unfortunately also limited by the low permeability of the capillaries, the need for a high perfusion pressure and the limited time for the contact of the vector with the possible target cells [55]. The application into the pericardial space, however, can overcome some of the limitations inherent to the other gene transfer methods. However, the intrapericardial administration of naked DNA did not result in a significant transfection into the myocardium. Accordingly, Fromes at al. [53] used proteolytic enzymes to increase permeability of the peri- and epicardium. By this they were able to demonstrate, both in rats and mice, that the intrapericardial injection of recombinant adenovirus vectors was an efficient and safe strategy to deliver transgenes to the heart. To enable transfection through the peri-

cardium a mixture of collagenase and hyaluronidase together with the virus was applied, resulting in a large diffusion of the transgene activity, by reaching up to 40% of the myocardium. No functional or structural damage to the heart was detected in this experimental study, which is hardly believable.

Similarly, Lazarous et al. [56] have demonstrated an efficient intrapericardial adenoviral-mediated gene transfer in mongrel dogs, as well as the induction of sustained VEGF-165 expression in the pericardium. However, locally targeted pericardial VEGF delivery failed to improve myocardial collateral perfusion in this model.

In an attempt to improve the regional delivery of plasmid DNA by intrapericardial administration formulations based on a thermosensitive gel of Poloxamer 407 (copolymer of ethylene oxide and propylene oxide able to undergo a sol to gel transition at high concentration and at body temperature) were utilized by Roques et al. [54]. The intrapericardial injection of Poloxamer based formulations was possible with neither an ectopic expression of the transgene nor an extracardiac toxicity.

Intrapericardial Application of Growth Factors

Growth factor-induced angiogenesis was investigated in various studies as a potential perspective for extensive ischemic heart disease. Growth factors can induce the collateralization around sites of occlusion particularly in the epicardially situated major coronary arteries, or by inducing growth of small intramyocardial collaterals [57, 58]. Intracoronary and intravenous delivery of growth factors is technically the most practical application form, but unfortunately it is limited by a low myocardial uptake and a significant systemic recirculation. In the experimental pig model of ischemic heart disease, intrapericardial delivery of basic fibroblast growth factor FGF-2 provided a significantly higher myocardial deposition and retention and a lower systemic recirculation than the intracoronary or intravenous delivery route.

Systemic recirculation was markedly lower when 125I-FGF-2 was delivered intrapericardially. The liver accounted for less than 1% of administered

125I–FGF-2 at 1 and 24 hours in contrast to intra-coronary or intravenous delivery. Most of the administered growth factor remained in the pericardium, myocardium, and pericardial space with the total cardiac uptake of 30.9% after 1 hour. By intravascular delivery only 23.9% of the growth factor remained in the myocardium or pericardium after 24 hours [59].

Another growth factor that was investigated in an experimental intrapericardial delivery study is insulin-like growth factor I (IGF-I). Its intrapericardial application in a bovine model of ischemic congestive heart failure resulted in a rapid and sustained increase in left ventricular ejection fraction, which remained elevated 14 days after the cessation of treatment. In contrast, the subcutaneous IGF-I treatment did not affect left ventricular performance [60].

As in the study, which evaluated the intrapericardial application of paclitaxel, one of the potentially major limitations of the intrapericardial application of growth factors lies in the induction of pericardial inflammation and fibrosis that could lead to (peri) myocardial constriction. In addition, this mode of delivery requires the presence of an intact pericardial space, which is not the case in patients with previous coronary artery bypass surgery who are the most important potential group that could benefit from growth factor therapy.

Intrapericardial Application of Stem Cells

Until recently, myocardial regeneration was considered impossible and cardiomyocytes in adult mammalian heart were regarded as terminally differentiated and not capable of reentering the cell cycle [61]. However, evidence from confocal microscopy has identified cardiomyocyte division in the normal adult human heart, although at low rates (14/106 myocytes) [62]. Importantly, the number of dividing cardiomyocytes was found to increase approximately ten times in end-stage ischemic heart disease and in idiopathic dilated cardiomyopathy. The present evidence for cardiomyocyte division suggests that mature cardiomyocytes can re-enter the cell cycle and/or immature cells reside in the heart, similar to other tissues, and are capable of proliferation and differentiation into cardiomyocytes [63]. The potential for myocardial regeneration has been explored in several therapeutic studies based on stem/progenitor cells from skeletal muscle [64], bone marrow [65] and embryos [66]. The results appear promising. However, further studies are still needed to resolve the issue on the most suitable approach for cell delivery, homing, cell differentiation or proliferation [67, 68].

Although the intrapericardial route for the application of stem cells is potentially very attractive there is only one experimental study on this issue published so far. Steele et al. [69] developed an ex vivo culture system that promotes trafficking of progenitor-like cells from mouse ventricles to a culture surface. Cells that "trafficked" from cardiac tissue were phenotyped by flow cytometry and immunohistochemistry. Morphologically distinct cells spontaneously trafficked from mouse ventricular tissue, adhered in culture, and proliferated for up to 4 weeks in Dulbecco's minimal essential media supplemented with fetal calf serum. After 4 weeks in culture, the cell number declined. Co-culture with unfractionated bone marrow restored the proliferation of these trafficked cells. A significant population of the trafficked cells expressed a phenotype consistent with that of myo-

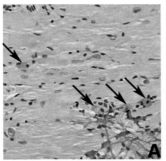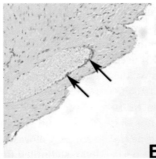

◘ **Fig. 12.6a,b.** Immunohistochemical evidence of the migration of intrapericardially applied GFP+ stem cells into mice heart tissue (magnification: x20; *arrows* in **a** and differentiation into endothelium in the Apo-E– deficient animals (magnification: x10; *arrows* in **b**. Reproduced with permission from Steele et al. (2002) [69]

genic progenitor cells. An expanded population of trafficked cells from ventricles of mice expressing green fluorescent protein (GFP+) and containing cardiac-derived progenitor cells were injected into the pericardial space of GFP-mice. GFP+ cells trafficked throughout the heart but retained a primitive undifferentiated morphology. However, when injected into the pericardial space of Apo-E-deficient mice with coronary vasculopathy, progenitor-like cells trafficked into myocardium, and GFP+ cells differentiated into vessel-lining endothelial cells and, rarely, smooth muscle and cardiomyocytes (Fig. 12.6).

Intrapericardial Treatment of Ventricular Rupture

Cardiac rupture is the second most frequent cause of in-hospital death after acute myocardial infarction. Its diagnosis may sometimes be challenging despite new imaging techniques and management can be even more difficult in hemodynamically unstable patients presenting with cardiac tamponade in hospitals without cardiac surgery.

Percutaneous intrapericardial fibrin-glue therapy was recently suggested as an alternative, less aggressive therapeutic option, as a final treatment or as a bridge to cardiac surgery [70]. Three successfully treated cases were reported so far and in all of them fibrin glue composed of 6–10 ml of solution A (800 mg human fibrinogen, 750 units coagulation factor VIII, and 10000 KIE aprotinin solution) and 6–10 ml of solution B (2500 units thrombin and 10 ml calcium chloride) was used. Solutions A and B were infused separately into the intrapericardial space through the drainage catheter. In all patients the hemopericardium resolved gradually. There was no need for surgical treatment. It should be stressed however, that all three cases were relatively stable, with no pseudo-aneurysms and that the extent of the rupture was certainly not too large.

Another type of glue (BioGlue® – a synthetic compound formed by mixing bovine albumin with glutaraldehyde, CryoLife, Kennesaw, GA) was tested in the experimental setting as a protective barrier after pericardiotomy, but no clinical experience in patients with cardiac rupture was gained so far [71].

In addition, Ogiwara et al. [72] examined the effectiveness of intrapericardial fibrin-glue fixation in an experimental canine model of left ventricular free wall rupture and found that this therapy prevented the progression of cardiac rupture and saved 66% of cases.

Hattori et al. [73] investigated the pharmacokinetics of fibrin-glue in the pericardial space of rats. After intrapericardial injection, a fibrin network is formed within one day and than eliminated within one week. In one of the cases reported by Murata et al. [70] autopsy performed few weeks after the treatment revealed that the site of rupture was completely covered by fibrin-glue without adhesion. However, the indication of intrapericardial fibrin-glue fixation therapy is probably limited to a small proportion of relatively stable patients with cardiac rupture and a high risk for cardiac surgery.

Ambulatory Pericardial Drainage Using a Permanent Port System

An alternative surgical concept for the management of recurring malignant pericardial effusions is the use of a permanently implanted port-system as suggested by Melfi et al. [74]. Using video-assisted thoracoscopy a port-system was implanted through the subxiphoid window in the pericardium of 40 patients with malignant effusion (Medi-Port MP-GS9 in 12 patients and IAP-HMP in 28 patients; Fig. 12.7).

The aim of the port implantation is to allow home management of pericardial effusion in patients with advanced malignancy and recurrent effusions. The reservoir body of the port system was placed in a subcutaneous pocket and the outlet catheter inserted into the pleural cavity, which allows aspiration of the effusion at home, when the patient starts experiencing the recurrence of symptoms.

The system was very efficient – no recurrent effusions were noted and the device was easily controlled at home in all cases. A certain disadvantage of this otherwise interesting concept in comparison to intrapericardial instillation of cytostatic agents is that it requires general anesthesia. The implantation of a permanent port system also imposes the risk of infection. Such complications, however, did not oc-

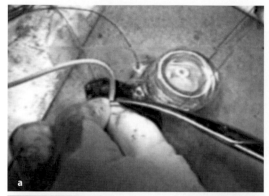

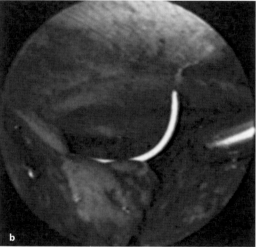

Fig. 12.7a,b. The implantation of the Medi-Port MP-GS9 system through the incision in the IV/V intercostal space (**a**). Video-assisted thoracoscopy showed the position of the outlet catheter in the pleura (**b**). Reproduced with permission from Melfi et al. (2002)[74]

cur in the study of Melfi et al. and the patients have used the system one to five times a week (mean 3 ± 1) [74].

The Heart-Lander® – Intrapericardial Crawling Robotic Device

The Heart-Lander is a miniature 2-footed crawling robot that navigates on the epicardium, recently developed at the Robotics Institute of the Carnegie Mellon University, Pittsburgh, PA, USA [75–84]. The device is now in the phase of 4th prototype and has successfully undergone experimental testing on beating porcine hearts. The pericardial access was obtained through a closed-chest video-pericardioscopy subxiphoid approach. The Heart-Lander consists of 2 modules that are connected by an extensible midsection (Fig. 12.8).

It adheres to the epicardium using vacuum suction pads. Locomotion and turning are accomplished by moving the two modules in an alternating fashion using wires that run through the midsection between them. The Heart-Lander can travel across the anterior and lateral surfaces of the beating heart without restriction, including locomotion forward, backward, and turning. No adverse hemodynamic or electrophysiologic events were noted during the trial. No epicardial damage was found on the excised heart after the porcine trial.

The potential future indication for clinical application of such a revolutionary device could address epicardial ablation procedures, local subepicardial application of drugs, gene and stem-cell therapy, but also, if the robotic device is further developed in this direction, a safe alternative for taking epicardial biopsies under endoscopic control.

Epicardial Mapping and Radiofrequency Ablation

Standard, endocardial radiofrequency ablation of malignant arrhythmias can be impossible in some patients due to the subepicardial location of the arrhythmogenic focus. Importantly, epicardial ventricular tachycardia circuits may occur in the wide range from 15% in patients with a prior myocardial infarction to 40% in patients with Chagas' disease [85–87]. Sosa et al. [18–20] did the pioneering work that demonstrated safety and feasibility of pericardial access for ventricular mapping and ablation of ventricular tachycardia in the absence of any pericardial effusion (see Chapter 6). Furthermore, Soejima et al. [88] have demonstrated that the subxiphoid surgical approach is possible for epicardial mapping and ablation in patients with prior cardiac surgery or difficult pericardial access. Using this approach, manual lysis of adhesions through the rather small subxiphoid pericardial window enabled free access to the epicardial surface and electrophysiological evaluation.

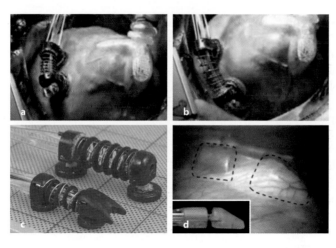

□ **Fig. 12.8a–d.** The first prototype of Heart-Lander on the epicardial surface of a beating porcine heart (**a,b**), the second prototype (**c**), and the fourth generation of the device (**d**). The second prototype features a retractable needle for myocardial injection. Reproduced with permission from Patronik et al. (2005) [82] and Ota et al. (2006) [76]

Furthermore, catheter ablation of atrial fibrillation may also be facilitated by the pericardial approach since the proximal ends of the pulmonary veins are situated inside the pericardial space [89, 90].

Depending on its location and the amount of the epicardial fat tissue, these conditions may either facilitate or diminish the efficacy and safety of epicardial catheter ablation procedures. Because of its usually extensive presence around the major coronary vessels, the risk of vascular damage during epicardial RF ablation is minimized [91]. On the other hand, the epicardial fat can act as an insulating layer and prevent ablation of an epicardial target site with RF energy. Indeed, the presence of epicardial fat interposed between the tip of the ablation catheter and the target tissue may be one of the reasons for failure of epicardial RF catheter ablation. No cases of pericardial fat necrosis following epicardial catheter mapping or ablation have been reported to date. Another technical improvement, "cooled-tip" RF ablation appears to be of particular benefit in ablating areas with overlying epicardial fat, and can generate epicardial lesions more effectively than standard RF ablation [92].

Although obstacles are not present during the mapping of the ventricular surface of the heart, the mapping of the atrial surface, particularly the left atrial surface, requires a careful negotiation into the pericardial sinuses. An 8-F Hemaquet is advanced intrapericardially and a 4-mm deflectable tip catheter can applied for epicardial mapping.

Zenati et al. [93] have recently reported on a novel subxiphoid video pericardioscopy approach for epicardial mapping that allows direct visualization of the epicardium with minimal use of fluoroscopy. The FLEXview system (Boston Scientific Cardiac Surgery, Santa Clara, CA), which is capable of a free navigation around the heart owing to its flexible neck, was inserted into the pericardial space through a small subxiphoid incision. A commercially available mapping catheter advanced through the working port of the device could be navigated around virtually the entire biventricular epicardial surface. The subxiphoid video pericardioscopy approach using the FLEXview system provided adequate visualization and access to the epicardium of both ventricles for electroanatomic mapping while minimizing surgical invasiveness.

In addition, direct epicardial ultrasound imaging was also evaluated for the guidance of complex epicardial ablation procedures [17]. Using a double-wire technique, two sheaths were placed in the pericardium, and a phased-array intracardiac ultrasound catheter was manipulated within the pericardial sinuses for imaging in order to facilitate catheter navigation and ablation. The procedure was performed in ten patients with no complications.

Importantly, pericarditis is a potential complication of catheter-based percutaneous epicardial mapping and ablation. In a porcine model of ablation-related pericarditis, intrapericardial instillation of 2 mg/kg of intermediate-acting corticosteroid triamcinolone effectively prevents post-procedure inflammatory adhesion formation [94].

Future Perspectives and Recommendations

The intrapericardial delivery of pharmacologic agents represents a promising novel route of administration in a variety of heart diseases. The possible benefits include reduced systemic absorption and prolonged exposure of the myocardium to the therapeutic material.

A potential intriguing application is the use of an intrapericardial cooling of the epicardial surface to reduce myocardial infarct size [95]. There are multiple advantages of the pericardial drug delivery, including the following:

1. the pericardial space appears to be the only natural drug receptacle able to restrict drug delivery to the heart;
2. because effective pericardial doses are approximately 5- to 10-fold lower than systemic doses, there is a minimal concern regarding systemic drug exposure with pericardial drug dosing. However, higher pericardial drug doses could in some instances produce also systemic drug exposure.
3. Once in the pericardial space, the substances have access to a number of cardiac structures, including the intracardiac autonomic nerves, epicardial coronary arteries, and atrial and ventricular myocardial tissue.

Finally, there appears to be a significant role for cardiac resynchronization therapy ion the treatment of patients with congestive heart failure and conduction system disease. However, technical difficulties are frequently encountered when attempting to place the intravascular pacing leads into the appropriate branch of the coronary sinus. This may be surmountable by using the pericardial approach to place epicardial biventricular or left ventricular pacing leads in these patients.

Indeed, the pericardial space seems to be the only natural drug receptacle to restrict drug delivery to the heart and may be used with a number of intrinsic advantages. The intrapericardial route permits delivery of a high concentration of compounds into a low-turnover chamber with a minimum of loss into the circulation. However, at the present stage of clinical cardiology, the most solid indication for access to the normal pericardial space is percutaneous mapping and ablation from within the pericardial space since it provides an important option for the management of otherwise potentially fatal arrhythmias.

References

1. Stoll HP, Carlson K, Keefer LK, Hrabie JA, March KL. Pharmacokinetics and consistency of pericardial delivery directed to coronary arteries: direct comparison with endoluminal delivery. Clin Cardiol 1999; 22 (1 Suppl 1): I10–16
2. Ware JA, Simons M. Angiogenesis in ischemic heart disease. Nat Med 1997; 3: 158–164
3. Lewis BS, Flugelman MY, Weisz A, Keren-Tal I, Schaper W. Angiogenesis by gene therapy: a new horizon for myocardial revascularization? Cardiovasc Res 1997; 35: 490–497
4. Waltenberger J. Modulation of growth factor action: implications for the treatment of cardiovascular diseases. Circulation 1997; 96: 4083–4094
5. Lazarous DF, Shou M, Stiber JA, Dadhania DM, Thirumurti V, Hodge E, Unger EF. Pharmacodynamics of basic fibroblast growth factor: route of administration determines myocardial and systemic distribution. Cardiovasc Res 1997; 36: 78–85
6. Howell SB, Chu BB, Wung WE, Metha BM, Mendelsohn J. Long-duration intracavitary infusion of methotrexate with systemic leucovorin protection in patients with malignant effusions. J Clin Invest 1981; 67: 1161–1170
7. Arndt JO, Pasch U, Samodelov LF, et al. Reversible blockade of myelinated and non-myelinated cardiac afferents in cats by instillation of procaine into the pericardium. Cardiovasc Res 1981; 25: 61–67
8. Samodelov LF, Pohl M, Arndt JO. Reversible blockade of cardiac efferents with procaine instilled into the pericardium of cats. Cardiovasc Res 1982; 16: 187–193
9. Dorward PK, Flaim M, Ludbrook J. Blockade of cardiac nerves by intrapericardial local anesthetics in the conscious rabbit. Aust J Exp Biol Med Sci 1983; 61(pt 2): 219–230
10. DiCarlo SE, Bishop VS. Regional vascular resistance during exercise: role of cardiac afferents and exercise training. Am J Physiol 1990; 258: H842–847
11. Miyazaki T, Pride HP, Zipes DP. Modulation of cardiac autonomic neurotransmission by epicardial superperfusion: effects of hexamethonium and tetrodotoxin. Circ Res 1989; 65: 1212–1219
12. O'Donnell CP, Scheuer DA, Keil LC, et al. Cardiac nerve blockade by infusion of procaine into the pericardial space of conscious dogs. Am J Physiol 1991; 260: R1176–1182
13. Evans RG, Hayes IP, Ludbrook J, et al. Factors confounding blockade of cardiac afferents by intrapericardial procaine in conscious rabbits. Am J Physiol 1993; 264: H1861–1870
14. Waxman S, Moreno R, Rowe KA, et al. Persistent primary coronary dilation induced by transatrial delivery of nitroglycerin into the pericardial space: a novel approach for local cardiac drug delivery. J Am Coll Cardiol 1999; 33: 2073–2077

15. Rodrigues AC, d'Avila A, Houghtaling C, Ruskin JN, Picard M, Reddy VY. Intrapericardial echocardiography: a novel catheter-based approach to cardiac imaging. J Am Soc Echocardiogr 2004; 17(3): 269–274

16. Rodrigues AC. Intrapericardial echocardiography: a novel catheter-based approach to cardiac imaging. In: Natale A (ed) Intracardiac echocardiography in interventional electrophysiology. Abingdon [U.K.]: Informa Healthcare, 2006, pp 88–94

17. Horowitz BN, Vaseghi M, Mahajan A, et al. Percutaneous intrapericardial echocardiography during catheter ablation: a feasibility study. Heart Rhythm 2006; 3(11): 1275–1282

18. Sosa E, Scanavacca M, d'Avila A, Pilleggi F. A new technique to perform epicardial mapping in the electrophysiology laboratory. J Cardiovasc Electrophysiol 1996; 7(6): 531–536

19. Sosa E, Scanavacca M, d'Avila A.Different ways of approaching the normal pericardial space. Circulation 1999; 100(24): e115–116

20. Sosa E, Scanavacca M, d'Avila A. Gaining access to the pericardial space. Am J Cardiol 2002; 90(2): 203–204

21. Furnary AP, Siqueira C Jr, Lowe RI, Thigpen T, Wu Y, Floten HS. Initial clinical trial of substernal epicardial echocardiography: seeing a new window to the postoperative heart. Ann Thorac Surg 2001; 72: 1077–1082

22. Spodick DH. Intrapericardial therapy and diagnosis. Curr Cardiol Rep 2002; 4(1): 22–25

23. Willerson JT, Igo SR, Yao SK, Ober JC, Macris MP, Ferguson JJ. Localized administration of sodium nitroprusside enhances its protection against platelet aggregation in stenosed and injured coronary arteries. Tex Heart Inst J 1996; 23(1): 1–8

24. Kumar K, Nguyen K, Waxman S, et al. Potent antifibrillatory effects of intrapericardial nitroglycerin in the ischemic porcine heart. J Am Coll Cardiol 2003; 41(10): 1831–1837

25. Baek SH, Hrabie JA, Keefer LK, et al. Augmentation of intrapericardial nitric oxide level by a prolonged-release nitric oxide donor reduces luminal narrowing after porcine coronary angioplasty. Circulation 2002; 105: 2779–2784

26. Borer JS, Kent KM, Goldstein RE, Epstein SE. Nitroglycerin-induced reduction in the incidence of spontaneous ventricular fibrillation during coronary occlusion in dogs. Am J Cardiol 1974; 33: 517–520

27. Kent KM, Smith ER, Redwood DR, Epstein SE. Beneficial electrophysiologic effects of nitroglycerin during acute myocardial infarction. Am J Cardiol 1974; 33: 513–516

28. Dashkoff N, Roland J-MA, Varghese PJ, Pitt B. Effect of nitroglycerin on ventricular fibrillation threshold of nonischemic myocardium. Am J Cardiol 1976; 38: 184–188

29. Stockman MB, Verrier RL, Lown B. Effect of nitroglycerin on vulnerability to ventricular fibrillation during myocardial ischemia and reperfusion. Am J Cardiol 1979; 43: 233–238

30. Engelman DT, Watanabe M, Maulik N, et al. L-arginine reduces endothelial inflammation and myocardial stunning during ischemia/reperfusion. Ann Thorac Surg 1995; 60: 1275–1281

31. Hoelzer M, Schaal SF, Leier CV. Electrophysiologic and antiarrhythmic effects of nitroglycerin in man. J Cardiovasc Pharmacol 1981; 3: 917–923

32. Bussmann WD, Neumann K, Kaltenbach M. Effects of intravenous nitroglycerin on ventricular ectopic beats in acute myocardial infarction. Am Heart J 1984; 107: 940–944

33. Margonato A, Bonetti F, Mailhac A, Vicedomini G, Cianflone D, Chierchia SL. Intravenous nitroglycerin suppresses exercise-induced arrhythmias in patients with ischaemic heart disease: implications for long-term treatment. Eur Heart J 1991; 12: 1278–1282

34. Armstrong JA, Slaughter SE, Marks GS, Armstrong PW. Rapid disappearance of nitroglycerin following incubation with human blood. Can J Physiol Pharmacol 1980; 58: 459–462

35. Fei L, Baron AD, Henry DP, et al. Intrapericardial delivery of L-arginine reduces the increased severity of ventricular arrhythmias during sympathetic stimulation in dogs with acute coronary occlusion. Nitric oxide modulates sympathetic effects on ventricular electrophysiological properties. Circulation 1997; 96: 4044–4049

36. Ayers GM, Rho TH, Ben-David J, et al. Amiodarone instilled into the canine pericardial sac migrates transmurally to produce electrophysiologic effects and suppress atrial fibrillation. J Cardiovasc Electrophysiol 1996; 7: 713–721

37. Miyazaki T, Zipes DP. Pericardial prostaglandin biosynthesis prevents the increased incidence of reperfusion-induced ventricular fibrillation produced by efferent sympathetic stimulation in dogs. Circulation 1990; 82: 1008–1019

38. Avitall B, Hare J, Zander G, et al. Iontophoretic transmyocardial drug delivery: a novel approach to antiarrhythmic drug therapy. Circulation 1992; 85: 1582–1593

39. Moreno R, Waxman S, Rowe K, Verrier RL. Intrapericardial beta-adrenergic blockade with esmolol exerts a potent antitachycardic effect without depressing contractility. J Cardiovasc Pharmacol 2000; 36(6): 722–727

40. Lew MJ, Ludbrook J, Pavia JM, et al. Selective manipulation of neurohumoral control of the cardiac pacemaker by drugs given intrapericardially. J Pharmacol Meth 1987; 17: 137–148

41. Wiest D. Esmolol. A review of its therapeutic efficacy and pharmacokinetic characteristics. Clin Pharmacokinet 1995; 28: 190–202

42. Takada M, Dohi S, Akamatsu S, Suzuki A. Effects of pericardial lidocaine on hemodynamic parameters and responses in dogs anesthetized with midazolam and fentanyl. J Cardiothorac Vasc Anesth 2007; 21(3): 393–399

43. Kolettis TM, Kazakos N, Katsouras CS, et al. Intrapericardial drug delivery: pharmacologic properties and long-term safety in swine. Int J Cardiol 2005; 99(3): 415–421

44. Gillis AM, Duff HJ, Mitchell LB, Wyse DG. Myocardial uptake and pharmacodynamics of procainamide in patients with coronary heart disease and sustained ventricular tachyarrhythmias. J Pharmacol Exp Ther 1993; 266: 1001–1006

45. Ujhelyi MR, Hadsall KZ, Euler DE, Mehra R. Intrapericardial therapeutics: a pharmacodynamic and pharmacokinetic comparison between pericardial and intravenous procainamide delivery. Cardiovasc Electrophysiol 2002; 13: 605–611

46. Greene M, Newman D, Geist M, Paquette M, Heng D, Dorian P. Is electrical storm in ICD patients the sign of a dying heart? Outcome of patients with clusters of ventricular tachyarrhythmias. Europace 2000; 2: 263–269

47. Hou D, Rogers PI, Toleikis PM, et al. Intrapericardial paclitaxel delivery inhibits neointimal proliferation and promotes arterial enlargement after porcine coronary overstretch. Circulation 2000; 102: 1575–1581

48. Heldman AW, Cheng L, Jenkins GM, et al. Paclitaxel stent coating inhibits neointimal hyperplasia at 4 weeks in a porcine model of coronary restenosis. Circulation 2001; 103(18): 2289–2295

49. Lansky AJ, Costa RA, Mintz GS, et al. Non-polymer-based paclitaxel-coated coronary stents for the treatment of patients with de novo coronary lesions: angiographic follow-up of the DELIVER clinical trial. Circulation 2004; 109(16): 1948–1954

50. Hou D, Zhang P, Marsh AE, March KL. Intrapericardial ethanol delivery inhibits neointimal proliferation after porcine coronary overstretch. J Chin Med Assoc 2003; 66(11): 637–642

51. French B, Mazur W, Geske R, Bolli R. Direct in vivo gene transfer into porcine myocardium using replication-deficient adenoviral vectors. Circulation 1994; 90: 2414–2424

52. Kypson AP, Peppel K, Akhter SA, et al. Ex vivo adenovirus-mediated gene transfer to the adult rat heart. J Thorac Cardiovasc Surg 1998; 115(3): 623–630

53. Fromes Y, Salmon A, Wang X, et al. Gene delivery to the myocardium by intrapericardial injection. Gene Ther 1999; 6(4): 683–688

54. Roques C, Salmon A, Fiszman MY, Fattal E, Fromes Y. Intrapericardial administration of novel DNA formulations based on thermosensitive Poloxamer 407 gel. Int J Pharm 2007; 331(2): 220–223

55. Donahue JK, Kikkawa K, Johns DC, Marban E, Lawrence JH. Ultrarapid, highly efficient viral gene transfer to the heart. Proc Natl Acad Sci USA 1997; 94(9): 4664–4668

56. Lazarous DF, Shou M, Stiber JA, et al. Adeno-viral-mediated gene transfer induces sustained pericardial VEGF expression in dogs: effect on myocardial angiogenesis. Cardiovasc Res 1999; 44(2): 294–302

57. Schaper W, Ito W. Molecular mechanisms of collateral vessel growth. Circ Res 1996; 79: 911–919

58. Simons M, Laham RJ. Therapeutic angiogenesis in myocardial ischemia. In: Ware J, Simons M (eds) Angiogenesis and cardiovascular disease. Oxford University Press, New York, 1999, pp 289–320

59. Laham RJ, Rezaee M, Post M, Xu X, Sellke FW. Intrapericardial administration of basic fibroblast growth factor: myocardial and tissue distribution and comparison with intracoronary and intravenous administration. Catheter Cardiovasc Interv 2003; 58(3): 375–381

60. Matthews KG, Devlin GP, Stuart SP, et al. Intrapericardial IGF-I improves cardiac function in an ovine model of chronic heart failure. Heart Lung Circ 2005; 14(2): 98–103

61. Soonpaa MH, Kim KK, Pajak L, et al. Cardiomyocyte DNA synthesis and binucleation during murine development. Am J Physiol 1996; 271: H2183–2189

62. Anversa P, Leri A, Kajstura J, et al. Myocyte growth and cardiac repair. J Mol Cell Cardiol 2002; 34: 91–105

63. Young HE. Existence of reserve quiescent stem cells in adults, from amphibians to humans. Curr Top Microbiol Immunol 2004; 280: 71–109

64. Hutcheson KA, Atkins BZ, Hueman MT, et al. Comparison of benefits on myocardial performance of cellular cardiomyoplasty with skeletal myoblasts and fibroblasts. Cell Transplantation 2000; 9: 359–368

65. Orlic D, Kajstura J, Chimenti S, et al. Bone marrow stem cells regenerate infarcted myocardium. Pediatr Transplant 2003; 7(Suppl 3): 86–88

66. Nir SG, David R, Zaruba M, et al. Human embryonic stem cells for cardiovascular repair. Cardiovasc Res 2003; 58: 313–323

67. Menasche P. Myoblast transplantation: feasibility, safety and efficacy. Ann Med 2002; 34: 314–315

68. Murry CE, Soonpaa MH, Reinecke H, et al. Haematopoietic stem cells do not transdifferentiate into cardiac myocytes in myocardial infarcts. Nature 2004; 428: 664–668

69. Steele A, Jones OY, Gok F, et al. Stem-like cells traffic from heart ex vivo, expand in vitro, and can be transplanted in vivo. J Heart Lung Transplant 2005; 24(11): 1930–1939

70. Murata H, Masuo M, Yoshimoto H, et al. Oozing type cardiac rupture repaired with percutaneous injection of fibrin-glue into the pericardial space: Case report. Jpn Circ J 2000; 64: 312–325

71. Wang ND, Doty DB, Doty JR, Yuksel U, Flinner R. BioGlue: a protective barrier after pericardiotomy. J Card Surg 2007; 22(4): 295–299

72. Ogiwara M. Treatment of left ventricular free wall rupture with fibrin-glue in dogs. Jpn J Cardiovasc Surg 1995; 24: 18–23

73. Hattori R, Otani H, Omiya H, et al. Fate of fibrin sealant in pericardial space. Ann Thorac Surg 2000; 70: 2132–2136

74. Melfi FM, Menconi GF, Chella A, Angeletti CA. The management of malignant pericardial effusions using permanently implanted devices. Eur J Cardiothorac Surg 2002; 21(2): 345–347

75. Patronik NA, Ota T, Zenati MA, Riviere CN. Improved traction for a mobile robot traveling on the heart. Conf Proc IEEE Eng Med Biol Soc 2006; 1: 339–342

76. Ota T, Patronik N, Riviere C, Zenati MA. Percutaneous subxiphoid access to the epicardium using a miniature crawling robotic device. Innovations 2006; 1(5): 227–231

77. Razjouyan F, Patronik NA, Zenati MA, Riviere CN. Enhancing the locomotion of an in vivo robot for cardiac surgery. Proceedings of the IEEE 32nd Annual Northeast Bioengineering Conference, April, 2006, pp 97–98

78. Patronik NA, Riviere CN, El Qarra S, Zenati MA. "The HeartLander: a novel epicardial crawling robot for myocardial injections". Proceedings of the 19th International Congress of Computer Assisted Radiology and Surgery, Elsevier 2005; 1281C: 735–739

79. Patronik NA, Zenati MA, Riviere CN. Preliminary evaluation of a mobile robotic device for navigation and intervention on the beating heart. Comput Aided Surg 2005; 10(4): 225–232

80. Patronik NA, Zenati MA, Riviere CN. A miniature cable-driven robot for crawling on the heart. Conf Proc IEEE Eng Med Biol Soc 2005; 6: 5771–5774

81. Patronik NA, Riviere CN, Qarra SE, Zenati MA. The Heart-Lander: A Novel Epicardial Crawling Robot for Myocardial Injections. Proceedings of the 19th International Congress of Computer Assisted Radiology and Surgery, Elsevier, Vol. 1281C, June, 2005, pp 735–739

82. Ota T, Patronil NA, Schwarzman D, Riviere CN, Zenati MI. Minimally invasive epicardial injections using a novel semiautonomous robotic device. Circulation 2008; 118 (14 Suppl): 115–120

83. Riviere CN, Patronik NA, Zenati MA. Prototype epicardial crawling device for intrapericardial intervention on the beating heart. Heart Surg Forum 2004; 7(6): E639–643

84. Patronik NA, Zenati MA, Riviere CN. Development of a tethered epicardial crawler for minimally invasive cardiac therapies. IEEE 30th Annual Northeast Bioengineering Conference, IEEE, April, 2004, pp 239–240

85. Sosa E, Scanavacca M, d'Avila A, Oliveira F, Ramires JAF. Nonsurgical transthoracic epicardial catheter ablation to treat recurrent ventricular tachycardia occurring late after myocardial infarction. J Am Coll Cardiol 2000; 35: 1442–1449

86. d'Avila A, Scanavacca M, Sosa E. Transthoracic epicardial catheter ablation of ventricular tachycardia. Heart Rhythm 2006; 3(9): 1110 1111

87. d'Avila A, Splinter R, Svenson RH, et al. New perspectives on catheter-based ablation of ventricular tachycardia complicating Chagas' disease: experimental evidence of the efficacy of near infrared lasers for catheter ablation of Chagas' VT. J Interv Card Electrophysiol 2002; 7(1): 23–38

88. Soejima K, Couper G, Cooper JM, Sapp JL, Epstein L M, Stevenson WG. Subxiphoid surgical approach for epicardial catheter-based mapping and ablation in patients with prior cardiac surgery or difficult pericardial access. Circulation 2004; 110(10): 1197–1201

89. Shivkumar K. Percutaneous epicardial ablation of atrial fibrillation. Heart Rhythm 2008; 5(1): 152–154.

90. Wudel JH, Chaudhuri P, Hiller JJ. Video-assisted epicardial ablation and left atrial appendage exclusion for atrial fibrillation: extended follow-up. Ann Thorac Surg 2008; 85(1): 34–38

91. d'Avila A, Gutierrez P, Scanavacca M, et al. Effects of radio-frequency pulses delivered in the vicinity of the coronary arteries: Implications for nonsurgical transthoracic epicardial catheter ablation to treat ventricular tachycardia. Pacing Clin Electrophysiol 2002; 25: 1488–1495

92. d'Avila A, Houghtaling C, Gutierrez P, et al. Catheter ablation of ventricular epicardial tissue: a comparison of standard and cooled-tip radiofrequency energy. Circulation 2004; 109(19): 2363–2369

93. Zenati MA, Shalaby A, Eisenman G, Nosbisch J, McGarvey J, Ota T. Epicardial left ventricular mapping using subxiphoid video pericardioscopy. Ann Thorac Surg 2007; 84(6): 2106–2107

94. d'Avila A, Neuzil P, Thiagalingam A, et al. Experimental efficacy of pericardial instillation of anti-inflammatory agents during percutaneous epicardial catheter ablation to prevent postprocedure pericarditis. J Cardiovasc Electrophysiol 2007; 18(11): 1178–1183

95. Hale SL, Kloner RA. Myocardial temperature in acute myocardial infarction: protection with mild regional hypothermia. Am J Physiol 1997; 273: H220–H227

Subject Index

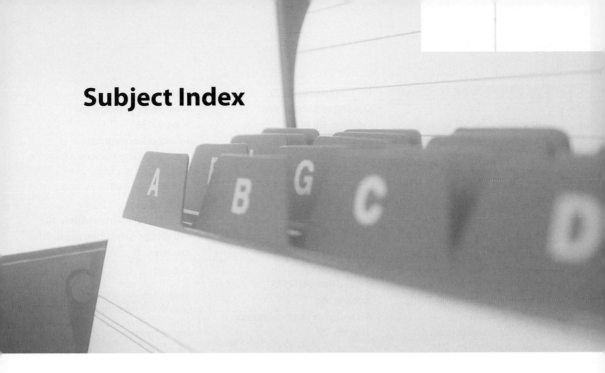